IMAGING CASE STUDIES IN PEDIATRIC NEUROLOGY 2026

A Clinical Reference and Guide to Neuroradiologic Pattern Recognition, Diagnostic Correlation, and Decision-Making for Neuroradiology Trainees

Ramon C. Henson, MD

TABLE OF CONTENTS

PREFACE

Why a Clinical-Imaging Crosswalk

A child arrives with a clinical sign, not a clinical scan. The neurology resident on service sees a bulging fontanelle, an asymmetric grasp, a first afebrile seizure, or a plateau in developmental milestones before any image exists to explain it. The neuroimaging findings that eventually confirm or redirect that clinical impression are learned, in most training pathways, from a separate literature organized around the finding rather than the presentation: a chapter on periventricular leukomalacia, a chapter on holoprosencephaly, a chapter on posterior fossa malformations, each comprehensive and each silent on how the child arrived in the room. The result is a durable and well-documented gap between the clinical service and the reading room, one that widens further in pediatrics, where a normal developmental structure can closely mimic disease and a genuinely pathologic finding can hide behind an unremarkable-sounding history.

This book is built to close that gap directly. Every chapter opens where the patient opens: with a presentation, an examination finding, or a clinical question that a child neurology resident, pediatric radiology fellow, or general pediatric neurologist actually confronts. From there, the text moves outward into the imaging correlate that confirms or excludes the leading possibilities, the mimics and normal variants that must be actively ruled out before a diagnosis is accepted, and the decision that the crossing of clinical and imaging information is meant to produce, whether that decision is a diagnosis, a change in management, or the choice of the next study to order.

Who This Book Is For

The primary reader is the child neurology resident or fellow who needs to read an MRI or CT independently well enough to counsel a family, direct the next step in a workup, and communicate precisely with a neuroradiology colleague. The text is equally built for the pediatric radiology fellow developing the clinical fluency to understand why a study was ordered and what decision hangs on the answer, and for the general pediatric neurologist in community practice who wants a case-anchored refresher rather than a shelf reference to be consulted only when a diagnosis is already suspected. General radiology residents rotating through pediatric neuroradiology, pediatric emergency medicine physicians who order and triage initial neuroimaging, and advanced practice clinicians in child neurology will find the same clinically-anchored structure useful, because the organizing question throughout is never simply what does this image show, but what does this child have, and what happens next.

How This Book Is Organized

The text opens with three foundational chapters covering imaging technique, normal neurodevelopmental appearance across the pediatric age range, and the evidence base for deciding when imaging is and is not indicated in the first place, a decision that published data show is made inconsistently even among experienced clinicians. The chapters that follow are organized by clinical domain, moving from the neonatal and perinatal period through congenital and developmental disorders, epilepsy, neuro-oncology and the neurocutaneous syndromes, acquired and inflammatory disease, and vascular and traumatic disease, closing with a presentation-based chapter on headache, macrocephaly, microcephaly, and developmental regression that draws directly on the imaging-ordering reasoning developed early in the book.

Every chapter carries the Clinical-Imaging Crosswalk System, a five-part structure repeated at each major clinical topic: The Crossing names the clinical-imaging correlation under discussion; the Presentation Signature describes the recognizable clinical profile; the Imaging Correlate specifies the pattern and sequence findings that confirm it; Trap Logic names the mimics and normal variants that must be discriminated before the diagnosis is accepted; and the Crossing Anchor states the single decision the crossing resolves, whether a diagnostic threshold, a next imaging step, or a management pivot. Each chapter closes with a Crosswalk Synthesis Recap that consolidates every crossing introduced in that chapter into a single scannable reference.

Using the Pediatric Neuroimaging Crosswalk Atlas

The Atlas at the close of this book indexes every crossing introduced across all twenty chapters, dual-indexed by presenting complaint and by imaging pattern, so the reader can enter from either direction: from a clinical sign encountered on rounds, or from an imaging finding encountered on a rotation through the reading room. Each Atlas entry cross-references its home chapter for the full clinical and imaging discussion, so the Atlas functions as a rapid point-of-care lookup rather than a substitute for the chapter narrative.

A Note on Scope

This text is a clinical reference, not an examination-preparation workbook. It contains no practice questions, review items, or quizzes of any kind; every page is written as the connected clinical prose of an authoritative reference, because the goal is durable clinical reasoning rather than short-term recall. Drug and dosing information is presented as guidance to be confirmed against current formulary and institutional protocol at the time of use, and imaging findings are described as they are understood at the time of writing, in a field where technique and evidence continue to evolve. It is offered in the hope that it will make the space between the bedside and the reading room a little narrower for the clinicians who work in both.

CHAPTER 1: PRINCIPLES OF PEDIATRIC NEUROIMAGING AND THE CLINICAL-IMAGING CROSSWALK

Learning Objectives

1. Select the appropriate imaging modality for a given pediatric neurologic presentation, weighing diagnostic yield against radiation exposure, sedation risk, and availability.
2. Construct or critique an MRI protocol for a stated clinical question rather than defaulting to a generic brain protocol.
3. Apply age-appropriate sedation and motion-reduction strategies, recognizing when sedation can be avoided altogether.
4. Describe the five-part Clinical-Imaging Crosswalk structure used throughout this book and explain its diagnostic rationale.
5. Compose a structured, clinically actionable report and communicate an unexpected or urgent finding appropriately.

Imaging Modalities in Infants, Children, and Adolescents

The choice of imaging modality in child neurology is rarely a question of which study is best in the abstract; it is a question of which study answers the specific clinical question in front of the clinician, at the specific age of the child, with the least cumulative risk. Because the developing brain is more radiosensitive than the adult brain and because children have more remaining years of life over which a stochastic radiation effect could manifest, modality selection carries a weight in pediatrics that it does not carry in adult neurology. This chapter establishes the modality landscape and the sequence-selection logic that every later chapter assumes.

The radiosensitivity difference is not merely theoretical. Epidemiologic cohort data following children exposed to diagnostic CT radiation have demonstrated a measurable, dose-dependent association with subsequent hematologic and central nervous system malignancy, an association strong enough to have driven a decade-long, coordinated campaign across pediatric radiology to reduce CT utilization and dose per study wherever an equivalent-yield alternative exists. This history explains why a specialty that once used CT liberally for head trauma and headache evaluation now reserves it for a narrower set of indications, and why the clinician ordering a study bears real responsibility for confirming that the question at hand actually requires ionizing radiation to answer.

Magnetic Resonance Imaging as the Primary Modality

Magnetic resonance imaging is the primary modality for essentially all nonemergent pediatric neuroimaging because it provides superior soft-tissue contrast without ionizing radiation, and because the pediatric central nervous system, with its evolving myelination pattern and higher water content, is particularly well suited to the contrast mechanisms MRI exploits. The tradeoff is acquisition time, which in turn drives the need for sedation or motion-reduction strategies discussed later in this chapter, and susceptibility to motion artifact, which can itself mimic pathology if not recognized.

The physical basis of this superior soft-tissue contrast lies in the differential T1 and T2 relaxation behavior of tissues with differing water and lipid content, a behavior that changes systematically as the pediatric brain myelinates, meaning the same sequence produces a different normal appearance at different ages. This age-dependence, developed fully in Chapter 2, is the single most important source of interpretive error for clinicians trained primarily on adult imaging, because a signal pattern that would be unambiguously abnormal in a ten-year-old may be entirely expected in a four-month-old.

Figure 1.1: Normal Neonatal Brain MRI Sequence Panel

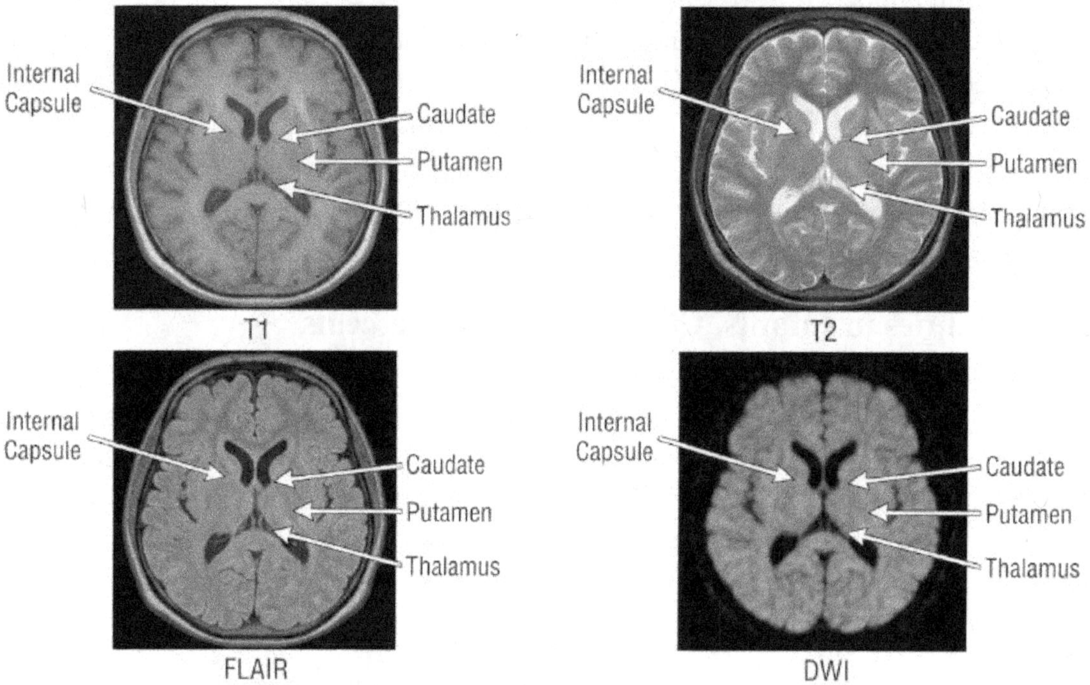

Figure 1.1: Normal Neonatal Brain MRI Sequence Panel

Fetal MRI as an Extension of Pediatric Neuroimaging

Fetal MRI, performed as an adjunct to prenatal ultrasound when a suspected central nervous system anomaly is identified, extends the principles of this chapter into the prenatal period and is increasingly encountered by the child neurologist as a component of the prenatal counseling team. The technique relies on single-shot, motion-robust sequences acquired rapidly enough to freeze ongoing fetal movement, since the fetus cannot be sedated or positioned in the way a born infant can, and interpretation requires familiarity with the markedly different, still-lissencephalic normal cortical appearance of the fetal brain relative to the postnatal brain, a distinction that becomes directly relevant to the malformations of cortical development discussed in Chapter 7.

The clinical value of fetal MRI lies chiefly in its superior soft-tissue resolution relative to prenatal ultrasound for posterior fossa, cortical, and midline structures, findings that can meaningfully change delivery planning, family counseling, and postnatal management planning before birth; a fetal MRI finding is nonetheless understood as provisional, since a substantial minority of prenatally suspected abnormalities are revised, either upgraded or downgraded in severity, once postnatal imaging with its superior resolution and absence of fetal motion becomes available.

Computed Tomography — Indications and Radiation Stewardship

Computed tomography retains a defined and important role despite its radiation dose, principally in three circumstances: the acute trauma setting, where speed and the detection of acute hemorrhage or fracture outweigh the radiation concern; the evaluation of bony anatomy, including craniosynostosis and skull base anomalies, where CT remains superior to MRI; and settings in which MRI is unavailable or the child cannot be adequately sedated in a timely fashion. Radiation stewardship in children follows the as-low-as-reasonably-achievable principle, which in practice means pediatric-specific dose protocols, weight- or age-based technique charts, and a low threshold to substitute MRI or ultrasound whenever either can answer the same clinical question.

Applying this principle at the point of care means the ordering clinician asks a second question after the first: not only whether this child needs imaging, addressed later in Chapter 3, but whether this specific imaging question requires CT, or would MRI or ultrasound answer it equally well. In the setting of suspected abusive head trauma, discussed fully in Chapter 19, CT remains the acute first-line study because of its speed and sensitivity for acute hemorrhage in an unstable or uncooperative infant, but a follow-up MRI is frequently obtained days later once the child is stable, both to characterize injury age and extent with greater sensitivity and to avoid a second CT-radiation exposure for the same clinical question.

KEY POINT: A noncontrast head CT obtained to rule out something without a specific clinical question in mind is the single most common source of low-yield pediatric neuroimaging; the question should be defined before the study is ordered, not after the images are reviewed.

Cranial Ultrasound in the Neonate and Young Infant

Cranial ultrasound occupies a unique niche made possible by the open anterior fontanelle, which serves as an acoustic window into the neonatal brain. It is inexpensive, requires no sedation, can be performed at the bedside in a critically ill infant, and is the first-line modality for screening preterm infants for germinal matrix hemorrhage and periventricular leukomalacia, both discussed in detail in Chapter 5. Its principal limitation is a restricted field of view that favors the periventricular and deep structures over the peripheral cortex and posterior fossa, and its utility declines as the fontanelle narrows over the first year of life.

Because cranial ultrasound can be repeated serially at the bedside without the logistical burden of transport or sedation, it is particularly well suited to longitudinal monitoring of a known process, such as tracking the evolution of a germinal matrix hemorrhage or following ventricular size after a documented intraventricular hemorrhage, roles in which its lower sensitivity for subtle cortical or extra-axial pathology is an acceptable tradeoff against the clinical value of frequent, low-burden reassessment.

Figure 1.2: Cranial Ultrasound Acoustic Windows and Fontanelle Anatomy

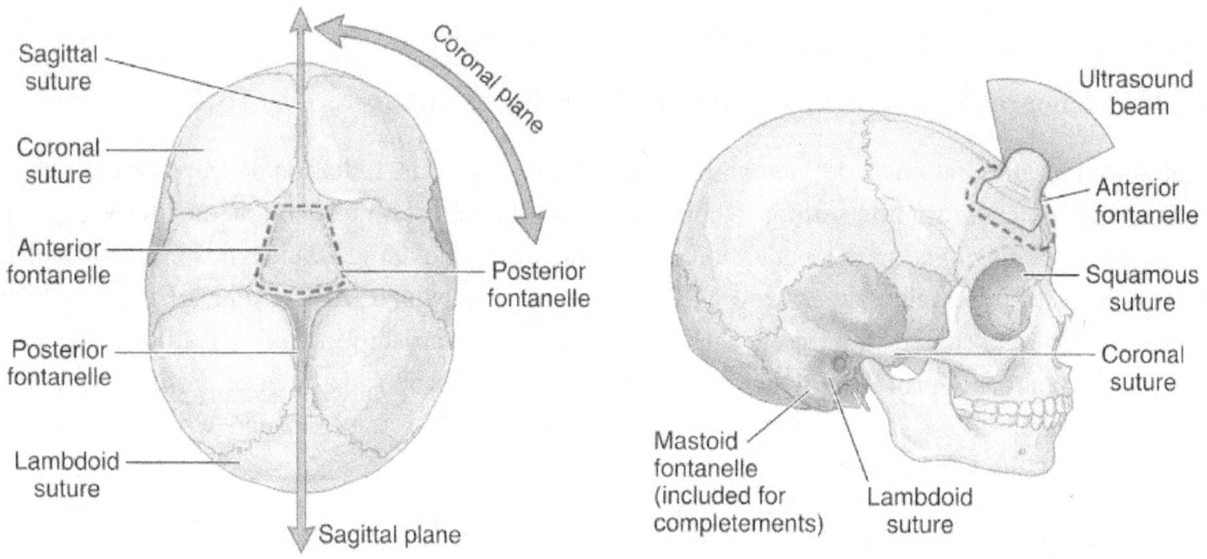

Superior and lateral schematic views of the neonatal skull demonstrating the anterior fontanelle acoustic window and standard coronal and sagittal ultrasound scan planes.

Ultrasound Beyond the Neonatal Period: Doppler and Adjunct Roles

Beyond gray-scale cranial ultrasound in the open-fontanelle period, Doppler ultrasound retains a role in monitoring cerebral blood flow velocity in specific clinical circumstances, most notably transcranial Doppler screening for stroke risk in children with sickle cell disease, discussed in Chapter 18, where elevated flow velocities identify a subgroup at meaningfully increased stroke risk who benefit from chronic transfusion therapy. Spinal ultrasound, performed through the still-unossified posterior elements in infants younger than approximately four to six months, offers a low-burden screening tool for occult spinal dysraphism in infants with a concerning cutaneous marker, discussed further in Chapter 9, though a positive or equivocal finding is generally followed by MRI for definitive characterization.

Because transcranial Doppler screening depends on operator technique and requires an accessible acoustic bone window, results can vary meaningfully between examiners in the same child, which is why programs offering chronic sickle cell stroke-risk screening typically require sonographers to complete standardized, protocol-specific certification before their velocity measurements are used to guide transfusion decisions; a single, uncertified measurement suggesting an elevated velocity is generally confirmed by repeat, certified examination before a management change is made on that basis alone.

Cost-Effectiveness and Avoiding Redundant Imaging

Beyond the individual risk-benefit calculation for a single child, redundant imaging carries a system-level cost that a busy referral practice can lose sight of: a child transferred between institutions frequently arrives having already had an outside MRI that is technically adequate to answer the clinical question, yet a repeat study is sometimes obtained reflexively rather than after a deliberate review of the outside images and outside report. Requesting the actual outside images, not merely the outside report, and reviewing them before ordering a repeat study is both more cost-effective and, when sedation would otherwise be required, meaningfully reduces the child's cumulative anesthetic exposure; a repeat study is warranted when the outside images are technically inadequate, outdated relative to a changing clinical picture, or performed without the specific sequences the current question requires, not as a default response to any inter-institutional transfer.

Nuclear Medicine and Advanced Techniques

Nuclear medicine studies, including ictal and interictal single-photon emission computed tomography and fluorodeoxyglucose positron emission tomography, occupy a targeted role in presurgical epilepsy evaluation, discussed in Chapter 11, where they localize a seizure focus that structural imaging alone does not resolve. Advanced MRI techniques, including diffusion tensor imaging, magnetic resonance spectroscopy, and perfusion imaging, add physiologic and microstructural information beyond conventional sequences and are introduced where they change a specific clinical decision, rather than as routine additions to every protocol.

Ictal SPECT requires radiotracer injection at the moment of clinical seizure onset, a logistical demand that in practice confines the technique to inpatient video-electroencephalography monitoring units where the injection can be triggered promptly once seizure activity is confirmed; the resulting image of regional hyperperfusion is then subtracted from an interictal baseline study to localize the seizure onset zone, a technique whose value depends entirely on the precision of injection timing relative to seizure onset.

Contrast Agent Selection and Safety

Gadolinium-based contrast agents used in pediatric neuroimaging are selected in part on the basis of their macrocyclic versus linear chelate structure, since macrocyclic agents are associated with lower rates of free gadolinium release and are generally preferred in children, who may face a longer cumulative lifetime exposure across multiple studies than an adult patient with a similar diagnosis. Renal function is assessed before contrast administration in any child with known renal impairment, congenital heart disease with reduced renal perfusion, or critical illness, following the same nephrogenic systemic fibrosis precautions applied in adult practice, though the pediatric incidence of this complication is very low with modern macrocyclic agents.

Iodinated contrast for CT angiography or CT myelography follows an analogous weight-based dosing principle, with the additional consideration that a young child's smaller total blood volume narrows the margin between a diagnostic contrast bolus and a volume that risks transient hemodynamic effect, making precise, weight-based dose calculation, rather than a fixed adult-derived volume, a nonnegotiable step in pediatric contrast administration regardless of modality.

Intravenous Access and Practical Workflow Considerations

Establishing intravenous access before a sedated study, even when contrast is not anticipated, is common practice in many pediatric imaging centers, since sedation itself may require intravenous rescue medication and an unanticipated finding may prompt same-visit contrast administration; placing access after induction in an already-sedated child is technically easier than in an awake, anxious child, and coordinating the sequence of sedation induction and line placement is a routine part of the pediatric imaging workflow that distinguishes it meaningfully from adult imaging practice, where access is typically obtained before the patient ever enters the department.

Modality	Radiation	Sedation Typically Required	Primary Pediatric Neurology Role
MRI	None	Age-dependent (see below)	Primary modality for nearly all nonemergent indications
CT	Yes	Rarely (fast acquisition)	Acute trauma, bony anatomy, MRI unavailable
Cranial Ultrasound	None	Never	Neonatal/infant screening while fontanelle open
Nuclear Medicine (SPECT/PET)	Yes (lower than CT)	Often, by age	Presurgical epilepsy localization

MRI Sequence Selection and Protocol Design by Clinical Question

A protocol built for one clinical question is frequently the wrong protocol for another, even when both studies are labeled brain MRI. The sequences that best demonstrate an acute infarct are not the sequences that best characterize a suspected malformation of cortical development, and a protocol reflexively duplicated across every indication wastes scanner time, prolongs sedation exposure, and can miss the finding the clinician actually needed to see.

Core Sequence Building Blocks

T1-weighted imaging demonstrates anatomy and, in the pediatric brain, tracks the progression of myelination, which appears T1-hyperintense before it becomes T2-hyperintense, a sequence discussed further in Chapter 2. T2-weighted imaging is the primary sequence for detecting parenchymal signal abnormality, including edema, gliosis, and demyelination. Fluid-attenuated inversion recovery, or FLAIR, suppresses cerebrospinal fluid signal and is particularly useful for periventricular and cortical lesions, though it is used cautiously in children younger than two years, in whom incomplete myelination can produce a FLAIR appearance that mimics pathology.

Diffusion-weighted imaging with apparent diffusion coefficient mapping is the most sensitive sequence for acute infarction and for the restricted diffusion characteristic of pyogenic abscess and certain highly cellular tumors; the underlying mechanism, restriction of water molecule movement within densely packed cells or cytotoxic edema, applies identically in children and adults, but the differential diagnosis for a restricted-diffusion lesion shifts substantially by age, a distinction developed throughout this book. Susceptibility-weighted or gradient-echo imaging detects blood products, calcification, and mineralization, exploiting the local magnetic field distortion these substances produce, and is particularly valuable in the evaluation of prior hemorrhage, vascular malformation, and the mineralizing microangiopathy sometimes seen after radiation or chemotherapy. Postcontrast T1-weighted imaging is added when there is concern for tumor, infection, or an inflammatory or demyelinating process in which enhancement carries diagnostic or activity-staging significance, because gadolinium-based contrast agents enhance regions where the blood-brain barrier has been disrupted.

Field Strength: 1.5T Versus 3T in Children

Higher field strength, most commonly 3 Tesla in current pediatric practice, increases signal-to-noise ratio, which can be applied either to shorten acquisition time, a meaningful benefit when sedation duration is a limiting factor, or to increase spatial resolution for indications such as focal cortical dysplasia detection, where submillimeter resolution improves lesion conspicuity. The tradeoff at higher field strength includes increased susceptibility artifact, which can degrade image quality near the skull base and paranasal sinuses, and increased specific absorption rate, the radiofrequency energy deposited in tissue, which in practice is managed through vendor-specific sequence adjustments rather than by avoiding 3 Tesla imaging altogether. Neither field strength is categorically superior; the choice is made in the context of the specific clinical question, the child's size, and the anatomic region under evaluation.

Coil Selection and Positioning for Optimal Signal

Receive-coil selection matters more in pediatric imaging than in adult imaging because a coil sized and shaped for an adult head produces disproportionately reduced signal-to-noise when wrapped loosely around a much smaller pediatric head, and many pediatric imaging centers maintain a dedicated set of smaller, age-appropriate head and neonatal coils for this reason. Careful positioning, including symmetric head placement and, in an awake or lightly sedated child, immobilization padding to minimize the small residual motion that even a cooperative child produces, further protects image quality; a technically excellent sequence choice can still yield a nondiagnostic study if coil selection and positioning are treated as an afterthought rather than as an integral part of protocol execution.

Protocol Design by Clinical Question

Building a protocol begins with the question, not the anatomy. The following sequence reflects the reasoning applied throughout this book each time a study is ordered.

1. Define the leading clinical question: Is this a question of acute ischemia, a question of malformation, a question of mass, or a question of demyelination?
2. Select the sequence combination with the highest yield for that question first: diffusion-weighted imaging and susceptibility-weighted imaging for suspected acute stroke; thin-section, high-resolution T1 and T2 for suspected malformation; postcontrast T1 for suspected mass or infection.
3. Add adjunct sequences only when they will change management: spectroscopy when a mass has an atypical appearance, perfusion imaging when tumor grade is in question, susceptibility-weighted imaging when a vascular malformation is suspected.
4. Extend the field of view to the spine when the clinical question or an unexpected brain finding raises concern for a coexisting spinal process, such as a Chiari malformation with an associated syrinx.

Common Protocol Design Errors

Three protocol errors recur across referral practice with sufficient frequency to warrant explicit naming. The first is the reflexive substitution of a routine brain protocol for a question that requires dedicated sequencing, illustrated in the epilepsy-protocol Crossing below. The second is the omission of postcontrast sequencing when the clinical scenario, such as new headache with papilledema or a new focal deficit, carries a real prior probability of mass or infection, an omission that can necessitate a second study and a second sedation exposure. The third is over-inclusion of adjunct sequences that prolong acquisition time without changing management, which in a sedated child directly increases anesthetic exposure without a corresponding diagnostic benefit; the discipline of adding a sequence only because it will change a decision, not because it is available, is a recurring theme of this book.

A fourth, subtler error occurs at the interface between the ordering clinician and the imaging department: a vaguely worded order such as evaluate for pathology, without a stated leading diagnosis, forces the protocoling radiologist or technologist to guess at the intended clinical question, and a guess that differs from the ordering clinician's actual concern can result in a technically excellent but clinically unhelpful study. Stating the specific concern directly on the order, not merely the broad category of symptom, is itself a component of correct protocol design.

Vendor and Site Variation in Sequence Nomenclature

Sequence names vary between MRI vendors even when the underlying physics is equivalent, so that a fluid-attenuated inversion recovery sequence may appear under a different proprietary acronym depending on the scanner manufacturer; a clinician transferring a child between institutions or reviewing an outside study should confirm sequence identity by its underlying contrast behavior rather than by acronym alone, since assuming an unfamiliar acronym represents a sequence it does not is a preventable source of protocol confusion, particularly when comparing serial studies performed at different sites over the course of a child's care. This confusion compounds when a family transfers care between health systems using different MRI vendors mid-workup, making a clear, plain-language description of what each prior sequence actually showed, rather than reliance on the acronym alone, an important part of chart continuity.

Advanced and Adjunct Sequences

Diffusion tensor imaging characterizes white matter tract integrity and is used selectively in presurgical planning and in the evaluation of certain leukodystrophies discussed in Chapter 17. Magnetic resonance spectroscopy provides a biochemical profile of a region of interest and is most useful when a mass lesion or a metabolic disorder produces an ambiguous conventional appearance, since characteristic elevations or reductions in metabolites such as N-acetylaspartate, choline, and lactate can distinguish tumor from a nonneoplastic process. Arterial spin labeling perfusion avoids the need for gadolinium and is increasingly used in tumor grading and in the evaluation of vascular steal phenomena in moyamoya disease, discussed in Chapter 18.

THE CLINICAL-IMAGING CROSSWALK SYSTEM — Sequence Selection for an Ambiguous First-Seizure Presentation

The Crossing: A four-year-old presents with a first afebrile focal seizure and a nonfocal examination. The referring team orders a brain MRI, without further specification.

Presentation Signature: New-onset focal seizure, normal examination, no fever, no prior neurologic history; the clinical question is whether a structural, epileptogenic lesion is present.

Imaging Correlate: The correct protocol is not a routine brain MRI but a dedicated epilepsy protocol: thin-section, high-resolution T1 and T2/FLAIR through the temporal lobes with attention to hippocampal architecture, because the most common structural lesions producing new focal seizures in this age group, including focal cortical dysplasia and hippocampal abnormality, are frequently missed on a standard-resolution protocol.

Trap Logic: A standard brain protocol ordered without epilepsy-specific sequencing may be read as normal, falsely reassuring the family and delaying the correct diagnosis; subtle cortical dysplasia is among the most commonly missed findings on a non-dedicated protocol.

Crossing Anchor: Any new-onset focal seizure with a normal general neurologic examination should trigger a dedicated epilepsy MRI protocol, not a routine brain MRI, whenever epilepsy is a serious diagnostic consideration.

Sedation, Motion Control, and Safety in Pediatric Imaging

Because MRI acquisition times measured in tens of minutes are incompatible with a wakeful young child holding still, sedation and motion-reduction strategy is inseparable from pediatric MRI practice, and the decision to sedate carries its own risk-benefit calculation distinct from the imaging question itself.

Sedation Risk-Benefit and Alternatives

Sedation and general anesthesia in young children carry a small but real risk of airway compromise, cardiovascular instability, and, per an evolving body of preclinical and epidemiologic evidence, a theoretical concern regarding neurodevelopmental effects of repeated or prolonged anesthetic exposure in very young children, an association that remains under active investigation rather than firmly established. This risk is weighed against the diagnostic cost of a motion-degraded, nondiagnostic study that may require repeat imaging and repeat sedation. In practice, feed-and-wrap technique, in which a neonate or young infant is fed, swaddled, and imaged during natural sleep, avoids sedation entirely for infants younger than approximately three to six months and is the preferred approach whenever the clinical scenario allows the additional time required for feeding and settling.

Figure 1.3: Feed-and-Wrap Positioning for Infant MRI

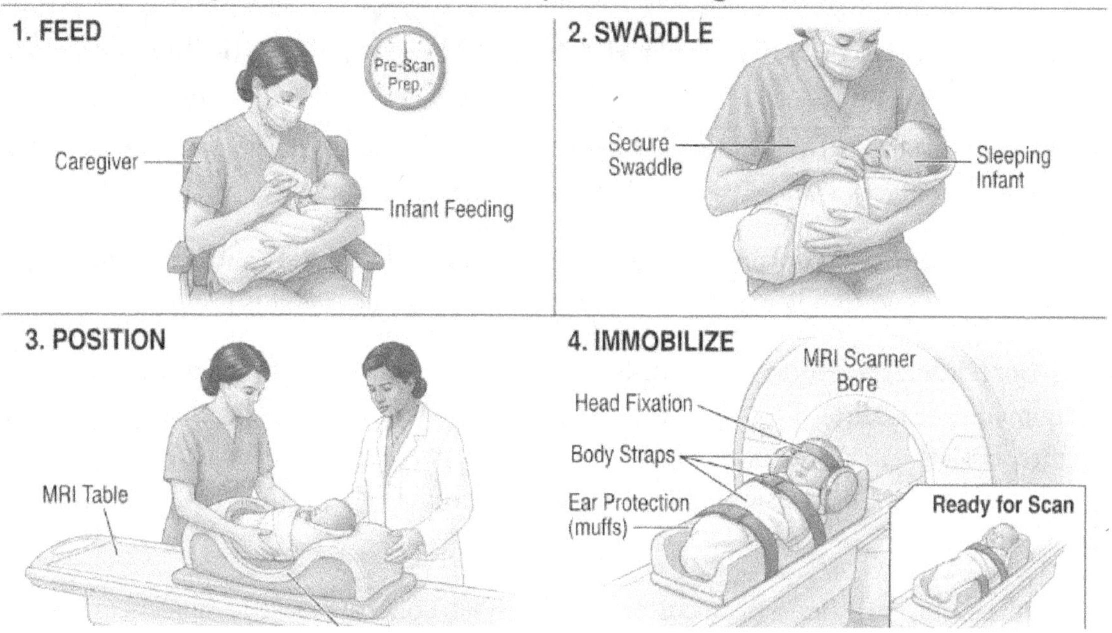

The Anesthesia Neurotoxicity Question in Context

The concern regarding anesthetic neurotoxicity originates from preclinical animal studies demonstrating neuronal apoptosis after exposure to common anesthetic agents during a critical developmental window, findings that prompted a regulatory advisory regarding prolonged or repeated anesthetic exposure in children younger than three years. Subsequent large human cohort studies of single, brief anesthetic exposures have been largely reassuring regarding long-term neurodevelopmental outcome, and the current clinical consensus is that a single, medically necessary anesthetic exposure of typical MRI duration should not be withheld out of neurotoxicity concern when the study is genuinely indicated; the concern carries more practical weight in the setting of anticipated multiple or prolonged exposures, in which the timing and consolidation of studies, discussed further below, becomes clinically relevant.

Motion Reduction Strategies

Beyond feed-and-wrap technique, motion reduction includes child-life specialist preparation and mock-scanner rehearsal for children old enough to cooperate, typically from approximately five to six years of age; shortened, motion-robust sequence variants that trade some spatial resolution for speed when full sedation is not warranted; and, for children in the intermediate age range who are too old for feed-and-wrap and too young to cooperate reliably, a frank discussion with the family regarding whether the clinical question truly requires imaging at that visit or can be deferred to an age at which sedation can be avoided.

Special Populations: Children With Neurodevelopmental or Behavioral Needs

Children with autism spectrum disorder, intellectual disability, or significant sensory sensitivity present a distinct motion-control challenge, since standard mock-scanner desensitization protocols may require substantially more preparation time or may not succeed regardless of preparation, and the threshold for proceeding directly to sedation is appropriately lower in this population. Coordination with a developmental-behavioral specialist or the family's existing behavioral team, when available, before the imaging visit itself frequently improves the likelihood of a successful, diagnostic-quality study on the first attempt, avoiding the added burden of a second visit and, if sedation is ultimately required, a second anesthetic exposure.

Environmental modifications, including dimmed lighting in the waiting and preparation areas, noise-reducing headphones during acquisition, weighted blankets for proprioceptive comfort, and permitting a preferred comfort item into the scan room when it contains no ferromagnetic material, can meaningfully improve tolerance in sensory-sensitive children without requiring escalation to sedation, and are increasingly incorporated as a standard first step before sedation is considered rather than as an occasional accommodation.

Pre-Procedure Fasting, Recovery, and Discharge Criteria

Standard pediatric anesthesia fasting guidelines, typically permitting clear liquids up to two hours before sedation and solids or non-clear liquids up to six to eight hours before, apply to sedated MRI as they do to any procedural sedation, and deviation from fasting guidelines is a common, avoidable cause of same-day cancellation. Recovery monitoring following sedation follows standard post-anesthesia discharge criteria, including return to baseline mental status, stable vital signs, and adequate oral intake tolerance, with the family counseled in advance that the child may remain drowsy or unsteady for several hours after discharge and should avoid activities requiring full coordination, such as bathing unsupervised or riding a bicycle, for the remainder of the day.

The Role of the Pediatric Anesthesiologist and Multidisciplinary Coordination

Involvement of a pediatric-trained anesthesiologist, rather than a general or adult-trained anesthesia provider, meaningfully reduces sedation-related complication rates in young children, particularly those with underlying airway anomalies, congenital heart disease, or craniofacial syndromes in whom airway management carries additional technical complexity. Coordinating the imaging order with the anesthesia team in advance, including flagging any anticipated need for concurrent contrast administration or an extended protocol, allows the anesthesia plan to be tailored to the expected study duration rather than adjusted reactively mid-procedure, which reduces both anesthetic time and the likelihood of a truncated, nondiagnostic study.

Institutional Protocols and Credentialing for Sedation Providers

Institutions vary in whether MRI sedation is provided by anesthesiology, a dedicated pediatric sedation service staffed by credentialed pediatric hospitalists or emergency physicians, or, in some community settings, the ordering clinician's own practice; regardless of which model is in place, institutional sedation credentialing typically requires documented competency in pediatric airway rescue, a defined emergency response pathway accessible from within the MRI suite despite the ferromagnetic environment, and a formal, monitored recovery area separate from the scanning room itself. A referring clinician working with an unfamiliar imaging center is well served by confirming which sedation model is in place before scheduling a study in a medically complex child, since the appropriate level of monitoring differs meaningfully between a straightforward, healthy toddler and a child with a complex cardiac or airway history.

Age Range	Preferred Approach	Key Consideration
Neonate to ~3-6 months	Feed-and-wrap, no sedation	Time natural sleep to the scan; avoid over-tiring before feeding
~6 months to 5 years	Sedation or general anesthesia, per institutional protocol	Weigh anesthetic risk against diagnostic urgency; consider deferral if nonurgent
~5-7 years and older (variable)	Awake with preparation, mock-scanner rehearsal	Child-life involvement substantially improves cooperation rates

MRI Safety in Children

Standard MRI safety screening for implanted devices, ferromagnetic foreign bodies, and cochlear implants applies to children as it does to adults, with the additional consideration that young children cannot reliably report a prior foreign body exposure or implanted device history themselves, placing greater weight on caregiver history and, where available, prior imaging or medical records. Ventriculoperitoneal shunt valves, common in the pediatric neurology population and discussed further in Chapter 10, require confirmation of MRI-conditional status and, for programmable valves, a post-scan settings check, since the magnetic field can alter valve programming.

CAUTION: Gadolinium-based contrast administration in children should follow weight-based dosing and current institutional and regulatory guidance regarding agent selection and the theoretical concern for gadolinium retention with repeated exposures; confirm current dosing and agent policy against institutional protocol before ordering contrast in a child with anticipated need for serial imaging.

The Clinical-Imaging Crosswalk: A Framework for This Book

The organizing structure of this book departs deliberately from the disease-first organization of most comprehensive pediatric neuroradiology references. That organization serves the reader who already suspects a diagnosis and wants to confirm the imaging appearance; it serves less well the reader standing at the bedside with a presentation and no diagnosis yet in hand. The Clinical-Imaging Crosswalk System is built to serve that second reader.

Historical Context: Why Existing Texts Are Organized by Finding

The disease-first, finding-organized structure of the major reference texts in this field reflects their origin and primary readership in diagnostic radiology, where the imaging finding is the starting point of the interpretive task and the clinical presentation arrives, if at all, as a brief history line accompanying the order. That structure is well matched to the radiologist confronting an unknown image and searching for the differential diagnosis that fits it. The child neurology trainee, by contrast, typically already has the clinical presentation in hand and needs the imaging correlate, not the reverse; a book organized to answer what a finding means answers a different question than what a clinician will see on a study about to be ordered, and the gap between the two organizational logics is, this book argues, a meaningful contributor to the persistent difficulty trainees report translating clinical findings into imaging fluency.

The Five-Part Crossing Structure

Each Crossing begins by naming the specific clinical-imaging correlation under discussion, then states the Presentation Signature, the recognizable clinical profile that should bring the crossing to mind at the bedside. The Imaging Correlate specifies the pattern and sequence findings that confirm the suspicion raised by the presentation. Trap Logic names the mimics, normal variants, or look-alike conditions that must be actively excluded before the diagnosis suggested by the crossing is accepted, addressing directly the pitfall most consistently identified in the pediatric neuroimaging literature as a source of diagnostic error. The Crossing Anchor closes each instance with a single, memorable decision rule: a diagnostic threshold, a next imaging step, or a management pivot that the crossing exists to produce.

How to Use the Crossings in Practice

A reader encountering an unfamiliar clinical scenario on service can locate the relevant Crossing directly within the chapter covering that clinical domain, using the Presentation Signature as the entry point; a reader instead confronted with an unexplained imaging finding can enter through the Pediatric Neuroimaging Crosswalk Atlas at the close of this book, which indexes every Crossing by imaging pattern as well as by presentation, allowing navigation from either direction depending on which piece of information the reader has in hand at that moment.

Why Clinical-First Organization Improves Diagnostic Reasoning

Clinical reasoning in practice runs from presentation to hypothesis to confirmatory or excluding data, not from an isolated image to a diagnosis. A text organized by imaging finding trains recognition of the finding in isolation; a text organized by presentation trains the full reasoning chain a clinician must actually execute, including the step, easy to omit in a finding-first text, of first deciding which findings are expected to be present at all before the image is obtained. The five-part Crossing structure makes each step in that chain explicit and repeatable across the entire book, so that by the closing chapters the structure itself becomes a transferable habit of reasoning, applicable to presentations this book does not specifically cover.

This transferability matters because no case-based text, however comprehensive, can enumerate every presentation a working clinician will eventually encounter; the intent of repeating the same five-part structure across twenty chapters and well over one hundred crossings is that the structure itself, rather than any single memorized crossing, becomes the durable clinical skill the reader carries forward.

Comparison to Traditional Disease-Based Texts: A Complementary Resource

This book is not offered as a replacement for the comprehensive, disease-organized references that remain the definitive shelf resource for exhaustive detail on any single diagnosis; rather, it is designed to sit alongside them, serving the specific moment of clinical uncertainty at the bedside or in the reading room when the reader has a presentation in hand and needs the fastest, clearest path to the imaging correlate, the mimics to exclude, and the decision that follows. A reader who identifies the likely crossing here is well served by then consulting a comprehensive disease-based reference for additional depth on a confirmed diagnosis; the two resource types answer different questions and are most effective used together.

Limitations of the Crossing Structure

The Crossing structure is a teaching framework, not a substitute for clinical judgment in an individual case; a real patient frequently presents with an atypical or incomplete signature that does not map cleanly onto a single named crossing, and the reader is expected to use the underlying reasoning pattern, not a lookup-table matching of symptoms to diagnosis, when the presentation in front of them departs from the textbook description. Similarly, a Crossing Anchor states the most common and best-supported decision rule for the scenario described, not an inflexible protocol that overrides individualized clinical judgment, local resource availability, or a family's specific circumstances.

THE CLINICAL-IMAGING CROSSWALK SYSTEM — Deferring an Elective Study Rather Than Sedating Unnecessarily

The Crossing: An eighteen-month-old with a single, brief breath-holding spell is referred for brain MRI, and the family is told sedation will be required given the child's age.

Presentation Signature: A toddler too old for feed-and-wrap and too young to cooperate with an awake study, referred for a presentation, breath-holding spells with a classic, stereotyped history, that carries a very low prior probability of structural brain pathology.

Imaging Correlate: Before scheduling sedation, the reasoning developed in Chapter 3 is applied first: a classic breath-holding spell history, with the stereotyped precipitant, color change, and rapid spontaneous recovery this presentation typically carries, does not meet an evidence-based threshold for neuroimaging at all, making the imaging correlate in this case simply that no study is indicated.

Trap Logic: Proceeding directly to scheduling a sedated MRI without first revisiting whether imaging is indicated exposes the child to anesthetic risk for a study unlikely to change management, and normalizes an imaging-first reflex this book is built to counter.

Crossing Anchor: The imaging-ordering decision precedes the imaging-technique decision; a child should never be scheduled for sedation before the underlying question of whether imaging is indicated at all has been explicitly revisited.

THE CLINICAL-IMAGING CROSSWALK SYSTEM — Recognizing a Motion Artifact Masquerading as Restricted Diffusion

The Crossing: A study performed without adequate motion control shows apparent diffusion restriction on a diffusion-weighted sequence that is not corroborated by the corresponding structural sequences.

Presentation Signature: A young, incompletely sedated or awake child, a study flagged as motion-degraded on technologist notes, and an isolated diffusion-weighted finding without a clinical picture that fits an acute ischemic event.

Imaging Correlate: True restricted diffusion from acute infarction shows a corresponding, anatomically concordant apparent diffusion coefficient signal drop and is reproducible across repeated diffusion directions; motion-related artifact tends to be inconsistent between diffusion directions, does not conform to a vascular territory, and frequently coincides with ghosting or blurring visible on the accompanying structural sequences.

Trap Logic: Accepting an isolated, artifact-degraded diffusion finding at face value risks a false diagnosis of acute stroke, with downstream consequences including unnecessary hematologic and cardiac workup and unwarranted parental alarm.

Crossing Anchor: Any diffusion-weighted finding that does not have a directly corresponding, vascular-territory-concordant signal change on the paired structural sequences should be treated as motion-suspect until a repeat, motion-free acquisition confirms it.

Figure 1.4: Motion Artifact Versus True Restricted Diffusion

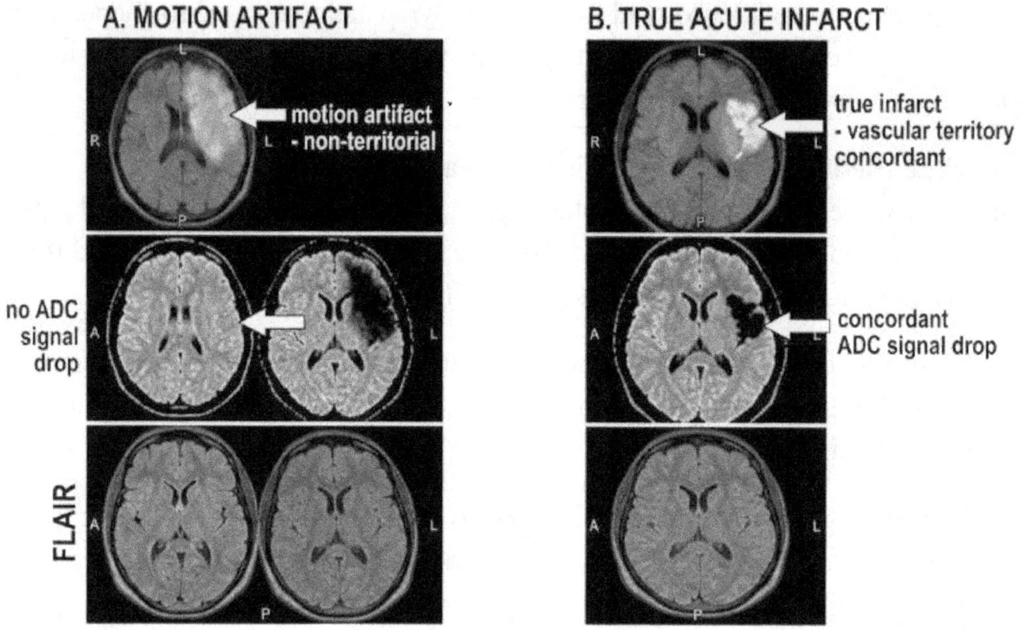

Figure 1.4: Motion Artifact Versus True Restricted Diffusion

DWI b=1000 (High Signal = Restricted Diffusion or Artifact)
ADC Map (Low Signal = True Restricted Diffusion)

Structured Reporting and Communication With Referring Clinicians

The value of a correctly interpreted study is realized only when the finding is communicated in a form the referring clinician can act on. Structured reporting and a clear communication pathway for urgent findings are therefore treated in this book as clinical skills, not administrative afterthoughts.

Elements of a Clinically Actionable Report

A clinically actionable report states the clinical question the study was intended to answer, addresses that question directly rather than burying the answer in a list of incidental observations, characterizes any abnormal finding with the specific descriptors that determine management, including size, location, signal characteristics, and enhancement pattern, and closes with an impression that translates the imaging language into a clinical recommendation the referring team can act on without independently reinterpreting the images.

Structured Reporting Templates and Structured Data

Institution-specific structured templates, in which standard fields for indication, technique, comparison, findings, and impression are consistently populated, improve the retrievability of prior information at follow-up imaging and reduce the likelihood that a clinically relevant negative finding, such as the absence of a mass in a headache workup, is omitted because it did not seem worth stating; a negative finding that answers the referring question is itself clinically actionable information and belongs explicitly in the impression, not only in the body of the findings.

Report Element	Purpose	Common Omission to Avoid
Clinical Indication	States the question the study must answer	Copying a vague referral reason verbatim without clarification
Technique	Documents sequences, contrast, and sedation used	Omitting whether a dedicated protocol (e.g., epilepsy) was actually performed
Comparison	Anchors interval change to a specific prior study	Comparing to "prior imaging" without date or modality specified
Findings	Full, systematic description of pertinent positives and negatives	Omitting a clinically relevant negative because it seemed obvious
Impression	Translates findings into an actionable clinical recommendation	Ending on a descriptive summary without a stated next step

Documenting Uncertainty and Recommending Follow-Up Imaging

Not every finding resolves cleanly into a confident diagnosis at the time of the initial study; an equivocal finding, such as a small focus of signal abnormality that could represent either a normal variant or an early demyelinating lesion, is better served by an explicit statement of the differential and a specific, time-bound follow-up recommendation than by a falsely definitive impression in either direction. A recommendation such as follow-up MRI in three months to assess for interval change, rather than a vague suggestion to correlate clinically, gives the referring clinician a concrete, schedulable action and reduces the risk that genuine uncertainty is lost in translation between the imaging report and the clinical note.

Legal and Documentation Considerations in Pediatric Neuroimaging Reports

Certain pediatric neuroimaging findings, most notably those raising concern for abusive head trauma, carry documentation obligations beyond routine clinical communication, since the written report may later be reviewed in a child protective services or legal proceeding; precise, objective, purely descriptive language regarding injury pattern, age estimation where the literature supports it, and explicit avoidance of unsupported causal attribution in the imaging report itself, with causal interpretation reserved for the multidisciplinary child abuse evaluation discussed in Chapter 19, protects both the accuracy of the medical record and the child's interests in any subsequent proceeding. The same discipline of precise, defensible language, understated rather than overstated, serves every report, not only those bound for legal review, since overstatement in either direction, false reassurance or false alarm, ultimately serves the family and referring clinician poorly.

Retention and accessibility of the original images themselves, not merely the text report, matters in this same context, since a subsequent independent expert review, whether for a legal proceeding or a second clinical opinion, depends on access to the actual images at native resolution; institutional imaging archives are generally built to retain studies far longer than the general medical record retention period specifically in anticipation of this need, and a clinician involved in a case with potential legal implications should confirm early that the imaging archive, not only the written report, has been appropriately preserved.

PATIENT EDUCATION: Families are best served when the ordering clinician explains, before the imaging visit, what the study is being obtained to look for and, in age-appropriate terms, what the child can expect during preparation and the scan itself; a family that understands the specific clinical question is better equipped to ask an informed question when the results are discussed, and a child who has been age-appropriately prepared is more likely to tolerate the study successfully.

Communicating Urgent and Unexpected Findings

An unexpected finding with immediate management implications, such as a new mass, an acute hemorrhage, or evidence suggestive of abusive head trauma, warrants direct verbal communication to the ordering clinician rather than reliance on the written report alone, both because the written report may not be reviewed promptly and because a direct conversation allows the imaging findings to be placed immediately into clinical context. In the specific circumstance of findings suggestive of abusive head trauma, communication responsibilities extend beyond the ordering clinician to institutional child protection reporting requirements, addressed in full in Chapter 19.

Case Presentation: A Structured Consult

A two-year-old is referred for evaluation of macrocephaly identified at a routine well-child visit, with a head circumference tracking above the ninety-seventh percentile and a normal developmental history. The consulting neurologist first applies the reasoning developed earlier in this chapter: the clinical question is not simply whether the brain is normal, but specifically whether the macrocephaly reflects a benign familial pattern, benign enlargement of the subarachnoid spaces, or a pathologic process requiring intervention, a distinction developed fully in Chapter 20. A brain MRI without contrast is selected, since the leading considerations at this age do not require postcontrast sequences, and family head circumference history is obtained before the study to inform interpretation. The study demonstrates mildly prominent frontal subarachnoid spaces with normal underlying brain parenchyma and no ventricular enlargement, a pattern discussed in the Crosswalk Atlas at the close of this book, and the imaging correlate, combined with a family history of similarly large head size in an asymptomatic parent, supports a diagnosis of benign enlargement of the subarachnoid spaces of infancy rather than a pathologic process. The report closes with a specific, actionable recommendation: routine head circumference and developmental follow-up without further imaging, distinguishing this pathway clearly from the pathologic macrocephaly pathway also detailed in Chapter 20.

Case Presentation: An Unexpected Finding

A seven-year-old undergoes brain MRI for evaluation of chronic, non-progressive headache, ordered after the clinical assessment described in Chapter 3 identified features warranting imaging despite the generally low yield of imaging in isolated headache. The study is unexpectedly notable for a well-circumscribed posterior fossa mass with associated obstructive hydrocephalus, a constellation discussed fully in Chapter 13. Rather than issuing only a written report, the interpreting radiologist telephones the ordering clinician directly before the family leaves the imaging center, allowing same-day neurosurgical consultation and avoiding the delay that would have resulted had the family departed and the written report been reviewed asynchronously the following day; this sequence illustrates concretely why the communication pathway described above is treated as a clinical safety mechanism rather than a courtesy.

Case Presentation: Communicating Diagnostic Uncertainty

A ten-year-old with new-onset optic neuritis undergoes brain and orbital MRI, which demonstrates a single small periventricular T2-hyperintense lesion without enhancement, a finding that could represent an isolated, nonspecific white matter focus or an early demyelinating event in the spectrum of pediatric multiple sclerosis or myelin oligodendrocyte glycoprotein antibody disease, discussed fully in Chapter 16. Rather than committing prematurely to either diagnosis, the report explicitly states the differential, recommends correlation with serum antibody testing already in progress, and specifies a follow-up MRI interval to assess for new lesion development, giving the referring neurologist a clear, actionable pathway despite the genuine diagnostic uncertainty present at this single time point.

Case Presentation: Serial Imaging and Longitudinal Comparison

A twelve-year-old with a known, previously stable low-grade glioma undergoes surveillance MRI as part of routine longitudinal follow-up. The interpreting radiologist explicitly compares the current study, sequence by sequence, against the two most recent prior studies rather than the single most recent study alone, a practice that allows a slow, cumulative growth trend spanning multiple intervals to be recognized even when the change between any two consecutive studies individually falls within normal measurement variability. This case illustrates why the comparison field of a structured report, named earlier in this section, functions best when it anchors to a defined baseline and tracks trajectory over time rather than treating each study as an isolated snapshot.

THE CLINICAL-IMAGING CROSSWALK SYSTEM — Foundational Technique and Reasoning Crossings

---

Crossing 1 Recap: New focal seizure with normal examination leads to a dedicated epilepsy protocol with high-resolution hippocampal sequencing, not a routine brain MRI.

Crossing 2 Recap: A classic, low-risk presentation such as a stereotyped breath-holding spell should prompt reconsideration of whether imaging is indicated at all before any sedation plan is scheduled.

Crossing 3 Recap: Isolated diffusion-weighted signal without structural-sequence concordance or vascular-territory pattern should raise suspicion for motion artifact, warranting repeat imaging before diagnosing infarction.

Chapter Anchor: Every imaging decision in this book begins with a defined clinical question; the modality, the protocol, and the interpretation that follow are only as sound as the question that generated them.

Summary and Key Concepts

MRI is the primary pediatric neuroimaging modality; CT is reserved principally for trauma, bony anatomy, and settings in which MRI is unavailable, reflecting the radiosensitivity of the developing brain.

Protocol design should follow the clinical question, not a default brain-MRI template; epilepsy, tumor, and stroke questions each demand distinct sequence selection, and unnecessary adjunct sequences prolong sedation exposure without clinical benefit.

Feed-and-wrap technique avoids sedation in young infants; sedation decisions in older infants and toddlers require an explicit risk-benefit discussion, with additional consideration for children with neurodevelopmental or behavioral needs.

The Clinical-Imaging Crosswalk System — Presentation Signature, Imaging Correlate, Trap Logic, and Crossing Anchor — provides the reasoning structure used throughout this book, organized clinically first rather than by imaging finding.

A clinically actionable report answers the referring question directly, states clinically relevant negatives and genuine uncertainty explicitly, anchors serial comparisons to a defined baseline, and is paired with direct verbal communication for any urgent or unexpected finding.

CHAPTER 2: NORMAL NEURODEVELOPMENTAL IMAGING — FETAL LIFE THROUGH ADOLESCENCE

Learning Objectives

1. Describe the normal sequence of cortical gyration and sulcation across gestational age and correlate it with expected imaging appearance at a given developmental stage.
2. Track the expected pattern and timing of myelination on T1- and T2-weighted imaging from birth through early childhood.
3. Recognize the common normal anatomic variants of the skull, ventricles, and posterior fossa that are frequently mistaken for pathology.
4. Identify the age-dependent interpretive pitfalls most likely to produce a false-positive reading in infants and young children.
5. Distinguish normal pubertal and adolescent structural change, particularly of the pituitary gland, from early pathology.

KEY POINT: Correct interpretation of any pediatric neuroimaging study begins with confirming the child's exact corrected age and matching the expected developmental appearance to that age before any structure is characterized as abnormal; this single habit prevents the majority of the pitfalls catalogued throughout this chapter.

Fetal and Neonatal Brain Development on Imaging

Every imaging appearance discussed in this chapter is a snapshot of a moving target. The pediatric brain is not a smaller, static version of the adult brain; it is a structure actively completing gyration, myelinating in a predictable sequence, and remodeling its proportions well into adolescence, and a signal pattern or structural appearance that is entirely normal at one age is frequently abnormal at another. This chapter establishes the normal developmental trajectory that every disease-focused chapter later in this book assumes as its baseline.

The clinical stakes of getting this baseline correct are not abstract. A normal developmental appearance mistaken for pathology triggers unnecessary follow-up imaging, unnecessary specialist referral, and, in a young child, unnecessary sedation exposure to obtain that follow-up study; conversely, a genuine abnormality mistaken for a normal developmental variant delays the diagnosis and management of a real disease process. The reasoning developed throughout this chapter is therefore not academic background but a direct, load-bearing component of the Clinical-Imaging Crosswalk System's Trap Logic element in nearly every subsequent chapter of this book, and the reader is encouraged to treat this chapter as a reference to revisit, not a chapter to read once and set aside.

Cortical Development and Gyral Maturation Timeline

Cortical gyration follows a predictable, well-characterized timeline beginning around the fourteenth gestational week with the appearance of the earliest primary sulci, most notably the sylvian fissure, and progressing through a defined sequence of secondary and tertiary sulcation that continues into the third trimester and, for the smallest tertiary sulci, into the early postnatal period. A brain that appears smooth, or lissencephalic, at twenty-four weeks gestation is developmentally appropriate; the identical smooth appearance at thirty-six weeks or at term is markedly abnormal and raises concern for a malformation of cortical development, discussed fully in Chapter 7. Correct interpretation therefore depends absolutely on knowing the gestational or corrected age of the child at the time of the study, information that must accompany every fetal or neonatal imaging request.

The sequence of sulcation proceeds broadly from the sylvian fissure and central sulcus toward the parietal, occipital, and finally frontal and temporal poles, a pattern that allows an experienced interpreter to estimate gestational age from the imaging appearance alone within a reasonably narrow range, a skill particularly relevant in fetal MRI when dating information is uncertain or when growth restriction raises the question of whether cortical maturation is proceeding appropriately for the pregnancy's true gestational age.

Figure 2.1: Cortical Gyration and Sulcation Timeline Across Gestational Age

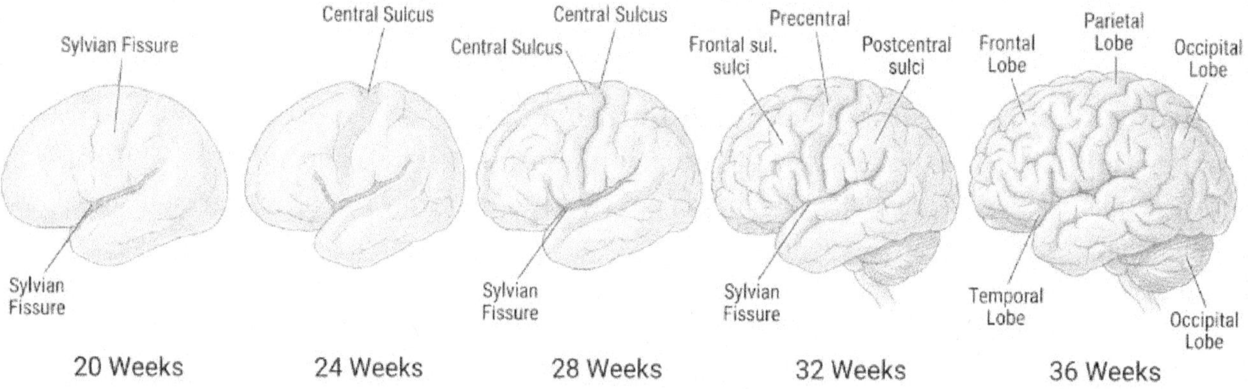

Germinal Matrix and Periventricular Zones in the Neonate

The germinal matrix, a highly cellular, richly vascularized region along the caudothalamic groove, is the source of neuronal and glial precursor cells during fetal development and remains present, though progressively involuting, through approximately thirty-two to thirty-four weeks gestation, after which it largely resolves. Its fragile, immature vasculature is the anatomic substrate for germinal matrix hemorrhage in the preterm infant, developed fully in Chapter 5, and its imaging appearance, a small, well-defined focus of T1 hyperintensity along the caudothalamic groove that should not be mistaken for hemorrhage or calcification, is itself a normal finding in an appropriately premature infant.

The progressive involution of the germinal matrix with advancing gestational age is itself clinically informative: its persistence beyond approximately thirty-four weeks in an infant born at term, or its unexpectedly early involution in a very premature infant, can signal an atypical developmental trajectory worth correlating with the broader clinical picture, though an isolated finding of this kind, without accompanying structural or clinical abnormality, does not by itself constitute a diagnosis.

Corpus Callosum Development and Normal Morphogenesis Timeline

The corpus callosum forms in a broadly anterior-to-posterior sequence beginning around the eighth to tenth gestational week, with the genu forming first, followed by the body, and the splenium and rostrum completing last, a sequence with direct clinical relevance because a callosal anomaly that spares only the posterior segment reflects a later developmental insult than one affecting the genu, information that can help date the timing of an underlying process. By term, the corpus callosum has achieved its complete anatomic configuration, though its thickness continues to increase gradually through infancy and early childhood in parallel with ongoing myelination, a normal thickening that should not be mistaken for a mass effect or thickening of pathologic significance.

Cerebellar Growth and Foliation in the Fetus and Neonate

The cerebellum undergoes a particularly rapid growth phase in the third trimester and continues substantial postnatal growth through the first two years of life, a trajectory that makes it disproportionately vulnerable to injury during the preterm period, discussed further in Chapter 5, and that produces a foliation pattern, the fine folding of the cerebellar cortex, that is visibly less mature on imaging in a preterm infant than in a term infant of otherwise similar overall brain maturity. Because cerebellar volume at a given gestational age correlates with subsequent motor and cognitive outcome in preterm infants, cerebellar growth assessment has become an increasingly emphasized component of preterm neuroimaging surveillance, addressed further in Chapter 5.

This vulnerability arises in part because the cerebellum's growth trajectory during the third trimester coincides directly with the period of greatest risk for preterm delivery, meaning an infant born prematurely is removed from the intrauterine environment at precisely the developmental window when cerebellar growth would otherwise be proceeding most rapidly; postnatal cerebellar growth outside the womb does not fully replicate the intrauterine trajectory, which is one proposed mechanism, among several under active investigation, for the disproportionate cerebellar volume reduction observed in some preterm cohorts relative to term-born peers assessed at the same corrected age.

Neonatal Brain Volume, Sulcation, and Ventricular Proportions

The term neonatal brain has a proportionally larger extra-axial cerebrospinal fluid space and proportionally larger ventricles relative to brain parenchyma than the brain will have at any later point in childhood, a normal proportion that narrows progressively over the first two years of life as brain volume increases; this normal proportion is the anatomic basis for the benign extra-axial fluid pattern discussed later in this chapter and must be distinguished from pathologic ventriculomegaly, a distinction developed fully in Chapter 10.

Ventricular Asymmetry as a Normal Variant

Mild asymmetry between the right and left lateral ventricles, typically involving the atrium or occipital horn and generally within a few millimeters of difference, is a common normal variant present in a meaningful proportion of healthy children and should not, in isolation, be equated with pathologic ventriculomegaly or a mass effect from an occult lesion; the distinguishing features that separate this normal asymmetry from a pathologic process are the absence of any associated periventricular signal abnormality, the absence of a mass effect displacing midline structures, and stability of the asymmetry when compared to any available prior imaging, none of which require the asymmetry itself to be perfectly symmetric before it can be called normal.

Quantifying ventricular size against an age-specific reference range, most commonly using the Evans index or a direct atrial width measurement compared to published pediatric norms, is more reliable than visual impression alone, particularly when the finding is borderline or when the interpreting clinician is comparing studies performed on different scanners or with different slice orientations; a single measurement obtained in isolation is nonetheless less informative than a trend, and whenever a prior study is available, tracking the measurement over time is the more clinically meaningful exercise than judging any single value in isolation against a population reference range.

Preterm Versus Term Brain Appearance

A preterm infant's brain, even when structurally normal for its gestational age, differs systematically from a term brain in gyral complexity, myelination stage, and germinal matrix prominence, and comparing a preterm infant's imaging directly against term-brain reference expectations, rather than against gestational-age-corrected expectations, is among the most common sources of false concern in neonatal neuroimaging. Reports on preterm infants should explicitly state both chronologic and corrected gestational age, and normal-appearance determinations should be made against corrected-age reference standards, not chronologic age alone.

Fetal MRI Timing and Gestational Age Considerations

Fetal MRI is generally most informative from approximately twenty to twenty-two weeks gestation onward, once fetal structures are large enough to resolve reliably against the motion-robust sequences the technique requires, and its interpretive value continues to increase through the third trimester as cortical symmetric, predominantly frontal distribution; a family history of similarly large head size in an otherwise asymptomatic parent further supports the diagnosis and is worth eliciting specifically.

The natural history of benign enlargement of the subarachnoid spaces is spontaneous resolution, typically by age two, as brain growth outpaces the extra-axial space, and this expected trajectory itself functions as a confirmatory feature: a family counseled about the benign, self-limited nature of the finding and followed with head circumference tracking alone, rather than repeat imaging, that subsequently shows the expected narrowing of the extra-axial space on any interval clinical imaging obtained for an unrelated reason, retrospectively confirms the original diagnosis was correct.

Cavum Septum Pellucidum and Cavum Vergae

A cavum septum pellucidum, a fluid-filled space between the leaflets of the septum pellucidum, and its posterior extension, the cavum vergae, are present in essentially all fetuses and neonates and remain a normal, incidental finding in a substantial proportion of the general population into adulthood; an isolated cavum septum pellucidum or cavum vergae, without associated abnormality of the corpus callosum or ventricular system, requires no further workup and should be reported as a normal variant rather than as an incidental finding of uncertain significance.

Choroid Plexus Cysts

Choroid plexus cysts, small cystic structures within the choroid plexus of the lateral ventricles, are identified on a meaningful proportion of second-trimester prenatal ultrasounds and, when isolated without other structural or soft marker abnormality, carry a benign prognosis with a very low residual association with chromosomal abnormality once other major markers have been excluded; postnatally, an incidental choroid plexus cyst identified on MRI performed for an unrelated indication is a normal finding requiring no follow-up, and the distinction between a prenatal choroid plexus cyst finding, which carries genetic counseling implications in the context of other markers, and a postnatal incidental finding, which generally does not, is worth making explicitly when counseling a family who recalls a prenatal ultrasound mention of this finding.

The great majority of prenatally identified choroid plexus cysts, whether isolated or accompanied by other soft markers ultimately assessed as low risk, resolve spontaneously by the third trimester and are no longer visible on postnatal imaging at all; a family counseled at the time of the original prenatal finding that the cyst itself was expected to resolve, and that its resolution or persistence carries no independent prognostic weight once other screening has been reassuring, generally experiences considerably less anxiety at the postnatal visit than a family for whom this natural history was not explained in advance.

Arachnoid Cysts as an Incidental Finding

A small, asymptomatic arachnoid cyst identified incidentally, most commonly in the middle cranial fossa, is common enough in the general pediatric population that its discovery on a study obtained for an unrelated reason does not by itself indicate pathology; the great majority of incidentally discovered arachnoid cysts remain stable in size and asymptomatic over long-term follow-up. A minority enlarge, become symptomatic through mass effect or, rarely, hemorrhage after minor trauma, or require neurosurgical evaluation, and this distinction between an incidental, stable arachnoid cyst and one requiring active management is developed fully in Chapter 10.

Persistent Falcine and Dural Venous Variants

Variations in dural venous sinus anatomy, including a hypoplastic or asymmetric transverse sinus, a persistent falcine sinus representing an embryonic venous channel that normally involutes, and prominent arachnoid granulations projecting into the dural venous sinuses, are common incidental findings on venous-phase imaging that should not be mistaken for venous sinus thrombosis, discussed in Chapter 6 and Chapter 18; the key distinguishing feature in each case is the absence of an expansile filling defect and the presence of normal flow-related signal, rather than the simple presence of asymmetry, since some degree of transverse sinus size asymmetry is itself a normal population variant present in a substantial minority of healthy individuals.

When genuine uncertainty remains after conventional venous-phase imaging, dedicated MR venography with flow-sensitive sequencing resolves the ambiguity more reliably than an isolated observation of asymmetry on a routine postcontrast sequence, since flow-related signal dropout at a site of normal anatomic narrowing can otherwise be mistaken for a filling defect; this distinction carries genuine clinical weight; because the management pathways for a confirmed venous sinus thrombosis and for a benign anatomic variant diverge substantially, the threshold for obtaining dedicated venographic confirmation should be low whenever the initial finding is anything short of unambiguous.

Posterior Fossa Normal Variants: Mega Cisterna Magna and Blake's Pouch Cyst

A mega cisterna magna, an enlarged but otherwise normal cisterna magna communicating freely with the fourth ventricle and subarachnoid space, and a Blake pouch cyst, a thin-walled, retrocerebellar cystic structure representing a persistent embryonic remnant, are both distinguished from the pathologic posterior fossa malformations discussed in Chapter 8 by the presence of a normal-appearing, normally positioned cerebellar vermis; the vermis, not the size of the retrocerebellar space alone, is the structure that determines whether a posterior fossa finding is a benign variant or a true malformation, a distinction developed at length in Chapter 8.

Skull Variants: Wormian Bones and Venous Lakes

Wormian bones, small accessory ossification centers within the cranial sutures, are a common incidental finding on CT or skull radiography and are typically benign in isolation, though numerous or unusually prominent wormian bones can be associated with certain skeletal dysplasias or connective tissue disorders and warrant consideration of the broader clinical picture rather than automatic dismissal. Venous lakes and arachnoid granulation-related calvarial lucencies represent normal venous drainage structures and should not be mistaken for a lytic bony lesion, a distinction aided by their characteristic location along known venous sinus and granulation sites and their smooth, well-corticated margins.

Physiologic Intracranial Calcifications

Physiologic calcification of the choroid plexus and, somewhat later in childhood, the pineal gland and habenular commissure, is a normal age-related finding on CT that becomes progressively more common through later childhood and adolescence and is essentially universal by adulthood; its presence in a young child before the typical age of onset, or an unusually dense or extensive pattern of intracranial calcification more broadly, can occasionally signal an underlying congenital infection or metabolic disorder, discussed further in Chapter 15 and Chapter 17, making the age at which physiologic calcification is first observed, and its distribution, clinically relevant details rather than an incidental finding to be dismissed without consideration of the child's age.

Basal ganglia calcification, most often involving the globus pallidus bilaterally and symmetrically, follows a somewhat later and more variable timeline than pineal or choroid plexus calcification and, when mild, symmetric, and identified as an incidental finding in an older child or adolescent without an associated movement disorder or endocrine abnormality, is generally a benign, physiologic finding; bilateral basal ganglia calcification that is unusually extensive for age, markedly asymmetric, or accompanied by a movement disorder, seizures, or endocrine dysfunction instead warrants evaluation for a calcifying microangiopathy or a metabolic or genetic calcification syndrome, a distinction made primarily on the basis of the accompanying clinical picture rather than the calcification pattern on CT alone.

Fontanelle and Suture Closure Timeline

The anterior fontanelle, palpable and imageable at birth, typically closes between approximately nine and eighteen months of age, a range wide enough that closure occurring at either edge of this window, in isolation, does not by itself indicate pathology; the posterior fontanelle closes considerably earlier, typically within the first two to three months. Premature suture fusion, or craniosynostosis, discussed fully in Chapter 8, is distinguished from normal, appropriately timed closure by the presence of an abnormal, characteristically asymmetric head shape, a palpable bony ridge along the fused suture on examination, and, when imaging is obtained, direct visualization of sutural fusion on CT rather than simple advanced closure timing alone; a family's report that a fontanelle feels small at a particular well-child visit is not, by itself, sufficient grounds for imaging in the absence of an abnormal head shape or a palpable ridge.

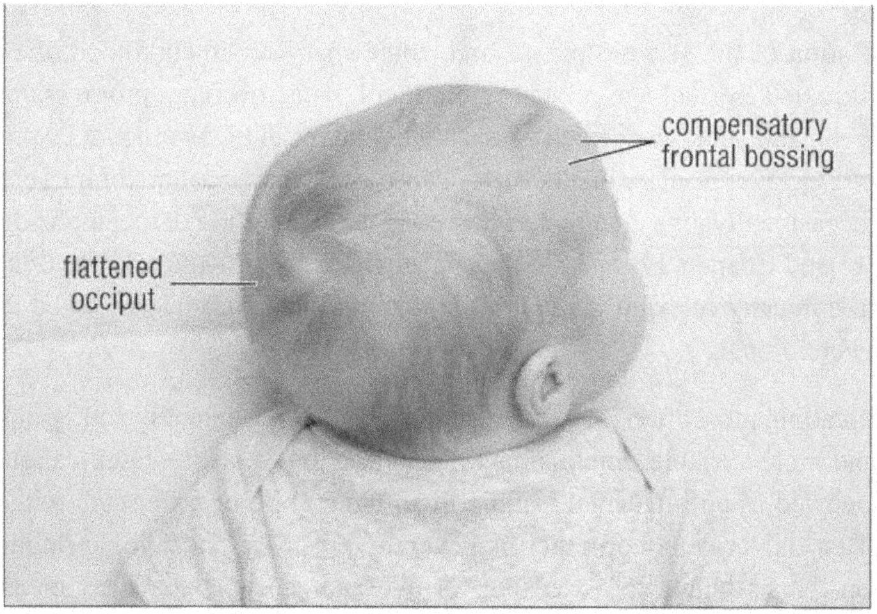

Figure 2.3 Physical Head-Shape Presentation of a Common Benign Skull Variant

Age-Dependent Pitfalls in Interpretation

Beyond the discrete normal variants named above, several broader interpretive pitfalls recur specifically because the pediatric brain's normal appearance changes continuously with age, and a finding that would be unambiguous in an adult carries genuine interpretive ambiguity in a child.

FLAIR Hyperintensity in the Infant Brain

Fluid-attenuated inversion recovery imaging in a child younger than approximately two years can show periventricular and deep white matter T2 hyperintensity that reflects normal, incomplete myelination rather than true pathology, because the FLAIR sequence's fluid-suppression mechanism behaves differently against the higher water content of unmyelinated white matter; this normal appearance is a well-documented source of false-positive concern for periventricular leukomalacia or demyelinating disease in young children and is a principal reason this book, in Chapter 1, cautions against reflexive FLAIR-based interpretation in this age group without correlating against the T1 and T2 myelination timeline established earlier in this chapter.

Pseudo-Subarachnoid Hemorrhage Sign in Infants

On CT, diffuse cerebral edema or, less commonly, the relatively higher density of unmyelinated white matter relative to cerebrospinal fluid in a young infant can produce an apparent increase in attenuation along the basal cisterns and cerebral sulci that mimics true subarachnoid hemorrhage, a phenomenon termed the pseudo-subarachnoid hemorrhage sign; distinguishing the true finding from the pseudo-finding relies on assessing whether the apparent hyperattenuation follows the expected gyral and sulcal pattern of true blood, correlating against the clinical scenario, and, when genuine uncertainty remains, obtaining MRI, which resolves the ambiguity far more reliably than CT alone in this specific age-dependent pitfall.

Terminal Zones of Myelination and Periventricular Signal

The terminal zones, small regions of persistent T2 hyperintensity typically located in the peritrigonal white matter, represent the last areas of the brain to complete myelination and can remain visible as a subtle, symmetric finding into later childhood and even young adulthood in some individuals; their symmetric distribution, characteristic peritrigonal location, and lack of associated volume loss or diffusion abnormality distinguish them from a pathologic process, and recognizing this specific, named normal variant prevents unnecessary additional workup for an otherwise incidental finding.

Apparent Diffusion Coefficient Values Change With Age

Quantitative apparent diffusion coefficient values in normal brain parenchyma are not static across childhood; unmyelinated white matter in a young infant shows higher baseline apparent diffusion coefficient values than the same region will show once myelination and the accompanying increase in tissue density and organization are complete, meaning a numeric apparent diffusion coefficient value considered abnormally elevated by adult reference ranges may fall entirely within the normal range for an infant of a given age. Applying adult apparent diffusion coefficient reference values to a pediatric study without age adjustment is a preventable source of both false-positive and false-negative interpretation of subtle diffusion abnormality.

Perivascular (Virchow-Robin) Spaces

Perivascular spaces, also known by the eponym Virchow-Robin spaces, are fluid-filled extensions of the subarachnoid space accompanying penetrating vessels into the brain parenchyma, most commonly visible in the basal ganglia and centrum semiovale, and follow cerebrospinal fluid signal on every sequence, a key feature distinguishing them from a true cystic lesion or lacunar infarct. They are typically small, round or linear along the course of the vessel, and multiple, and become more numerous and more conspicuous with age; prominent perivascular spaces in a child are usually an incidental normal finding, though unusually extensive or asymmetric perivascular space prominence occasionally warrants consideration of an underlying mucopolysaccharidosis or other metabolic process, discussed further in Chapter 17.

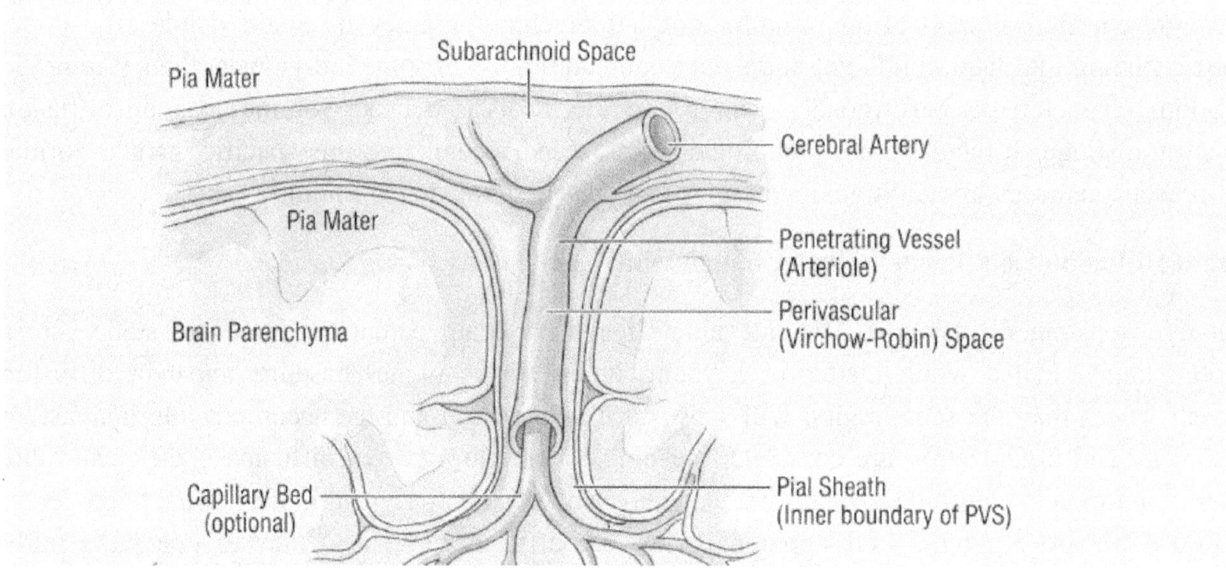

Pseudo-Pathology From Partial Volume and Motion in Young Children

Partial volume averaging, in which a thick imaging slice blends signal from adjacent structures of differing composition, is exaggerated in small pediatric structures relative to the larger equivalent adult structures, and can produce an apparent signal abnormality at a tissue boundary, such as the gray-white junction, that resolves on thinner-section imaging; combined with the motion artifact discussed in Chapter 1, this makes technically optimized, motion-free, appropriately thin-section acquisition a prerequisite for confident exclusion of subtle pathology in a young child, rather than a technical nicety.

Cerebellar Signal Variability in the Neonate

The neonatal cerebellum, still completing the rapid growth and foliation described earlier in this chapter, can show a mildly heterogeneous, less uniformly organized signal appearance on both T1- and T2-weighted imaging than the more homogeneous, fully organized appearance expected later in infancy, a normal transitional appearance that has occasionally been mistaken for cerebellar injury or hypoplasia by a reader unfamiliar with the expected neonatal cerebellar signal pattern; correlating the cerebellar appearance against gestational age and against the overall foliation pattern, rather than against an isolated signal impression, resolves this ambiguity in the great majority of cases and avoids an unwarranted diagnosis of cerebellar injury, discussed fully in Chapter 5, in a structurally normal neonate.

CLINICAL PEARL: When a finding in a young child looks unusual, the first question should be whether the finding fits a known age-dependent normal pattern before it is characterized as pathologic; the differential for an unusual-appearing but ultimately normal finding in pediatric neuroimaging is frequently broader than the differential for genuine pathology at the same location.

THE CLINICAL-IMAGING CROSSWALK SYSTEM — Prominent Perivascular Spaces Mistaken for Cystic Pathology

The Crossing: A three-year-old undergoes brain MRI for an unrelated indication, and the study incidentally shows multiple small, round, symmetric lesions in the basal ganglia bilaterally, prompting concern for a cystic or vacuolating process.

Presentation Signature: An asymptomatic child with a normal neurologic examination, in whom the finding is entirely incidental to the indication for the study, with no clinical features suggesting a metabolic or neurodegenerative process.

Imaging Correlate: The lesions follow cerebrospinal fluid signal on every sequence, including complete suppression on FLAIR, are round to linear in configuration following the expected course of penetrating lenticulostriate vessels, and are symmetric and multiple; these features are diagnostic of prominent, normal perivascular spaces rather than a cystic lesion, tumor, or vacuolating leukoencephalopathy.

Trap Logic: Failing to confirm complete FLAIR suppression, the single most reliable discriminating feature, risks mistaking prominent perivascular spaces for a genuinely pathologic cystic process and triggering an unnecessary metabolic workup in an asymptomatic child.

Crossing Anchor: Any small, round, symmetric basal ganglia or centrum semiovale lesion that fully suppresses on FLAIR and follows cerebrospinal fluid signal on every sequence is a perivascular space until proven otherwise, and does not require further workup in an asymptomatic child with a normal examination.

Puberty and Adolescent Structural Change

The final developmental transition covered in this chapter, and the one most likely to be misread as pathology by a clinician trained primarily on younger pediatric or adult imaging, is the structural remodeling that accompanies puberty, most notably of the pituitary gland.

Pituitary Gland Size and Signal Changes at Puberty

The pituitary gland undergoes a well-documented, hormonally driven increase in height during puberty, with the upper limit of normal gland height reaching approximately ten to twelve millimeters in pubertal girls, somewhat less in boys, and the gland frequently developing a convex, rather than flat or concave, superior margin during this period; this normal pubertal enlargement, sometimes accompanied by physiologic signal heterogeneity, is a well-recognized source of false concern for a pituitary adenoma or other sellar mass when the reader is unaware of the expected pubertal appearance and applies adult or prepubertal size thresholds instead.

Adolescent Female Pituitary Height Versus Adolescent Male

The pubertal pituitary height threshold differs meaningfully by sex, with adolescent girls, particularly around the time of menarche, showing a more pronounced and slightly higher normal upper limit than adolescent boys undergoing an equivalent pubertal stage, a difference attributable to the greater hormonal stimulation of gonadotroph and lactotroph cell populations during female pubertal maturation; applying a single, sex-nonspecific size threshold across all adolescents therefore risks both under-calling a genuine finding in a boy, whose normal upper limit is lower, and over-calling a normal finding in a girl, whose normal upper limit is higher, making explicit documentation of the patient's sex and pubertal stage a necessary component of correctly interpreting pituitary size in this age group.

Gray and White Matter Volume Trajectories in Adolescence

Neuroimaging-based developmental cohort studies have consistently demonstrated that gray matter volume follows an inverted-U trajectory through childhood and adolescence, increasing through mid-childhood and then declining gradually through adolescence as synaptic pruning proceeds, while white matter volume increases steadily and roughly linearly through adolescence as myelination continues to mature into the third decade of life; these population-level trends are relevant chiefly as context for understanding that continued structural change through adolescence is itself the normal pattern, not evidence of an evolving pathologic process, when a study performed at two different adolescent time points shows subtle volumetric difference.

Pineal Gland Cysts as a Normal Adolescent Finding

Small pineal cysts, generally under one centimeter, thin-walled, and without solid enhancing components, are a common incidental finding in adolescents and young adults, identified on a substantial proportion of brain MRIs performed for unrelated indications in this age group, and require no follow-up imaging when they meet these benign size and morphology criteria; a larger cyst, one with a thickened or nodular wall, solid enhancing components, or associated hydrocephalus from aqueductal compression, falls outside this benign pattern and warrants the pineal region tumor evaluation detailed in Chapter 12.

Skull Base and Paranasal Sinus Pneumatization Changes at Puberty

The paranasal sinuses, particularly the frontal and sphenoid sinuses, undergo substantial pneumatization during the pubertal growth period, changing markedly in size and shape between a pre-adolescent and a late-adolescent study of the same individual; an adolescent skull base and sinus appearance that would be considered underdeveloped in an adult is entirely expected earlier in this pneumatization sequence, and this same growth process explains why skull base imaging performed for an unrelated indication, such as a headache evaluation, can appear to change substantially between two studies obtained several years apart in the same patient without any pathologic process having occurred.

This same pneumatization process has practical relevance beyond incidental comparison: an incompletely pneumatized, still-marrow-filled sphenoid bone in a younger adolescent can show T1 and T2 signal characteristics that differ from the fully aerated adult pattern and should not be mistaken for a skull base marrow-replacing process, a distinction made by correlating the signal pattern against the child's pubertal stage and by confirming the absence of any expansile or destructive component to the finding.

Distinguishing Normal Adolescent Change From Early Pathology

The general principle that distinguishes normal adolescent structural change from early pathology throughout this section is symmetry and smooth, expected morphology: normal pubertal pituitary enlargement is symmetric and smoothly convex rather than focally nodular or asymmetric; normal adolescent volumetric change is gradual and diffuse rather than focal; and a benign pineal cyst is thin-walled and non-enhancing rather than thick-walled or solid. Any finding that departs from the expected symmetric, smooth pattern for its structure warrants the same disease-specific evaluation that would be applied at any other age, rather than being attributed reflexively to normal adolescent change. Applied consistently, this symmetry principle, together with the corrected-age framework established at the start of this chapter, gives the reader a durable method for judging normal developmental appearance at any age covered in the chapters that follow, rather than a fixed list of findings to memorize in isolation.

Feature	Normal Pubertal Pituitary	Concerning for Pathology
Gland margin	Smooth, symmetric convexity	Focal bulge or nodularity
Height	Up to ~10-12 mm (girls), slightly less (boys)	Height exceeding sex- and stage-adjusted upper limit
Enhancement	Homogeneous	Focal non-enhancing or differentially enhancing region
Stalk	Midline, undeviated	Deviated or thickened stalk

THE CLINICAL-IMAGING CROSSWALK SYSTEM — Pubertal Sinus Pneumatization Mistaken for a Skull Base Lesion

The Crossing: A sixteen-year-old undergoes brain MRI for headache evaluation, and comparison to a study performed at age eleven shows a markedly different sphenoid bone appearance, prompting concern for an interval skull base process.

Presentation Signature: An adolescent with a comparison study obtained several years earlier, before substantial pubertal sinus pneumatization had occurred, now showing a sphenoid sinus that appears dramatically larger and more aerated than on the prior study.

Imaging Correlate: The current study shows a well-aerated, normally marginated sphenoid sinus with expected fatty marrow signal in the surrounding skull base bone and no soft tissue mass, enhancing lesion, or bone destruction; the appearance is fully explained by normal pubertal sinus pneumatization progressing between the two study dates, exactly the process described earlier in this chapter.

Trap Logic: Comparing an adolescent skull base study to a pre-pubertal comparison without accounting for expected pneumatization change risks describing a normal developmental process as an interval finding requiring further workup.

Crossing Anchor: Any interval skull base or sinus change identified when comparing a pre-pubertal study to a later adolescent study should be evaluated first against expected pubertal pneumatization before any additional workup is pursued.

Case Presentation: An Adolescent With Incidental Pituitary Enlargement

A fourteen-year-old girl undergoes brain MRI for evaluation of chronic headache, and the study incidentally demonstrates a pituitary gland measuring eleven millimeters in height with a smoothly convex superior margin and homogeneous enhancement. Applying the reasoning developed in this section, the interpreting radiologist recognizes this appearance as within the expected range for a pubertal girl at Tanner stage matching her reported menarche, rather than a pituitary microadenoma, and the report explicitly states that the finding is consistent with normal pubertal pituitary enlargement, recommending no dedicated pituitary follow-up imaging on this basis alone; the headache workup proceeds using the presentation-based reasoning developed in Chapter 20, unaffected by this incidental, benign finding.

Case Presentation: A Toddler With an Isolated Cavum Septum Pellucidum

A fifteen-month-old undergoes brain MRI for evaluation of a single febrile seizure, discussed further in Chapter 11, and the study incidentally demonstrates a cavum septum pellucidum with a small cavum vergae extension, an otherwise entirely normal corpus callosum, ventricular system, and cortical mantle. The report explicitly names the finding as a normal anatomic variant requiring no further workup or follow-up imaging, illustrating the broader principle developed throughout this chapter: a normal variant, once correctly recognized, is reported as a normal variant, not carried forward as an incidental finding of uncertain significance that generates unwarranted follow-up.

Case Presentation: An Infant With an Incidental Choroid Plexus Cyst and Prior Prenatal Marker History

A four-month-old undergoes brain MRI for evaluation of positional head shape concern, and the study incidentally identifies a small choroid plexus cyst. The family reports that a choroid plexus cyst had also been noted on a second-trimester prenatal ultrasound, prompting significant anxiety at the time regarding chromosomal risk. Applying the distinction developed earlier in this chapter, the interpreting clinician explains that the prenatal finding, once other soft markers and formal aneuploidy screening were reassuring, and given the infant's subsequently normal development, carried a low residual risk that has now been further reassured by a normal postnatal examination and development, and that the postnatal choroid plexus cyst finding itself is incidental and requires no follow-up; this case illustrates the value of explicitly distinguishing prenatal counseling implications from postnatal incidental-finding management when a family carries anxiety forward from an earlier prenatal finding.

Case Presentation: A Febrile Infant With an Apparent Pseudo-Subarachnoid Hemorrhage Sign on CT

A seven-month-old presents to the emergency department with fever, irritability, and a bulging fontanelle, and an urgent noncontrast head CT is obtained to evaluate for possible meningitis-related complication before lumbar puncture. The study shows subtle, diffuse hyperattenuation along the basal cisterns that the covering clinician initially interprets as possible subarachnoid hemorrhage. Applying the age-dependent pitfall reasoning developed in this chapter, the pediatric radiologist recognizes the pattern as consistent with the pseudo-subarachnoid hemorrhage sign, likely related to diffuse cerebral hyperemia and edema accompanying the infant's acute febrile illness rather than true hemorrhage, and confirms this impression by noting that the apparent hyperattenuation does not conform precisely to the expected gyral and sulcal pattern of true subarachnoid blood; the report explicitly names the pseudo-finding, recommends correlation with the ongoing infectious workup, and avoids triggering an unnecessary hematologic and vascular hemorrhage evaluation in a child whose presentation is otherwise fully explained by the infectious process already under evaluation.

THE CLINICAL-IMAGING CROSSWALK SYSTEM — Normal Development and Age-Dependent Variant Crossings

---

Crossing 1 Recap: Myelination status must always be read against the specific structures expected to be myelinated at the child's exact corrected age, never against a generic adult-pattern expectation.

Crossing 2 Recap: A small, round, symmetric lesion that fully suppresses on FLAIR and follows cerebrospinal fluid signal on every sequence is a perivascular space, not a cystic pathology, in an asymptomatic child.

Crossing 3 Recap: An interval skull base or sinus change between a pre-pubertal and adolescent study should be evaluated against expected pubertal pneumatization before further workup is pursued.

Chapter Anchor: Every apparent abnormality in a pediatric study should first be checked against the age-expected developmental timeline established in this chapter before it is characterized as pathologic.

Summary and Key Concepts

Cortical gyration, germinal matrix involution, corpus callosum morphogenesis, and cerebellar foliation all follow predictable developmental timelines that must be correlated against corrected, not chronologic, age in preterm infants.

Myelination proceeds center-to-periphery and follows separate T1 and T2 timelines, with T1 reaching the adult pattern by approximately one year and T2 by approximately eighteen to twenty-four months; diffusion tensor imaging offers a complementary quantitative measure via fractional anisotropy.

Benign enlargement of the subarachnoid spaces, cavum septum pellucidum, choroid plexus cysts, incidental arachnoid cysts, dural venous variants, mega cisterna magna, and Blake pouch cyst are among the most common normal variants generating unnecessary referral when unrecognized.

FLAIR hyperintensity and elevated apparent diffusion coefficient values in infants, the pseudo-subarachnoid hemorrhage sign, terminal zones of myelination, and perivascular spaces are age-dependent findings whose normal appearance must be actively distinguished from pathology.

Pubertal pituitary enlargement is symmetric and smoothly convex, with sex-specific normal height thresholds; asymmetric or nodular enlargement, and thick-walled or solid pineal cysts, fall outside the normal pattern and warrant dedicated evaluation.

CHAPTER 3: IMAGING-ORDERING DECISIONS IN CHILD NEUROLOGY

Learning Objectives

1. Apply evidence-based appropriateness criteria to determine whether neuroimaging is indicated for a given pediatric presentation.
2. Select the correct imaging modality among MRI, CT, ultrasound, and nuclear medicine for a defined clinical question, applying the framework introduced in Chapter 1.
3. Identify common pediatric neurologic presentations for which imaging is typically low-yield and can reasonably be deferred or omitted.
4. Communicate radiation risk, sedation risk, and diagnostic uncertainty to families in a way that supports informed, shared decision-making.

Appropriateness Criteria and Evidence-Based Thresholds

The decision to obtain neuroimaging at all is, in most pediatric neurologic presentations, a more consequential decision than the choice of which specific modality or protocol to use, and it is a decision the published literature shows clinicians make inconsistently even when working from the same evidence base. This chapter addresses that decision directly, extending the sequence-and-protocol reasoning developed in Chapter 1 one full step earlier in the clinical process, and closing the loop between the ordering decision and the interpretation skills built throughout the rest of this book.

The ACR Appropriateness Criteria as a Framework

The American College of Radiology Appropriateness Criteria provide condition-specific, evidence-graded guidance on which imaging study, if any, is generally appropriate for a defined clinical scenario, ranking modality options rather than issuing a single binary imaging-or-no-imaging verdict; for pediatric neurologic presentations, the criteria address scenarios including focal and generalized seizure, headache, and developmental delay, each stratified by specific clinical features that shift the recommendation, and each cross-referenced within the relevant disease-specific chapter later in this book. Using this framework as a starting point, rather than personal habit or the imaging pattern of a prior training program, anchors an individual clinician's threshold to a defensible, updated evidence base rather than to idiosyncratic practice.

The criteria are updated periodically as new evidence accumulates, and a clinician who last reviewed the relevant criteria during training may be working from a threshold that has since shifted; periodically revisiting the current criteria for the presentations encountered most frequently in one's own practice, rather than assuming a threshold learned years earlier remains current, is a component of maintaining an evidence-based imaging practice over the course of a career. Many institutions embed the relevant criteria directly into the electronic order-entry workflow through clinical decision support, presenting the evidence-graded appropriateness rating for a given indication at the point of ordering rather than requiring the clinician to consult an external reference separately; where available, this point-of-care integration measurably reduces low-yield ordering by surfacing the evidence at the exact moment the ordering decision is made.

Documented Variability in Imaging Thresholds

Published survey data examining physician imaging-ordering thresholds for pediatric recurrent headache found no consensus among pediatric neurologists, radiologists, and neurosurgeons regarding the risk level at which imaging became appropriate, with the proportion of physicians recommending imaging varying from near-universal at the highest documented risk category to a small minority at the lowest, illustrating that even among specialists working from the same underlying evidence, individual threshold varies substantially. Similar variability has been documented in the evaluation of children with autism spectrum disorder, where the diagnostic yield of brain MRI obtained for autism alone, without an additional red-flag feature such as regression, seizure, or an abnormal neurologic examination, has been shown in published cohort data to be low enough that routine imaging in this isolated presentation is not broadly supported.

This documented variability matters clinically because it means an individual clinician's personal threshold, however confidently held, may not reflect the best available evidence, and the deliberate goal of this chapter is to replace habit-based ordering with a reproducible, evidence-anchored decision process that a reader can apply consistently rather than reinvent for each new presentation. Variability of this kind also has a training-pathway origin worth naming directly: a clinician trained in a practice environment with a historically low imaging threshold internalizes that threshold as normal, and absent deliberate exposure to the published appropriateness literature, may carry that threshold forward into independent practice without ever having compared it explicitly against the evidence base this chapter presents.

Diagnostic Yield Data and How to Interpret It

Diagnostic yield, the proportion of studies obtained for a given indication that identify a clinically significant abnormality, is the central quantitative concept underlying every appropriateness recommendation in this chapter, and interpreting it correctly requires distinguishing yield for any abnormality, which is frequently higher and includes incidental findings without management implications, from yield for a clinically significant, management-changing abnormality, the more relevant figure for an ordering decision. A presentation with a reported ten percent yield for any abnormality may carry a yield below one percent for a finding that actually changes management, and a clinician citing yield data to a family or to a referring colleague should be precise about which figure is being used, since conflating the two overstates the practical value of imaging in a low-yield scenario.

Yield figures reported in the published literature are also population-level estimates, derived from cohorts that may not precisely match an individual child's specific combination of history and examination findings, and applying a population-level yield figure to an individual clinical decision requires judgment about how closely that individual child's presentation matches the cohort from which the figure was derived, including its age range, symptom duration, and examination criteria; a child whose presentation includes even one feature outside the low-risk profile described in a given study should not be assumed to carry that study's reported low yield, since the yield figure specifically describes the population meeting the stated low-risk criteria, not any child presenting with a superficially similar complaint.

A further, related consideration is publication and referral bias in the source data itself: yield studies conducted at tertiary academic centers, where a disproportionate share of genuinely complex or atypical presentations are ultimately referred, may report a somewhat higher baseline yield than would be observed in a general community pediatric or primary care population evaluating the identical presenting complaint, since the tertiary cohort has already been pre-selected, whether consciously or not, for cases a referring clinician found sufficiently concerning to send onward. Recognizing this referral-pattern effect helps explain why a yield figure drawn from a single-center tertiary study should be applied with appropriate caution to a general outpatient population, and reinforces the value of seeking multicenter or population-based yield data, when available, over a single institution's experience.

The Cost of False Reassurance and False Alarm

An evidence-based imaging threshold is sometimes mischaracterized as a cost-cutting exercise rather than what it actually is: a clinical tool for minimizing two distinct, opposing harms simultaneously. Imaging obtained beyond what the evidence supports carries the harms already discussed throughout this chapter, radiation, sedation risk, cost, and delay to definitive care elsewhere in the system; imaging withheld when a genuine red-flag feature was present, or when a clinician's threshold was set too conservatively out of an overcorrection to the low-yield reasoning developed in this chapter, carries the distinct harm of a missed or delayed diagnosis. The appropriateness framework developed in this chapter exists specifically to minimize the sum of both harms, not to minimize imaging utilization as an end in itself, a distinction worth stating explicitly because a clinician who internalizes only the low-yield half of this chapter's reasoning, without the equally important red-flag half, has misapplied the framework.

A useful discipline for holding both halves of this framework in mind simultaneously is to ask, before finalizing any imaging-ordering decision, not only whether the evidence supports imaging in this scenario, but whether this specific child's presentation has been actively and deliberately screened against the full red-flag list relevant to the presenting complaint, rather than assumed to fall into a low-yield category by superficial resemblance to a textbook description; a clinician who has performed this active screening and still concludes imaging is not indicated is applying the framework correctly, while a clinician who defers imaging without having actively screened for red-flag features has skipped the step that makes the deferral evidence-based rather than merely convenient.

Clinical Decision Rules Beyond ACR Criteria

Beyond the general appropriateness criteria, several validated, presentation-specific clinical decision rules exist for pediatric neuroimaging, most notably the PECARN head trauma decision rules discussed fully in Chapter 19, which stratify a child's risk of clinically important traumatic brain injury based on a defined set of history and examination variables and have been prospectively validated across large multicenter pediatric cohorts. Where a validated decision rule exists for the specific presentation under consideration, applying that rule directly, rather than relying on general appropriateness guidance alone, offers the most precise, evidence-anchored threshold available, and this book directs the reader to the relevant validated rule within each disease-specific chapter where one exists.

A validated decision rule differs from a general appropriateness guideline in an important respect: it has been prospectively tested against a real-world cohort and its sensitivity and specificity for the outcome of interest are known and published, giving the clinician a quantifiable sense of how much diagnostic certainty the rule provides and, equally important, what residual risk remains even when the rule suggests imaging is not required. Communicating this residual risk honestly, rather than presenting a validated decision rule as an infallible guarantee, is part of applying these tools correctly, since even a highly sensitive decision rule will, by definition, miss a small proportion of true positive cases, and a family should understand that a rule-based recommendation to defer imaging reflects a favorable probability, not an absolute certainty.

International and Regional Variation in Appropriateness Guidance

Appropriateness guidance is not fully uniform across countries and health systems; European and British guidance bodies, for example, have in some instances reached somewhat different thresholds than American guidance for comparable presentations, reflecting differences in underlying health system structure, resource availability, and, in some cases, genuine differences in expert interpretation of the same evidence base. A clinician training internationally, or reviewing imaging obtained under a different health system's guidance, benefits from recognizing this genuine variation rather than assuming a single universal threshold exists; the appropriateness framework developed in this chapter draws primarily on American guidance sources as its reference standard, consistent with this book's primary audience, while acknowledging that a clinician practicing elsewhere should confirm the specific guidance in force in that setting.

Shared Decision-Making When Evidence Is Ambiguous

Not every presentation resolves cleanly into a clear appropriateness verdict, and for the substantial minority of presentations in which the evidence is genuinely mixed or the individual child's features fall in an intermediate risk zone, shared decision-making, in which the clinician presents the estimated yield, the risks of imaging, and the risks of deferral in plain language and incorporates the family's own risk tolerance and preferences, is the appropriate response rather than a unilateral decision in either direction; this approach is developed further in the final section of this chapter.

Revisiting Thresholds as New Evidence Emerges

The appropriateness thresholds presented throughout this chapter reflect the evidence available at the time of writing and, consistent with the nature of an evolving evidence base, are expected to shift over the professional lifetime of any reader of this book as new outcome data, new decision rules, and revised society guidance accumulate; treating the specific thresholds in this chapter as a fixed, permanently correct answer rather than as the current best application of an evolving evidence base misunderstands the deeper skill this chapter is intended to teach. The durable skill is the three-question framework itself, red-flag assessment, yield-data awareness, and management-changing potential, which the reader can and should reapply to updated evidence throughout a career, rather than a fixed list of presentations to memorize as permanently low- or high-yield.

Figure 3.1: Evidence-Based Imaging Decision Framework

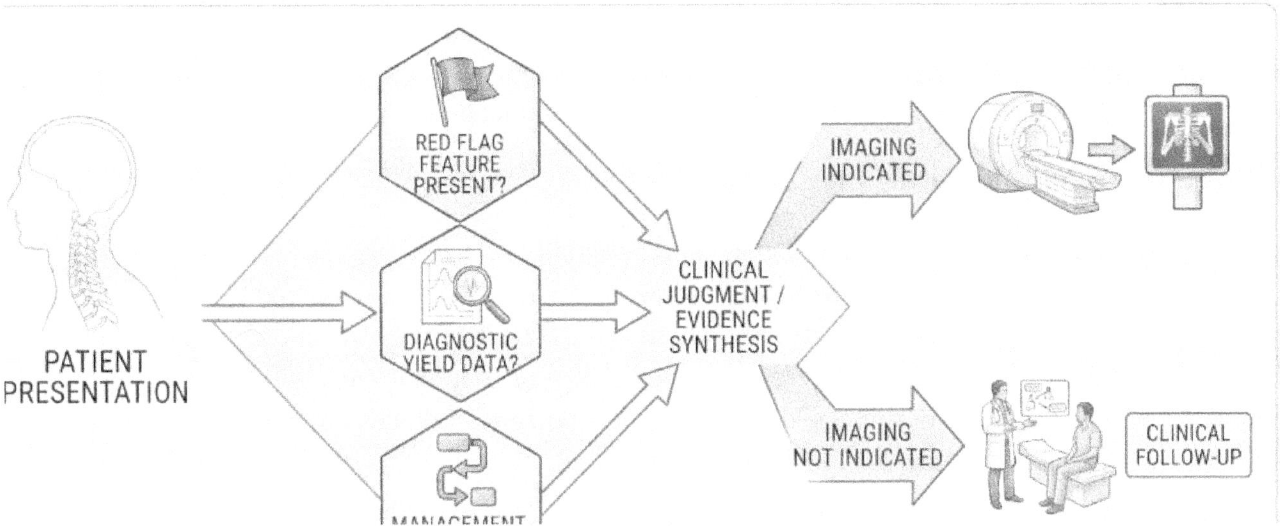

Modality Selection — MRI, CT, Ultrasound, and Nuclear Medicine

Once the decision to image has been made, the modality-selection reasoning introduced in Chapter 1 is applied here specifically to the ordering decision itself, before any protocol detail is considered, since the modality decision and the protocol decision are sequential, not simultaneous, steps.

A Decision Framework for Modality Selection

Applying a consistent sequence to modality selection reduces the likelihood of a reflexive, default choice that does not fit the specific clinical question.

1. Determine urgency: an acute, potentially time-sensitive presentation such as a new focal deficit or suspected acute stroke favors the fastest available modality that can answer the question, frequently CT in the acute setting even when MRI would ultimately be preferred for full characterization.
2. Determine the anatomic target: a bony or skull base question favors CT; a soft-tissue parenchymal question favors MRI; a question specific to the neonatal period with an open fontanelle favors ultrasound as a first-line screening tool.
3. Determine whether radiation avoidance is a priority that can be satisfied without sacrificing diagnostic yield, favoring MRI or ultrasound whenever either can answer the same question as CT.

4. Confirm modality availability and turnaround time against the clinical urgency established in step one, since the theoretically preferred modality is not the correct choice if it cannot be obtained within a clinically appropriate window.

Special Circumstances Favoring CT Despite Radiation

Beyond the acute trauma and bony-anatomy indications discussed in Chapter 1, CT retains a preferred first-line role in the setting of suspected acute hydrocephalus with a rapidly deteriorating clinical status, where the speed of acquisition and the ability to obtain the study without sedation in an unstable child outweighs the radiation concern, and in postoperative neurosurgical monitoring in the immediate perioperative period, where rapid detection of a surgical complication such as acute hemorrhage takes priority over radiation stewardship for that specific, narrow clinical window.

Special Circumstances Favoring Ultrasound

Beyond routine neonatal screening, ultrasound is preferentially selected for serial monitoring of a known process in a child with an accessible acoustic window, for rapid bedside assessment of ventricular size in a critically ill infant with a ventriculoperitoneal shunt and a concern for malfunction, discussed further in Chapter 10, and, in the intraoperative setting, for real-time neurosurgical guidance, a specialized application beyond the scope of this book's presurgical and diagnostic focus but worth acknowledging as part of the full modality landscape.

When Advanced or Nuclear Medicine Imaging Is Warranted

Nuclear medicine and advanced MRI techniques, introduced in Chapter 1, are ordered as second-line studies once conventional imaging has established a specific, narrower clinical question that the advanced technique is positioned to answer, such as seizure focus localization after conventional MRI has failed to identify a clear structural lesion in a child being evaluated for epilepsy surgery, rather than as an initial, first-line study for an undifferentiated presentation.

Cost and Resource Stewardship in Modality Selection

Modality selection carries a cost dimension distinct from, though related to, the radiation and sedation risk considerations already discussed: an advanced or nuclear medicine study is substantially more resource-intensive than a conventional MRI or CT, both in direct cost and in the specialized personnel and scheduling coordination it requires, and ordering an advanced study before conventional imaging has been obtained and reviewed, rather than sequentially as described above, both delays care and consumes a scarce resource for a question conventional imaging might resolve on its own. Responsible resource stewardship, understood correctly, is not a rationale for withholding an indicated study but a further argument for the same sequential, question-driven ordering discipline this chapter advocates throughout.

Modality Selection in Resource-Limited Settings

The decision framework presented in this chapter assumes access to the full range of modalities discussed, an assumption that does not hold in every practice setting; a clinician practicing where MRI access requires significant delay or transfer, discussed briefly in Chapter 1, applies the same underlying question-driven reasoning but must weigh the diagnostic cost of using an available, imperfect modality against the clinical cost of delay more heavily than a clinician working in a fully resourced tertiary center. In this circumstance, explicit communication with the receiving center before transfer, describing the specific clinical question and any imaging already obtained, allows the receiving team to plan the most efficient possible imaging pathway rather than repeating studies unnecessarily once the child arrives.

Telemedicine consultation with a pediatric neurology or neuroradiology specialist before a transfer decision is finalized, where available, can itself change the modality-selection calculus, since a specialist reviewing the available clinical information remotely may determine that a study already obtainable locally, even if not the theoretically ideal modality, is sufficient to answer the immediate clinical question and avoid transfer altogether, reserving transfer specifically for children whose clinical picture genuinely requires a modality or expertise unavailable locally; this kind of remote pre-transfer consultation has become an increasingly important tool for extending the reasoning developed in this chapter into settings that do not have every modality on site.

Protocol Coordination With the Radiology Department

Modality selection does not end with the ordering clinician's decision; effective coordination with the radiology department, including a clear statement of the clinical question on the order itself, consistent with the structured-reporting discipline introduced in Chapter 1, and, for an unusual or complex clinical question, a direct conversation with the interpreting radiologist before the study is performed, meaningfully improves the likelihood that the study obtained actually answers the question the ordering clinician intended. A referral pattern in which the same ordering clinician and the same imaging department repeatedly communicate directly for complex cases tends, over time, to produce better-protocoled, higher-yield studies than a purely transactional ordering relationship in which the clinical question is inferred from a brief order text alone.

Documenting the Modality-Selection Rationale

Just as the appropriateness decision itself benefits from explicit documentation, discussed later in this chapter, the specific reasoning behind a modality choice that departs from the most commonly expected option, such as selecting CT over MRI in a stable child specifically for a bony-anatomy question, or choosing a rapid, motion-robust MRI protocol over a standard CT in an unstable child, is worth stating explicitly in the clinical note; a future clinician reviewing the chart, or a quality-review process examining imaging utilization patterns, is better served by a note that states the specific reasoning for an atypical modality choice than by one that leaves the reader to infer the rationale after the fact.

Clinical Scenario	First-Line Modality	Rationale
Acute focal deficit, unstable child	CT	Speed, availability, sensitivity for acute hemorrhage
New focal seizure, stable child	MRI (epilepsy protocol)	Superior soft-tissue detail for epileptogenic lesion
Suspected shunt malfunction, known VP shunt	Rapid MRI sequence or CT per institutional protocol	Speed and ventricular size assessment
Preterm infant, open fontanelle	Cranial ultrasound	No sedation, bedside, first-line screening
Presurgical epilepsy focus localization	Ictal SPECT or PET (adjunct to MRI)	Localizes focus not resolved by structural imaging alone

THE CLINICAL-IMAGING CROSSWALK SYSTEM — Choosing the Fastest Adequate Modality in an Unstable Child

The Crossing: A six-year-old with a known ventriculoperitoneal shunt presents with vomiting, lethargy, and signs of rising intracranial pressure; the on-call team must decide between an immediate CT and an MRI that would require a longer wait for sedation availability.

Presentation Signature: An acutely deteriorating child with a known shunt, signs concerning for acute shunt malfunction and rising intracranial pressure, and a clinical status that does not allow for a delay to arrange sedated MRI.

Imaging Correlate: A rapid, sedation-free CT or a fast, motion-robust MRI sequence protocol, whichever is available soonest at the treating institution, is obtained to assess ventricular size and shunt hardware position, prioritizing speed over the superior soft-tissue detail MRI would otherwise provide for this question.

Trap Logic: Waiting for the theoretically preferred modality in an acutely deteriorating child risks a delay in diagnosing a surgical emergency; the correct modality in this scenario is defined by what can be obtained fastest without sacrificing the ability to answer the specific question of ventricular size and shunt position, not by which modality is generally preferred for shunt evaluation in a stable outpatient.

Crossing Anchor: In an acutely deteriorating child, modality selection is governed first by acquisition speed and availability, not by which modality would be preferred under nonurgent circumstances.

When Not to Image — Low-Yield Presentations

The single most common source of low-value pediatric neuroimaging is not a technically incorrect study but an unnecessary one, obtained for a presentation whose published diagnostic yield does not support routine imaging. This section names the specific, evidence-supported presentations for which imaging deferral, not imaging, is the appropriately evidence-based default.

Developmental Delay Without Focal Findings

Isolated developmental delay, without an abnormal neurologic examination, a specific dysmorphic feature, a concerning growth trajectory, or an additional red-flag finding such as regression or seizure, has a documented low diagnostic yield on brain MRI, and several published institutional protocols explicitly do not consider developmental delay in isolation an indication for imaging; this same reasoning applies to isolated autism spectrum disorder without an additional red-flag feature, discussed earlier in this chapter, where published cohort data similarly support a low routine imaging yield. Genetic and metabolic evaluation, rather than neuroimaging, is generally the higher-yield initial workup for isolated global developmental delay, a sequencing decision that belongs to the broader developmental evaluation literature but is worth naming explicitly here, since a family expecting imaging as the natural first test is often unaware that genetic and metabolic testing carries a higher diagnostic yield for this specific presentation.

Simple Febrile Seizures

A simple febrile seizure, defined as a generalized, brief seizure occurring with fever in a neurodevelopmentally normal child between six months and five years of age, without a focal component, without prolonged duration, and without recurrence within the same illness, is not an indication for neuroimaging, a position supported by consistent evidence that the diagnostic yield of imaging in this specific, well-defined scenario is essentially negligible; a complex febrile seizure, by contrast, one with a focal component, prolonged duration, or recurrence within twenty-four hours, shifts the evaluation toward the reasoning developed in Chapter 11.

Uncomplicated Primary Headache

A headache with features consistent with a primary headache disorder, migraine or tension-type, a normal neurologic examination, a normal growth trajectory, and no red-flag feature such as a headache that wakes the child from sleep, worsens with Valsalva maneuver, is accompanied by early-morning vomiting, or occurs alongside a new focal deficit, has a low diagnostic yield on imaging and does not routinely require neuroimaging, a specific application of the general reasoning developed in this chapter that is revisited in full, alongside its exceptions, in Chapter 20.

Benign Paroxysmal Conditions Mimicking Seizure

A cluster of benign, self-limited paroxysmal events, including breath-holding spells, benign paroxysmal vertigo of childhood, and typical, stereotyped shuddering attacks, are frequently referred for imaging out of diagnostic uncertainty regarding whether the event represents a seizure, when the correct next step in a classic, well-described presentation is careful clinical characterization of the event, not imaging; imaging is reserved for atypical features, an abnormal interictal examination, or genuine diagnostic uncertainty after clinical assessment, not applied reflexively to any paroxysmal event a family or referring clinician labels a possible seizure.

Uncomplicated Concussion Without Red-Flag Features

A child with a witnessed, low-mechanism head injury, a brief or absent loss of consciousness, a normal neurologic examination, and resolving symptoms consistent with an uncomplicated concussion does not routinely require neuroimaging, since the diagnostic yield of CT for a clinically important traumatic brain injury in this specific, low-risk presentation is well documented as low by the validated pediatric head trauma decision rules discussed fully in Chapter 19; a child instead meeting one of the specific higher-risk criteria defined by those validated rules, such as a severe mechanism, a palpable skull fracture, or a persistently altered mental status, shifts appropriately into the imaging-indicated pathway.

Persistent post-concussive symptoms beyond the typical expected recovery window, most commonly a headache pattern, cognitive complaints, or vestibular symptoms lasting beyond several weeks, represent a distinct clinical scenario from the acute presentation addressed by the validated head trauma decision rules, and the decision to obtain delayed imaging in this scenario is generally governed by the same headache- and focal-deficit-based reasoning developed elsewhere in this chapter and in Chapter 20, rather than by the acute-injury decision rules, since conventional structural imaging remains characteristically normal in prolonged post-concussive symptoms without a new red-flag feature having emerged.

Tics and Stereotypies

Motor and vocal tics, and stereotyped repetitive movements without an associated regression, focal neurologic sign, or abnormal examination, are common, typically benign neurodevelopmental findings that do not, by themselves, warrant neuroimaging; a family alarmed by a new tic and requesting imaging to rule something out is well served by an explanation, using the communication framework developed later in this chapter, that isolated tics and typical stereotypies have an established clinical diagnosis made on history and examination alone, without a role for structural imaging in the great majority of cases.

An exception worth naming explicitly is the sudden, abrupt onset of a complex tic or stereotypy in a previously unaffected child, particularly when accompanied by other new neuropsychiatric features, a presentation pattern that shifts consideration toward the autoimmune and postinfectious mechanisms discussed in Chapter 16 rather than a typical, gradual-onset primary tic disorder; the distinguishing feature between the two scenarios is less the movement itself than its tempo of onset and the presence or absence of accompanying neuropsychiatric change, both of which should be specifically elicited before a family is reassured that no further evaluation is needed.

Sports-Related Concussion and the Return-to-Play Imaging Myth

A persistent misconception among coaches, athletic trainers, and some families holds that a normal brain MRI or CT is required before a child can safely return to sports participation after a concussion, a belief without evidentiary support, since conventional structural imaging is characteristically normal in concussion by definition, given that concussion is a functional rather than a structural injury; return-to-play decisions are instead governed by a graduated, symptom-based clinical protocol, addressed fully in Chapter 19, and neuroimaging obtained solely to satisfy this misconception, in a child who does not otherwise meet imaging criteria, exposes the child to unnecessary risk for a study that cannot answer the return-to-play question in the first place. Correcting this specific misconception directly, using the family-communication approach developed later in this chapter, is a recurring and clinically important task in a general or sports-adjacent child neurology practice.

When a Family History Changes the Calculus

The low-yield presentations catalogued in this section describe the default, evidence-based threshold for a child without additional risk-modifying history; a strong family history of a specific structural or genetic neurologic condition, such as a first-degree relative with a known cerebral vascular malformation or a hereditary tumor predisposition syndrome, can appropriately shift an individual child's threshold even when the presenting complaint alone would otherwise fall into a low-yield category, since the relevant prior probability calculation is being made for that specific child's risk profile, not for the general population from which the published low-yield data was derived. Eliciting a focused, relevant family history as part of the standard evaluation, rather than treating the presenting complaint in isolation, is therefore a necessary component of applying this chapter's framework correctly.

Figure 3.2: Diagnostic Yield of Brain MRI by Presentation

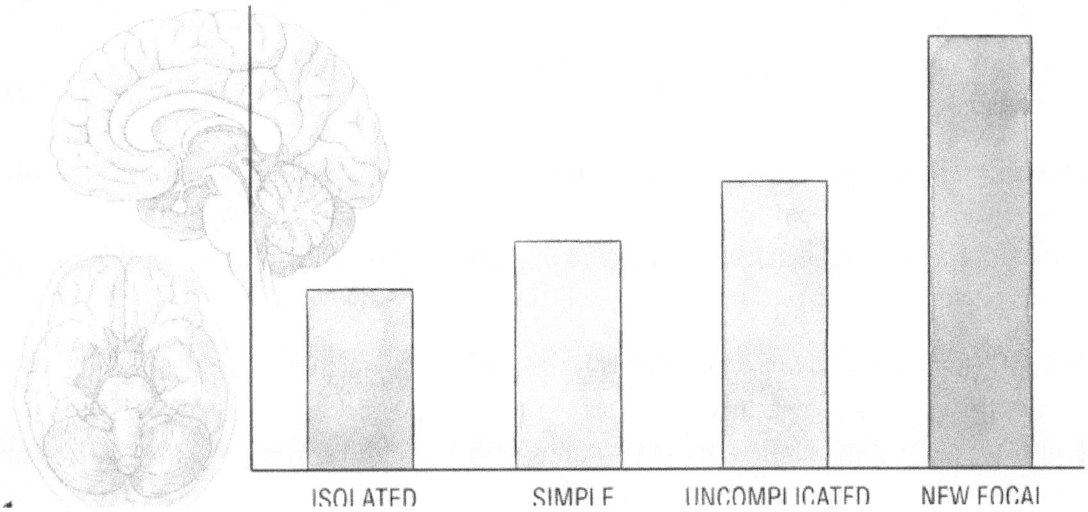

THE CLINICAL-IMAGING CROSSWALK SYSTEM — Recognizing When the Correct Next Step Is Not Imaging

The Crossing: A three-year-old with normal development, a normal examination, and a single simple febrile seizure during a documented viral illness is brought to clinic by a family requesting an MRI to be safe.

Presentation Signature: A neurodevelopmentally normal toddler, a classic simple febrile seizure history with no focal component and no recurrence, and a family whose primary driver is anxiety rather than a specific clinical concern raised by the examination.

Imaging Correlate: Applying the reasoning developed in this section, the correct imaging correlate for a true simple febrile seizure is the absence of an indication for imaging at all; the evaluation instead centers on confirming the seizure meets simple febrile seizure criteria and addressing the source of the fever.

Trap Logic: Ordering an MRI in response to parental anxiety alone, without a clinical indication, exposes the child to unnecessary sedation risk for a study with a well-documented negligible yield in this specific scenario, and can inadvertently reinforce a family's belief that imaging was medically necessary rather than reassure them that it was unnecessary.

Crossing Anchor: A true simple febrile seizure in a neurodevelopmentally normal child is not an indication for neuroimaging; the correct clinical response is evidence-based reassurance, communicated using the family-communication approach developed later in this chapter, not a deferential imaging order.

THE CLINICAL-IMAGING CROSSWALK SYSTEM — A Family History That Shifts a Low-Yield Presentation

The Crossing: An eight-year-old presents with a new, isolated headache pattern that otherwise fits the uncomplicated primary headache profile described earlier in this chapter, but the family mentions, when specifically asked, a first-degree relative with a known hereditary cerebral cavernous malformation syndrome.

Presentation Signature: A headache presentation that, absent the family history, would fall squarely into the low-yield category, combined with a specific, relevant hereditary vascular malformation syndrome in a first-degree relative.

Imaging Correlate: Brain MRI including susceptibility-weighted or gradient-echo sequencing, the sequence most sensitive for the cavernous malformations characteristic of this syndrome, is obtained despite the otherwise low-yield headache presentation, because the relevant prior probability for this specific child has been shifted upward by the family history.

Trap Logic: Applying the general low-yield headache threshold without eliciting the family history would miss the specific, individualized risk this child carries; the published low-yield data for uncomplicated headache describes a general population that does not include this child's specific genetic risk profile.

Crossing Anchor: A relevant family history of a hereditary structural or vascular neurologic condition shifts an individual child's imaging threshold even when the presenting complaint alone would otherwise fall into a low-yield category; family history must be actively elicited, not assumed absent.

Communicating Risk, Radiation, and Sedation to Families

An evidence-based imaging threshold is only as effective in practice as the clinician's ability to communicate it persuasively to a family who may arrive with a strong prior expectation that imaging equals thoroughness; this final section addresses that communication directly, since a technically correct decision to defer imaging that is poorly explained frequently results in the family seeking a second opinion or an emergency department visit specifically to obtain the imaging that was appropriately deferred.

Explaining Radiation Risk in Understandable Terms

Radiation risk is best communicated using concrete, comparative framing rather than abstract statistical language a family cannot readily interpret; explaining that a single head CT delivers a radiation dose comparable to a defined, familiar reference point, and that the radiation-associated cancer risk from a single, medically indicated study is small in absolute terms but is not zero, particularly across a child's remaining lifetime, gives a family an honest, proportionate basis for understanding why a clinician might prefer an alternative modality when one is available, without either minimizing or exaggerating the actual risk involved.

A family that has read alarming information online about radiation risk sometimes arrives already anxious about a CT that is, in fact, clearly indicated, and the same comparative, proportionate framing used to explain why radiation avoidance is preferred when possible is equally useful in the reverse direction, reassuring a family that a specific, indicated CT carries a small enough absolute risk that its diagnostic benefit clearly outweighs it; the communication skill developed throughout this section is fundamentally about proportionate, honest framing in either direction, not a one-directional argument for always avoiding radiation regardless of clinical context.

Age-Specific Communication: Involving the Child Directly

Beyond communicating with the parent or guardian, an age-appropriate explanation directed at the child themselves, particularly a school-age child or adolescent capable of understanding a simplified version of the clinical reasoning, both respects the child's own developing autonomy and frequently improves cooperation with the imaging visit itself; a ten-year-old told honestly, in age-appropriate language, why a test is or is not being recommended is generally a more cooperative participant in the visit and any subsequent imaging than one who is discussed about, rather than with, throughout the encounter. This practice becomes particularly important in adolescence, where involving the patient directly in the shared decision-making conversation, alongside the parent, is both developmentally appropriate and, in many jurisdictions, increasingly reflected in evolving standards around adolescent involvement in their own medical decision-making.

Discussing Sedation Risk and Alternatives

When MRI is recommended over CT specifically to avoid radiation, and sedation is anticipated as part of that MRI, the family is best served by an honest acknowledgment that this substitution trades one risk category for another rather than eliminating risk altogether, incorporating the sedation-risk discussion developed in Chapter 1 directly into this conversation; framing the decision as a genuine tradeoff, rather than implying MRI is simply the safer choice in every respect, builds trust and more accurately reflects the actual clinical reasoning.

Shared Decision-Making Tools and Documentation

For the intermediate-risk presentations discussed earlier in this chapter, in which the evidence does not clearly mandate imaging or clearly support deferral, structured shared decision-making, in which the estimated yield, the risks of each path, and the family's own preferences are explicitly discussed and the resulting decision is documented in the clinical note, both improves the quality of the decision itself and protects the clinical record should the decision be revisited later; a note stating simply imaging deferred, without documenting the reasoning and the family's informed agreement, is less defensible and less useful to a future clinician than one that captures the actual shared decision-making conversation.

A structured documentation template for this conversation, whether built into the electronic health record or applied consistently as a personal practice habit, typically captures four elements: the specific red-flag features actively assessed and found absent, the estimated yield discussed with the family, the specific risks of the alternative path (imaging or deferral) that were explained, and the family's stated understanding and agreement with the plan, including any explicit return-precautions given; a documentation habit built around these four elements produces a note that is both clinically useful on future review and defensible as evidence of a genuinely informed, shared decision rather than a unilateral one. Building this four-element structure into a reusable note template, rather than composing the language freely at each encounter, both saves time in a busy clinical practice and ensures no element is inadvertently omitted under time pressure.

Special Considerations: When the Referring Clinician Disagrees

A consulting neurologist who concludes, after full evaluation, that imaging is not indicated for a child referred specifically for imaging by another clinician faces a distinct communication task: explaining the evidence-based reasoning directly to the referring colleague, not only to the family, both as a matter of professional courtesy and because the referring clinician's own future threshold for similar presentations may shift as a result of a well-explained, evidence-cited response. A brief, specific explanation citing the relevant appropriateness criteria or diagnostic yield data, rather than a bare statement that imaging was not obtained, is more likely to be received as genuine clinical reasoning than as a dismissal of the referring clinician's concern, and over time, this kind of specific, collegial feedback measurably shifts referral patterns within a local practice community toward the evidence-based threshold this chapter advocates.

Addressing Parental Anxiety and the Just to Be Safe Request

A family's request to obtain imaging just to be safe, even when the clinical evidence does not support it, reflects genuine anxiety rather than a lack of trust in the clinician, and is best addressed by directly naming and validating that anxiety before presenting the evidence, rather than responding to the request with evidence alone; a clinician who says explicitly that the family's worry is completely understandable, and that the recommendation to defer imaging comes specifically because the evidence shows it would not change how the child is cared for, is more likely to be heard than one who responds to an emotional request with a purely clinical rebuttal.

Cultural and Health-Literacy Considerations in Risk Communication

The comparative-risk framing and shared decision-making approach developed throughout this section assume a baseline of health literacy and a cultural orientation toward individual, negotiated medical decision-making that does not hold uniformly across every family a clinician encounters; a family from a background in which medical authority is expected to direct care more directly, or a family with limited health literacy or limited proficiency in the language of care, may experience an open-ended, options-based conversation as confusing or as an abdication of the clinician's expertise rather than as respectful engagement. Adapting the communication approach, offering a clear recommendation alongside the supporting reasoning rather than presenting a menu of equally weighted options, while still ensuring the family's questions and concerns are genuinely heard and addressed, achieves the same goal of informed, trust-building communication across a wider range of family backgrounds and preferences than a single, fixed communication script could achieve alone. Engaging professional medical interpretation, rather than an ad hoc family member, whenever a language barrier is present is a further, frequently underused component of ensuring this communication genuinely reaches the family making the decision, and documenting that professional interpretation was used is itself part of a complete, defensible clinical record.

Case Presentation: Successful Shared Decision-Making

A five-year-old with three months of intermittent, non-progressive headaches, a normal neurologic examination, and a normal growth trajectory is evaluated in clinic. The family, having researched brain tumors online, requests an MRI. Applying the framework developed in this chapter, the clinician first validates the family's concern directly, then walks through the specific red-flag features that would change the recommendation, explaining that none are present in this child's history and examination, and explicitly states the estimated low yield of imaging in this scenario alongside the small but real sedation risk that would accompany it if imaging were pursued. The family, having understood the actual reasoning rather than simply being told no, agrees to a defined follow-up plan: return promptly if a specific red-flag feature develops, with a scheduled follow-up visit in six weeks regardless. This documented shared decision-making conversation, rather than either an unexamined imaging order or an unexplained refusal, resolves the encounter appropriately for both the clinical evidence and the family's genuine concern.

Case Presentation: When the Threshold Shifts Mid-Encounter

A seven-year-old initially presenting with headaches that appear consistent with the uncomplicated primary headache pattern discussed earlier in this chapter is further questioned during the visit, and the family mentions, only when specifically asked, that the headaches have recently begun waking the child from sleep and are accompanied by early-morning vomiting on two occasions. Applying the red-flag framework developed in this chapter, these two features shift the presentation out of the low-yield category and into a presentation warranting imaging, illustrating why the structured red-flag review developed in this chapter is applied actively through targeted questioning at every encounter, rather than passively accepting the presenting complaint at face value; a family does not always volunteer the specific detail that changes the clinical threshold unless directly asked.

Case Presentation: A Disagreement Resolved Through Explanation

A community pediatrician refers a nine-year-old with three isolated, brief episodes of eye fluttering during periods of quiet inattention, requesting brain MRI. On evaluation, the consulting neurologist recognizes a classic history for typical absence seizures, a presentation whose diagnostic evaluation centers on electroencephalography rather than structural imaging, discussed fully in Chapter 11. Rather than simply declining the imaging request, the neurologist calls the referring pediatrician directly, explains that the classic history strongly suggests a generalized, not focal, epilepsy syndrome for which electroencephalography, not MRI, is the appropriate next diagnostic step, and offers to coordinate that testing directly. The referring pediatrician, having received a specific, evidence-based explanation rather than a bare denial, both accepts the revised plan and reports finding the explanation useful for evaluating similar presentations in the future, illustrating the durable, practice-wide value of the collegial communication approach described earlier in this section.

Case Presentation: A Family Declining Recommended Imaging

A four-year-old presents with a new, persistent left-sided weakness and a headache that wakes the child from sleep, a presentation that clearly meets the red-flag criteria developed earlier in this chapter and warrants urgent brain MRI. The family, citing a prior difficult sedation experience with a sibling, initially declines imaging and requests to simply monitor the child at home. Rather than either accepting this decision without further discussion or responding with pressure alone, the clinician directly explores the specific source of the family's hesitation, addresses the sibling's prior sedation experience by explaining the specific motion-reduction and sedation-safety measures described in Chapter 1 that would apply to this child, and clearly explains the specific, concrete clinical risk of deferring imaging in the presence of this particular symptom combination, distinguishing it explicitly from the low-yield presentations discussed earlier in the chapter for which deferral would be entirely appropriate. Having understood both the specific plan to address their prior negative experience and the specific reason this presentation differs from a low-risk one, the family agrees to proceed, illustrating that the shared decision-making approach developed in this chapter applies as directly to overcoming appropriate resistance to an indicated study as it does to explaining an appropriate deferral. This closing case, paired with the chapter's opening case of successful deferral, frames the full range of this chapter's central skill: applying the same evidence-based, honestly communicated reasoning in either direction, toward more imaging or toward less, according to what the individual child's presentation actually warrants.

Synthesis: A Single Framework Applied in Both Directions

The four sections of this chapter, appropriateness thresholds, modality selection, low-yield presentations, and family communication, are not four independent skills but four facets of a single underlying discipline: matching the imaging-ordering decision precisely to the clinical question actually in front of the clinician, at the specific age, presentation, and risk profile of the specific child under evaluation, and being able to explain that match honestly to whoever needs to understand it, whether that is an anxious family, a referring colleague, or a future clinician reading the chart. A reader who has internalized this chapter correctly does not walk away with a fixed list of conditions to image or not image, but with a repeatable process for reaching that decision for any presentation, including the many presentations this chapter has not had space to name individually, and for explaining the resulting decision persuasively regardless of which direction it points. That same process, precise question-matching followed by honest explanation, reappears as the organizing logic of the Clinical-Imaging Crosswalk System across every remaining chapter of this book, making this chapter as much a methodological foundation for what follows as it is a stand-alone topic in its own right.

THE CLINICAL-IMAGING CROSSWALK SYSTEM — Imaging-Ordering Decisions and Their Communication

---

Crossing 1 Recap: In an acutely deteriorating child, modality selection is governed by acquisition speed and availability, not by the modality generally preferred under nonurgent circumstances.

Crossing 2 Recap: A true simple febrile seizure in a neurodevelopmentally normal child is not an indication for neuroimaging; evidence-based reassurance, not a deferential imaging order, is the correct response.

Crossing 3 Recap: A relevant family history of a hereditary structural or vascular condition shifts an individual child's imaging threshold even when the presenting complaint alone would otherwise be low-yield.

Chapter Anchor: The decision to image at all precedes and governs every downstream modality and protocol decision; applying a consistent, evidence-based threshold, and communicating it honestly, is as much a clinical skill as interpreting the resulting study.

Summary and Key Concepts

Evidence-based appropriateness criteria, such as the ACR Appropriateness Criteria and validated decision rules like PECARN, anchor imaging-ordering decisions to a defensible, updateable standard rather than to individual habit, addressing documented, substantial variability in physician imaging thresholds.

Modality selection in the acute setting is governed first by acquisition speed and availability; CT, ultrasound, and advanced or nuclear medicine imaging each retain defined, narrower roles alongside MRI as the general first-line modality, with resource stewardship and setting-specific access shaping the practical decision.

Isolated developmental delay, simple febrile seizures, uncomplicated primary headache, uncomplicated concussion, typical tics, and classic benign paroxysmal events are well-documented low-yield presentations for which imaging deferral is the evidence-based default, unless a relevant family history shifts the individual child's risk profile.

Communicating radiation and sedation risk in concrete, comparative terms, structuring shared decision-making documentation around four defined elements, adapting communication style to the family's health literacy and cultural context, and explicitly naming parental anxiety before presenting evidence, improves the likelihood that an appropriately conservative imaging decision is accepted by families and referring colleagues alike.

A structured red-flag review, applied actively through targeted questioning at every encounter, is necessary because families do not always volunteer the specific detail that shifts a presentation from low-yield to imaging-indicated; the same active-screening discipline protects against both unnecessary imaging and missed pathology.

CHAPTER 4: NEONATAL ENCEPHALOPATHY AND HYPOXIC-ISCHEMIC INJURY

Learning Objectives

1. Recognize the clinical staging criteria for neonatal encephalopathy and correlate severity with expected imaging findings.
2. Describe the distinct patterns of hypoxic-ischemic brain injury seen in the term versus the preterm infant and explain the pathophysiologic basis for each pattern.
3. Apply the correct imaging timing relative to therapeutic hypothermia to maximize prognostic yield while avoiding premature or falsely reassuring early imaging.
4. Identify the specific imaging features most strongly associated with adverse neurodevelopmental outcome after hypoxic-ischemic encephalopathy.

Clinical Recognition and Staging of Neonatal Encephalopathy

Neonatal encephalopathy is a clinical syndrome, diagnosed at the bedside before any imaging is obtained, and the imaging findings discussed throughout this chapter are interpreted against, not in place of, the clinical staging established in the first hours of life; a clinician who orders imaging without first anchoring the clinical severity assessment risks misreading an imaging finding's prognostic weight, since the same imaging pattern can carry different implications depending on the clinical context in which it occurs.

Epidemiology and Risk Factors for Neonatal Encephalopathy

Neonatal encephalopathy affects a well-documented proportion of term live births, with moderate to severe hypoxic-ischemic encephalopathy occurring less commonly but carrying disproportionate long-term morbidity; recognized risk factors include intrapartum events such as placental abruption, uterine rupture, cord prolapse, and prolonged or difficult delivery, as well as antepartum factors including maternal hypertensive disease, growth restriction, and chorioamnionitis, each of which can compromise fetal oxygenation through a distinct mechanism. A meaningful proportion of cases, however, occur without a clearly identifiable sentinel event on retrospective review, underscoring that the absence of an obvious intrapartum complication does not exclude a hypoxic-ischemic mechanism and that the multiorgan and biochemical evidence discussed later in this section carries independent diagnostic weight.

The Sarnat Staging System

The Sarnat staging system, the most widely used clinical framework for neonatal encephalopathy, classifies severity into three stages based on level of consciousness, tone, primitive reflexes, autonomic function, and seizure activity: stage one, mild encephalopathy, features hyperalertness, mild hypertonia, and an intact suck reflex without seizures; stage two, moderate encephalopathy, features lethargy, hypotonia, a weak or absent suck, and frequently accompanying seizures; and stage three, severe encephalopathy, features stupor or coma, flaccid tone, absent primitive reflexes, and profound autonomic dysfunction. This staging, performed clinically within the first hours to days of life, is the single most important determinant of both the decision to proceed with therapeutic hypothermia, discussed later in this chapter, and the baseline against which subsequent imaging findings are interpreted.

Sarnat staging is dynamic in the acute period, and a neonate can evolve between stages over the first day of life as the underlying injury process unfolds; documenting stage serially, rather than relying on a single assessment, gives a more complete clinical picture and is standard practice in most neonatal intensive care units managing suspected hypoxic-ischemic encephalopathy. A modified version of the original Sarnat system, incorporating a more granular assessment of specific examination findings, is used at many centers to standardize scoring across multiple examiners and shifts, since inter-examiner variability in an unstructured clinical assessment can meaningfully affect both the eligibility determination for therapeutic hypothermia and the baseline severity documentation against which recovery or deterioration is later tracked.

Electroencephalographic Correlation With Clinical Stage

Continuous electroencephalographic monitoring, increasingly standard practice in neonates undergoing therapeutic hypothermia, provides a complementary, continuous physiologic correlate to the intermittent clinical examination that anchors Sarnat staging; background patterns ranging from normal continuity through discontinuous, burst-suppression, and ultimately isoelectric patterns correlate with increasing clinical severity and carry independent prognostic value, while electrographic seizures, which in the neonate frequently occur without an obvious clinical correlate, are identified reliably only through continuous monitoring rather than clinical observation alone. A neonate with a reassuring examination between clinical assessments but a severely abnormal background pattern or frequent electrographic seizures on continuous monitoring should not be assumed to have a milder injury than the electroencephalographic picture suggests, since the continuous physiologic data captures information the intermittent clinical examination alone cannot.

Distinguishing Hypoxic-Ischemic Encephalopathy From Other Causes of Neonatal Encephalopathy

Neonatal encephalopathy is a clinical syndrome with a broad differential diagnosis, and hypoxic-ischemic injury, while the most common and most extensively studied cause, is not the only one; metabolic disease, discussed further in Chapter 17, congenital infection, discussed in Chapter 15, and a primary structural brain malformation, discussed in Chapters 7 and 8, can each present with a clinical picture that overlaps substantially with hypoxic-ischemic encephalopathy in the first hours of life. A history of a defined perinatal sentinel event, such as a placental abruption, uterine rupture, prolonged fetal heart rate decelerations, or a need for prolonged neonatal resuscitation, together with objective evidence of fetal acidosis on cord blood gas analysis, supports a hypoxic-ischemic etiology, while the absence of such a history should prompt active consideration of the alternative causes named above rather than a default assumption of hypoxic-ischemic injury.

The Role of Cord Blood Gas and Apgar Scores

Objective biochemical evidence of fetal acidosis, most commonly a cord arterial pH below 7.0 or a base deficit exceeding a defined threshold, together with a low Apgar score persisting beyond the first several minutes of life, forms part of the standard multiorgan criteria used to establish a hypoxic-ischemic etiology and to determine eligibility for therapeutic hypothermia; a normal cord blood gas in the setting of a clinically encephalopathic neonate should prompt reconsideration of the alternative diagnoses named above, since normal cord gas values argue against acute peripartum hypoxic-ischemic injury as the primary cause, though they do not entirely exclude a more remote or antepartum injury.

Multiorgan Involvement as a Supporting Clinical Feature

Because hypoxic-ischemic injury affects organ systems beyond the brain, evidence of concurrent renal, hepatic, cardiac, or hematologic dysfunction in the immediate newborn period supports a systemic hypoxic-ischemic process and adds diagnostic confidence when the neurologic presentation alone is ambiguous; a neonate with encephalopathy but entirely normal renal function, liver enzymes, and cardiac function on the first day of life presents a somewhat less typical picture for hypoxic-ischemic injury and, per the reasoning developed above, warrants a broader diagnostic consideration rather than an assumption that the multiorgan pattern will simply emerge later.

The specific pattern of multiorgan involvement can itself carry additional clinical information: acute tubular injury reflected in rising creatinine and oliguria reflects the same relative redistribution of blood flow away from peripheral organs toward the brain and heart that characterizes the fetal diving reflex during acute hypoxic-ischemic stress, while elevated troponin and echocardiographic evidence of transient myocardial dysfunction reflect direct cardiac hypoxic injury; documenting the full multiorgan picture, not the neurologic findings in isolation, therefore supports both diagnostic confidence and a more complete understanding of the acute physiologic insult the neonate experienced.

Neonatal Seizures as a Component of the Clinical Picture

Seizures occurring in the setting of moderate to severe hypoxic-ischemic encephalopathy are common and are incorporated directly into the Sarnat staging framework described above, but neonatal seizures present a specific clinical challenge because a substantial proportion are electrographic only, occurring without an accompanying clinical correlate visible to bedside observation, a phenomenon termed electroclinical dissociation that is particularly pronounced in neonates who have received antiseizure medication, which can suppress the clinical manifestation of a seizure while leaving the underlying electrographic seizure activity unchanged. This dissociation is a primary rationale for the continuous electroencephalographic monitoring discussed above, since a management strategy relying on clinical seizure observation alone in a hypoxic-ischemic encephalopathy population will systematically underestimate true seizure burden, with direct implications for antiseizure medication dosing and for prognostic counseling, since seizure burden itself has been independently associated with adverse outcome in published cohorts.

Differentiating Hypoxic-Ischemic Encephalopathy From Neonatal Stroke

Focal neonatal arterial ischemic stroke, discussed fully in Chapter 6, can present with encephalopathic features overlapping those of diffuse hypoxic-ischemic injury, particularly in the first day of life before the focal nature of a stroke-related deficit becomes clinically apparent; the key distinguishing clinical feature is often the presence of focal, lateralized seizure activity or a lateralized examination finding in a neonate who otherwise lacks the systemic multiorgan and biochemical evidence of a global hypoxic-ischemic insult described earlier in this section, a distinction that is often definitively resolved only once imaging is obtained, underscoring why the imaging patterns developed in the next section of this chapter are interpreted alongside, not as a simple confirmation of, the initial clinical impression.

Timing of Initial Clinical Assessment Relative to Resuscitation

Because the immediate postresuscitation period can itself produce a transient depression in level of consciousness, tone, and reflexes independent of any underlying brain injury, particularly in a neonate who received prolonged positive-pressure ventilation, chest compressions, or emergency medications during resuscitation, formal Sarnat staging is generally most reliable once this immediate peri-resuscitation period has passed, typically by one to several hours of age, rather than in the first minutes after birth; a low initial Apgar score and depressed immediate examination, while important supporting evidence for a hypoxic-ischemic mechanism, are distinguished from the formal encephalopathy staging that determines therapeutic hypothermia eligibility, and conflating the two can lead to either premature over-staging in a neonate who is still recovering from acute resuscitation or, conversely, a missed opportunity to identify evolving encephalopathy in a neonate whose immediate postresuscitation examination was reassuring but who develops clear encephalopathic features over the following hours.

Amplitude-Integrated EEG as a Bedside Screening Adjunct

Amplitude-integrated electroencephalography, a simplified, continuous bedside monitoring technique distinct from full conventional electroencephalography, is used at many centers as a rapid, accessible screening tool to support the eligibility determination for therapeutic hypothermia in the critical early hours after birth, when a full conventional electroencephalographic study may not be immediately available; a moderately or severely abnormal background pattern on amplitude-integrated electroencephalography within the first hours of life correlates with, and supports, the clinical Sarnat staging already established, while a normal background in a clinically encephalopathic neonate should prompt reconsideration of the staging and the underlying diagnosis, consistent with the general principle that multiple, converging sources of evidence, not any single data point, support a confident hypoxic-ischemic encephalopathy diagnosis and appropriate treatment decision.

Interdisciplinary Communication at the Time of Initial Diagnosis

The initial hours after a neonate is identified as potentially eligible for therapeutic hypothermia typically involve rapid, time-pressured communication among the delivering obstetric team, the neonatology team, and, once cooling has been initiated, the child neurology consultant, and clear, structured handoff communication at this stage, explicitly conveying the specific perinatal history, the cord gas and Apgar data, and the evolving Sarnat stage, meaningfully reduces the risk that a critical detail is lost in the transition between teams during what is often a chaotic, urgent clinical period. Institutions with a standardized, structured handoff tool or checklist specifically for this transition have reported improved consistency in the completeness of information available to the team making the final cooling-eligibility determination.

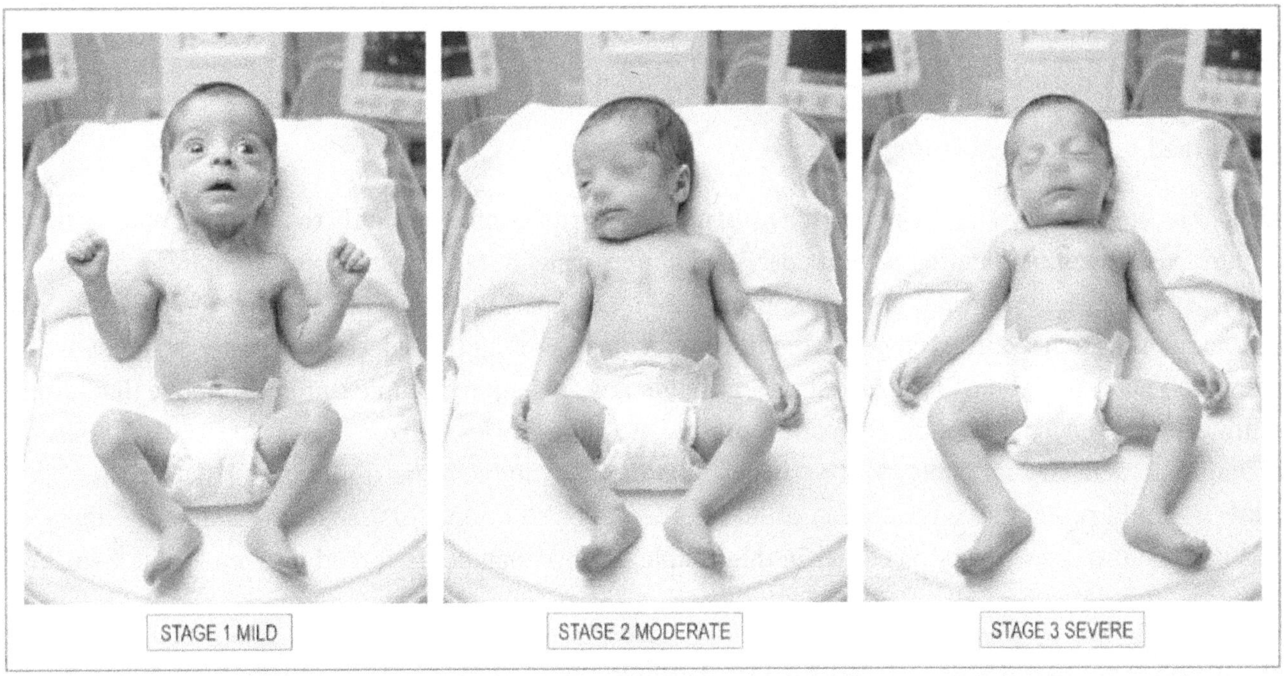

Figure 4.1: Sarnat Staging Clinical Features

Patterns of Hypoxic-Ischemic Injury by Gestational Age

The pattern of hypoxic-ischemic brain injury on imaging is determined jointly by the severity and duration of the hypoxic-ischemic insult and by the gestational age of the brain at the time of injury, since different brain regions are maximally vulnerable at different developmental stages; recognizing which pattern is present, and matching it against the clinical history, is one of the highest-yield skills in neonatal neuroimaging.

The Watershed (Partial Prolonged) Pattern

A partial, prolonged hypoxic-ischemic insult, in which cerebral perfusion is reduced but not entirely interrupted over a sustained period, produces injury preferentially in the arterial border-zone, or watershed, regions between the major cerebral artery territories, most classically the parasagittal cortex and subjacent white matter; this pattern reflects the physiologic redistribution of blood flow toward the brainstem and deep gray structures that occurs during a sustained partial insult, at the relative expense of the watershed cortical regions, and is the pattern most classically associated with a prolonged labor complicated by sustained, incomplete placental insufficiency.

The Basal Ganglia-Thalamic (Acute Profound) Pattern

A severe, acute, near-total interruption of cerebral perfusion, by contrast, preferentially injures the deep gray matter structures with the highest metabolic demand at the time of injury, most characteristically the posterior putamen, ventrolateral thalamus, hippocampi, and perirolandic cortex, sparing the watershed cortical regions relatively more than the acute profound pattern spares the deep gray structures; this pattern reflects the high metabolic rate of these deep gray structures during an acute, near-total insult, such as a placental abruption or uterine rupture, in which the brain has no opportunity to redistribute flow protectively as it does during the more gradual partial-prolonged pattern.

Combined and Atypical Injury Patterns

A meaningful proportion of hypoxic-ischemic injuries do not conform cleanly to either the pure watershed or pure basal ganglia-thalamic pattern described above, instead showing combined features of both, most often when a sustained partial insult is complicated by a superimposed acute, more profound event, such as a sudden placental abruption occurring during an already-complicated, prolonged labor; recognizing a combined pattern is clinically important because it suggests a more complex injury timeline than a single sentinel event and, correspondingly, carries prognostic implications spanning both the motor and cognitive domains associated separately with each pure pattern. An atypical distribution that fits neither classic pattern should prompt reconsideration of an alternative or additional diagnosis, including the metabolic and infectious causes discussed earlier in this chapter, rather than being forced into one of the two classic categories by default.

Diffusion-Weighted Imaging Timing and Pseudonormalization

Diffusion-weighted imaging is the most sensitive sequence for detecting acute hypoxic-ischemic injury in the first several days of life, typically showing restricted diffusion within the injured regions by twenty-four to forty-eight hours after the insult, but the apparent diffusion coefficient signal undergoes a well-documented phenomenon of pseudonormalization between approximately the fifth and tenth day after injury, in which the diffusion abnormality transiently normalizes despite ongoing, evolving tissue injury, before conventional T1 and T2 signal changes and volume loss become apparent later; imaging obtained during this pseudonormalization window can therefore substantially underestimate the true extent of injury if diffusion-weighted imaging alone is relied upon, a pitfall developed further in the Crossing below.

MR Spectroscopy as an Adjunct Prognostic Tool

Proton MR spectroscopy, obtained from the basal ganglia and, when feasible, additional regions of interest at the time of the primary prognostic MRI, adds quantitative biochemical information that complements the qualitative and semiquantitative signal-based assessment described above; an elevated lactate peak, reflecting anaerobic metabolism in injured tissue, and a reduced N-acetylaspartate-to-choline ratio, reflecting neuronal loss or dysfunction, have each been independently associated with adverse outcome in published cohorts, and a spectroscopy-based severity assessment obtained alongside conventional imaging can refine prognostic precision in cases where the conventional imaging findings alone leave meaningful uncertainty. Spectroscopy findings are interpreted as an adjunct to, not a replacement for, the conventional sequence findings and the established clinical severity, consistent with the general principle developed throughout this book that no single data source is interpreted in isolation from the full clinical and imaging picture.

Preterm-Specific Injury Patterns

The preterm brain responds to hypoxic-ischemic insult with a pattern distinct from the term patterns described above, reflecting the different regional vulnerabilities of the immature brain; periventricular white matter, discussed fully in Chapter 5 as periventricular leukomalacia, is the region of greatest vulnerability in the preterm infant, in contrast to the cortical and deep gray predominant patterns characteristic of term hypoxic-ischemic injury, a distinction that reflects the differing maturational state and metabolic demand of periventricular white matter relative to cortical gray matter at preterm gestational ages.

This age-dependent shift in regional vulnerability reflects the underlying biology of oligodendrocyte precursor cell maturation, which is maximally vulnerable to hypoxic-ischemic and inflammatory injury during a specific preterm developmental window and substantially less vulnerable once oligodendrocyte maturation has progressed further by term; a clinician evaluating a late-preterm or early-term infant with hypoxic-ischemic injury should recognize that the imaging pattern may reflect a transitional mixture of preterm periventricular vulnerability and term cortical or deep gray vulnerability, rather than fitting cleanly into either the classic preterm or classic term pattern alone.

Total Asphyxia and the Near-Total Global Pattern

At the most severe end of the injury spectrum, a truly global, near-total interruption of cerebral perfusion sustained long enough produces a diffuse pattern of injury affecting the entire brain relatively uniformly, sometimes described separately from the classic basal ganglia-thalamic pattern as a total or global pattern, in which diffusion restriction and eventual volume loss are seen throughout the cerebral hemispheres rather than confined to the specific deep gray and perirolandic regions characteristic of the acute profound pattern in its more typical, less extreme form. This global pattern carries the most severe prognostic implications of any hypoxic-ischemic injury pattern discussed in this chapter and is associated with the highest rates of both death and severe combined motor and cognitive disability among survivors, information that shapes the urgency and content of the family counseling conversation from the earliest post-injury discussion.

Cortical Highlighting and the Evolving Signal Appearance Over Time

Beyond the acute diffusion and early T1 and T2 changes discussed above, a characteristic pattern termed cortical highlighting, in which the injured cortical ribbon becomes abnormally T1-hyperintense relative to the underlying white matter, typically emerges over the first one to two weeks after injury and reflects a combination of early laminar necrosis and associated microhemorrhage within the injured cortex; recognizing this evolving appearance as a marker of the same underlying injury process, rather than mistaking it for a new or superimposed process, requires the reader to hold the full injury timeline in mind rather than interpreting a single time-point study without reference to the expected evolution described throughout this section.

Imaging the Spine in Hypoxic-Ischemic Injury

Although hypoxic-ischemic injury is predominantly a cerebral process, a severe, sustained global insult can, less commonly, also affect the spinal cord, particularly in the watershed distribution of the anterior spinal artery territory, and a neonate with an unexpectedly severe or atypical distribution of weakness on examination relative to the cerebral injury pattern identified on brain MRI should prompt consideration of extending the imaging field of view to include the spine, applying the same field-of-view extension principle introduced in Chapter 1 for other clinical scenarios in which the brain findings alone do not fully explain the clinical picture.

Timing Injury Onset From the Imaging Appearance

Beyond identifying the anatomic pattern of injury, the specific signal characteristics present on a given study can help estimate the approximate timing of the underlying insult relative to the imaging date, information that carries both clinical and, at times, medicolegal significance when the precise timing of injury relative to a specific intrapartum event is in question; acute restricted diffusion without T1 or T2 signal change suggests a very recent insult, typically within the preceding one to two days, while established T1 and T2 signal change, volume loss, or gliosis suggests a substantially older, subacute to chronic process, and an experienced reader integrates the full constellation of sequence findings, rather than any single sequence in isolation, to arrive at the most defensible estimate of injury timing that the imaging can support.

Antenatal Onset Injury and Its Distinct Imaging Signature

A minority of neonates presenting with an imaging pattern superficially consistent with hypoxic-ischemic injury are found, on careful review, to show established, chronic-appearing signal change, encephalomalacia, or volume loss already present at birth, findings that indicate the underlying insult occurred well before the intrapartum period captured in the delivery history, sometimes weeks to months earlier in gestation; recognizing this antenatal-onset pattern, most reliably suggested by the presence of mature gliotic signal change or established volume loss rather than the acute, evolving signal pattern expected of a genuinely peripartum insult, meaningfully changes the etiologic discussion with the family, shifting it away from a peripartum causation narrative and toward the antenatal evaluation, including possible placental pathology review and antenatal infectious or vascular workup, that this distinct pattern warrants.

Pattern	Mechanism	Typical Regions Affected	Classic Clinical Scenario
Watershed (partial prolonged)	Sustained partial hypoperfusion, protective flow redistribution	Parasagittal cortex, watershed white matter	Prolonged labor, sustained fetal distress
Basal ganglia-thalamic (acute profound)	Near-total, acute interruption of perfusion	Posterior putamen, ventrolateral thalamus, hippocampi, perirolandic cortex	Placental abruption, uterine rupture, cord prolapse
Combined pattern	Sustained partial insult with superimposed acute event	Both watershed and deep gray regions	Complicated labor with a superimposed acute event
Preterm periventricular pattern	Vulnerability of immature periventricular white matter	Periventricular white matter	Preterm infant, see Chapter 5

THE CLINICAL-IMAGING CROSSWALK SYSTEM — Diffusion Pseudonormalization Masking True Injury Extent

---

The Crossing: A term neonate with moderate hypoxic-ischemic encephalopathy undergoes MRI on day seven of life, and diffusion-weighted imaging appears largely unremarkable, prompting the referring team to ask whether the injury was actually mild.

Presentation Signature: A neonate with a clinical history and Sarnat staging consistent with a real hypoxic-ischemic insult, imaged in the day five to ten window, with diffusion-weighted imaging that appears reassuringly normal or near-normal.

Imaging Correlate: The conventional T1 and T2 sequences, not diffusion-weighted imaging alone, are the more reliable indicator of injury extent in this specific timing window, since true injury may show early T1 signal change, subtle volume loss, or evolving signal abnormality on conventional sequences even as the diffusion-weighted sequence has pseudonormalized.

Trap Logic: Interpreting a normal-appearing diffusion sequence in this specific day five to ten window as evidence of mild or resolved injury, without carefully scrutinizing the conventional sequences and correlating with the clinical severity already established by Sarnat staging, risks substantially underestimating the true injury extent and delivering falsely optimistic prognostic counseling to the family.

Crossing Anchor: Diffusion-weighted imaging obtained between approximately day five and day ten of life should never be interpreted in isolation; conventional T1 and T2 sequences and the established clinical severity must be weighted more heavily during this specific pseudonormalization window.

Therapeutic Hypothermia and Imaging Timing

Therapeutic hypothermia has fundamentally changed both the management and the imaging timeline for neonatal hypoxic-ischemic encephalopathy over the past two decades, and correct imaging interpretation in a cooled neonate requires understanding how cooling itself alters the expected injury evolution timeline described in the previous section.

Evidence Base for Therapeutic Hypothermia

Therapeutic hypothermia is supported by multiple large, prospectively randomized controlled trials and their subsequent meta-analyses, which consistently demonstrated a significant reduction in the combined outcome of death or major neurodevelopmental disability at eighteen to twenty-four months in cooled infants compared to standard normothermic care among neonates meeting the trials' eligibility criteria; this robust evidence base is what established therapeutic hypothermia as the current standard of care for moderate to severe neonatal hypoxic-ischemic encephalopathy meeting the defined criteria, and understanding this evidence base allows a clinician to counsel families accurately regarding both the real, quantified benefit of cooling and the reality that cooling reduces, rather than eliminates, the risk of adverse outcome.

Eligibility Criteria and the Cooling Protocol

Therapeutic hypothermia, in which the neonate's core temperature is reduced to a defined target, typically around thirty-three to thirty-four degrees Celsius, and maintained for approximately seventy-two hours, is initiated within six hours of birth in eligible neonates meeting defined criteria combining gestational age, evidence of perinatal acidosis or a sentinel hypoxic-ischemic event, and moderate to severe encephalopathy by Sarnat staging; the six-hour window reflects the underlying neuroprotective mechanism, which acts during the secondary energy failure phase that follows the initial hypoxic-ischemic insult, and cooling initiated beyond this window has not demonstrated the same neuroprotective benefit in the trials that established the current standard of care.

How Cooling Alters the Injury Evolution Timeline

Therapeutic hypothermia slows the evolution of hypoxic-ischemic injury on imaging relative to the noncooled timeline described in the previous section, meaning the classic day-of-life imaging landmarks established in the pre-cooling literature, including the timing of diffusion pseudonormalization, are shifted somewhat later in a cooled neonate; imaging obtained at a day-of-life that would be appropriately timed in a noncooled neonate may be relatively early in a cooled neonate's true injury evolution, a distinction with direct implications for the timing guidance developed in the next section.

Optimal Imaging Timing in the Cooled Neonate

Current practice generally favors obtaining the primary prognostic MRI after rewarming is complete, typically around day of life four to seven, rather than during the active cooling period itself, both because injury evolution is still actively unfolding during cooling and because logistical factors, including the child's clinical instability and the practical challenges of transporting and imaging a cooled, critically ill neonate, generally favor imaging once the child is medically more stable; an earlier study obtained during active cooling, when clinically necessary to exclude an alternative or coexisting acute process such as hemorrhage, should be explicitly understood and communicated as a study with a different, more limited prognostic purpose than the definitive post-rewarming study.

Adjunctive and Emerging Neuroprotective Therapies

Beyond therapeutic hypothermia itself, several adjunctive neuroprotective strategies, including erythropoietin and other pharmacologic agents targeting the secondary and tertiary phases of hypoxic-ischemic injury, are under active investigation in clinical trials as potential additions to standard cooling therapy, reflecting the recognition that hypothermia alone, while effective, does not eliminate adverse outcome risk for every treated infant. A clinician working at a center participating in such a trial, or counseling a family about a child potentially eligible for an adjunctive investigational therapy, should be prepared to discuss the current, still-evolving state of this evidence honestly, distinguishing an established standard-of-care intervention like hypothermia itself from an investigational adjunct still under active study.

Coordinating Imaging With the Neonatal Care Team

Because the optimal imaging timing depends on the specific cooling protocol and rewarming schedule used at a given institution, close coordination between the ordering neonatologist and the imaging department, including explicit communication of the day of life, the cooling and rewarming timeline, and the specific prognostic question the family and care team need answered, is essential to avoid a study obtained at a timing that neither confirms an early complication nor provides the fullest prognostic information the definitive post-rewarming study would offer. A standardized, institution-specific protocol specifying the target imaging day relative to rewarming, developed collaboratively between neonatology and radiology, reduces the variability in imaging timing that can otherwise arise from ad hoc, case-by-case scheduling decisions made under the time pressure of a busy neonatal intensive care unit.

Imaging During Active Cooling for Specific Indications

Notwithstanding the general preference for post-rewarming timing described above, specific clinical scenarios warrant imaging during active cooling despite its more limited prognostic value: a neonate with a new, unexplained focal neurologic finding raising concern for a coexisting or complicating process such as acute hemorrhage or stroke, a neonate whose clinical course deteriorates unexpectedly during cooling in a way not explained by the known hypoxic-ischemic process alone, or a neonate in whom a structural malformation or alternative diagnosis is being actively considered, all warrant earlier imaging specifically to answer that narrower, time-sensitive clinical question, understanding explicitly that this earlier study will likely need to be supplemented by the definitive post-rewarming study for full prognostic characterization.

Transport and Logistical Considerations for Sedation-Free Cooled Imaging

A cooled, critically ill neonate undergoing MRI typically does not require pharmacologic sedation in the way an older infant might, given the combination of the child's clinical instability and the sedating effect of the underlying encephalopathy itself, but does require MRI-compatible temperature management equipment and continuous physiologic monitoring throughout transport and image acquisition, a logistical requirement that differs meaningfully from the routine feed-and-wrap or standard sedation pathways discussed in Chapter 1 for a stable, well infant. Coordinating this specialized transport and monitoring capability in advance, rather than improvising it at the time of an urgent imaging need, is a component of institutional readiness for managing this specific patient population.

Documenting the Rationale for Imaging Timing in the Clinical Record

Given the genuine complexity of the timing considerations developed throughout this section, explicitly documenting the rationale for the specific imaging timing chosen in an individual case, including whether the study was obtained during active cooling for a specific, narrower indication or as the definitive post-rewarming prognostic study, protects against a later misinterpretation of an early study as though it carried the same prognostic completeness as a properly timed post-rewarming study; a chart note that clearly labels an early study's limited, indication-specific purpose prevents a subsequent clinician from inadvertently over-interpreting its reassuring or concerning findings as definitive.

Passive Versus Active Cooling and Transport Considerations

A neonate born at a community hospital without on-site cooling capability who meets eligibility criteria for therapeutic hypothermia typically undergoes passive cooling, in which active warming measures are withheld and core temperature is allowed to drift downward under close monitoring, during transport to a tertiary center capable of initiating and maintaining active servo-controlled cooling; passive cooling without careful temperature monitoring carries a real risk of overshooting the target temperature range, and structured transport protocols specifying target temperature range and monitoring frequency during transport are an important, sometimes underappreciated component of ensuring a neonate arrives at the receiving cooling center within the appropriate therapeutic temperature range rather than either inadequately or excessively cooled.

Managing Family Expectations During the Cooling Period Itself

The seventy-two-hour cooling period itself, occurring before the definitive prognostic MRI has even been obtained, is frequently a period of acute parental distress during which families understandably seek early prognostic information the care team is often not yet in a position to provide with confidence; establishing clear, consistent communication early in the cooling period about the general timeline, including explicitly when the family should expect the prognostic MRI and the subsequent results discussion to occur, helps set realistic expectations and reduces the likelihood that a family interprets the natural absence of early prognostic detail as evasiveness rather than as the genuine, honest limitation of what can be known at that early stage.

Figure 4.2: Therapeutic Hypothermia Timeline and Imaging Windows

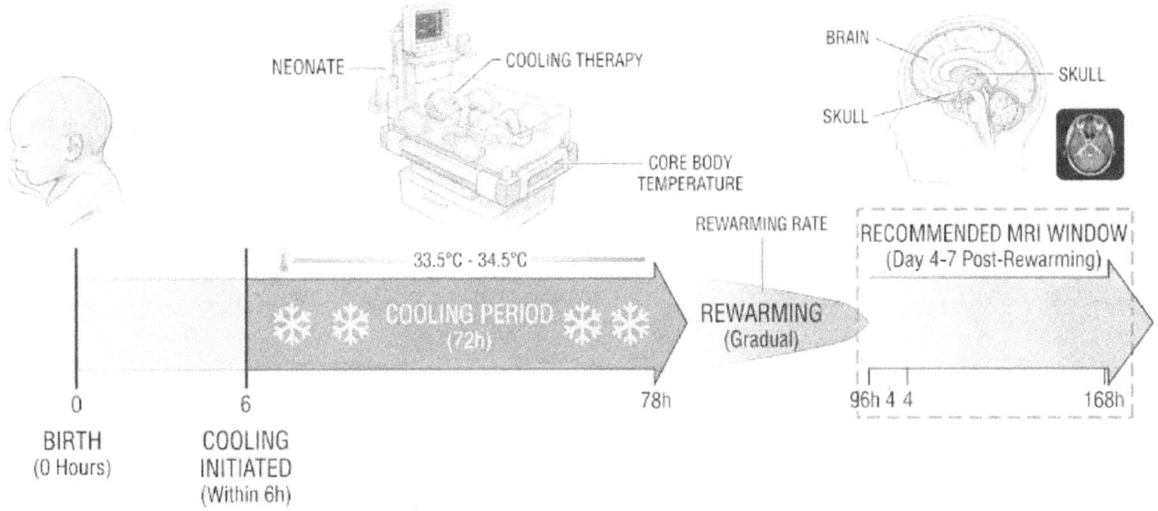

Prognostic Imaging Features

Families and referring clinicians alike look to the post-rewarming MRI as a central source of prognostic information following hypoxic-ischemic encephalopathy, and this final section addresses which specific imaging features carry the strongest evidence for predicting subsequent neurodevelopmental outcome, and how that information is appropriately communicated.

Basal Ganglia-Thalamic Injury as the Strongest Prognostic Marker

Involvement of the posterior limb of the internal capsule and the basal ganglia-thalamic structures, particularly when injury is bilateral and severe, is consistently identified across the published literature as the single strongest MRI predictor of adverse motor outcome, including cerebral palsy, reflecting the direct involvement of the corticospinal pathways traversing this region; an abnormal, absent, or asymmetric posterior limb of the internal capsule signal on the post-rewarming study is considered one of the most clinically significant individual findings a family and care team will discuss.

Watershed Injury and Cognitive Outcome

Watershed-pattern injury, by contrast, particularly when confined to the cortex and white matter without deep gray involvement, is more specifically associated with cognitive, language, and visuomotor outcome than with the motor outcome most strongly linked to basal ganglia-thalamic injury, reflecting the different functional territories affected by each pattern; a family counseled after a watershed-predominant injury pattern should understand that the prognostic implications, while still significant, differ in character from those of a basal ganglia-thalamic-predominant pattern, and combining both patterns in a single undifferentiated prognostic statement risks miscommunicating the specific nature of the expected outcome.

Cerebellar and Brainstem Injury

Injury to the cerebellum and brainstem, while less commonly the dominant feature than basal ganglia-thalamic or watershed cortical injury, occurs in a subset of severe hypoxic-ischemic encephalopathy cases and carries its own distinct prognostic weight, particularly for outcomes involving coordination, oromotor and feeding function, and, when brainstem involvement is severe, respiratory drive; brainstem signal abnormality on the post-rewarming study, though less frequently the primary focus of family counseling relative to the more commonly discussed basal ganglia-thalamic and watershed patterns, should be specifically assessed and reported, since its presence meaningfully shifts the anticipated clinical trajectory, including early feeding and respiratory support needs, in a direction distinct from a purely supratentorial injury pattern.

Grading Systems and Their Clinical Application

Several published MRI grading or scoring systems consolidate the injury features described above into a composite severity score correlated with outcome in published cohorts, and applying a validated, structured scoring approach, rather than an unstructured qualitative impression, both improves consistency of interpretation across readers and gives the family and care team a more precise, reproducible basis for prognostic discussion; using the same structured approach consistently across a practice also facilitates meaningful comparison between studies obtained on the same child over time or between children with differing injury patterns.

A structured grading system also serves an institutional quality-improvement function beyond the individual patient encounter, since consistent, reproducible scoring across a cooling program's patient population allows the program to track its own outcomes against the published literature and to identify any systematic drift in imaging timing, technique, or interpretation practice that might otherwise go unnoticed when each study is interpreted in isolation using an unstructured qualitative approach.

Inter-Reader Reliability and the Value of Structured Scoring

Published data examining agreement between different readers interpreting the same hypoxic-ischemic encephalopathy MRI have generally shown improved consistency when readers apply a validated structured scoring system compared to an unstructured qualitative overall impression, particularly for the more subtle, intermediate-severity injury patterns in which a purely qualitative read is more susceptible to genuine inter-observer disagreement; a family receiving prognostic counseling based on a structured, reproducible score can be given greater confidence that a second reader would likely reach a similar conclusion than a family counseled based on a single reader's unstructured qualitative impression alone.

Correlating Imaging Severity With Early Clinical Trajectory

The most robust prognostic counseling integrates the imaging severity score with the child's actual early clinical trajectory following the newborn period, including feeding competency, tone normalization, and early developmental milestone attainment over the first several months of life, rather than relying on the newborn imaging score in isolation; a child whose newborn imaging suggested a more severe injury pattern but who demonstrates an unexpectedly favorable early clinical trajectory, and conversely a child whose newborn imaging appeared relatively reassuring but who shows early clinical concern, both illustrate why ongoing clinical correlation, not a single newborn imaging score, ultimately governs the evolving prognostic conversation with the family over time.

The Role of Follow-Up Imaging Beyond the Newborn Period

A subset of children with significant newborn hypoxic-ischemic injury undergo follow-up brain MRI later in infancy or early childhood, typically to assess final volume loss and myelination pattern once the acute and subacute injury evolution described throughout this chapter has fully resolved, or to investigate a new clinical concern such as new-onset seizures or a significant change in the expected developmental trajectory; this later follow-up imaging is interpreted using the age-specific developmental framework established in Chapter 2, since a child imaged at eighteen months requires the same age-corrected interpretive discipline applied to any other pediatric neuroimaging study, not a hypoxic-ischemic-encephalopathy-specific exception to that general principle.

Prognostic Counseling in the Setting of Discordant Findings

Occasionally the imaging severity and the early clinical trajectory point in genuinely discordant directions, a scenario that requires particular care in family communication rather than a simple averaging of the two data sources; a structured approach acknowledges the discordance explicitly to the family, explains the specific reasons imaging and early clinical course do not always align perfectly, including the reality that imaging captures a single time-point anatomic snapshot while clinical trajectory reflects an integrated, ongoing functional assessment, and commits to closer, more frequent follow-up specifically because the usual concordance between these two data sources is not present in this particular child, rather than resolving the discordance prematurely in either the more optimistic or more pessimistic direction.

Integrating Placental Pathology Into the Full Diagnostic Picture

Placental pathology examination, when performed, frequently provides corroborating or, at times, unexpectedly discordant information relative to the presumed intrapartum mechanism suggested by the delivery history and imaging pattern; findings such as chronic villitis, maternal or fetal vascular malperfusion, or evidence of a more chronic placental insufficiency process can suggest that the injury process began well before the specific intrapartum sentinel event initially presumed to be causative, complementing the antenatal-onset imaging signature discussed earlier in this chapter, and a comprehensive etiologic discussion with the family, once all diagnostic information is available, ideally integrates the placental findings, the cord gas and multiorgan data, and the specific imaging pattern into a single coherent account of the injury timeline rather than treating each data source as an independent, unintegrated finding.

Long-Term Neurodevelopmental Follow-Up Beyond Imaging

The post-rewarming MRI is a single, time-limited data point in what is properly understood as a long-term neurodevelopmental surveillance process extending well beyond the newborn period; structured developmental follow-up through early childhood, incorporating standardized developmental assessment at defined intervals, captures functional outcome information that imaging alone cannot fully predict, particularly for cognitive and behavioral domains that may not manifest clearly until well beyond infancy. A family should understand from the outset that the newborn MRI, however informative, is the beginning of an ongoing surveillance and support process, not a single, final verdict on the child's eventual developmental trajectory, and structuring the family's expectations around this longitudinal framework from the earliest counseling conversation reduces the likelihood of later confusion or a sense of betrayal should the child's actual trajectory diverge, in either direction, from the newborn imaging-based prognosis.

Communicating Prognosis to Families

Prognostic communication after hypoxic-ischemic encephalopathy is among the most emotionally weighted conversations in child neurology, and the reasoning developed throughout this book regarding honest, proportionate, uncertainty-acknowledging communication applies with particular force here; imaging findings inform, but do not alone determine, an individual child's outcome, since clinical course, ongoing developmental assessment, and, for some outcome domains, the passage of time itself all contribute additional prognostic information beyond a single MRI, and a family is best served by an honest statement of what the imaging does and does not establish, framed alongside the plan for ongoing developmental follow-up, rather than either false reassurance or an unduly deterministic prognosis presented as certain.

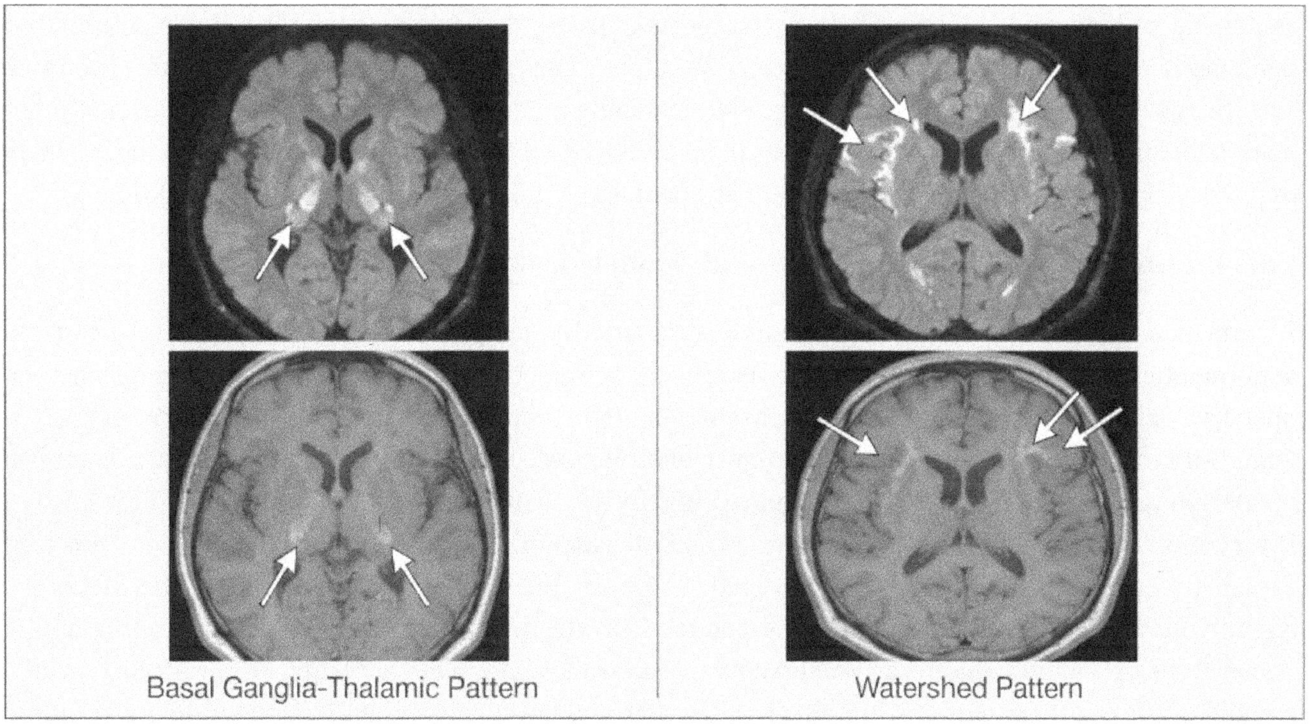

Figure 4.3: Basal Ganglia-Thalamic Versus Watershed Injury Pattern

Case Presentation: Severe Acute Profound Injury

A term neonate is born following an acute placental abruption with a cord pH of 6.8 and Apgar scores of 1 and 3 at one and five minutes, requiring prolonged resuscitation. Sarnat staging on admission is severe, and therapeutic hypothermia is initiated within two hours of birth. A post-rewarming MRI on day of life six demonstrates bilateral, symmetric restricted diffusion and T1 hyperintensity involving the posterior putamen, ventrolateral thalami, and perirolandic cortex bilaterally, with relative sparing of the watershed cortical regions, a classic acute profound pattern fully consistent with the acute, near-total nature of the perinatal insult described in the clinical history. Applying the reasoning developed in this chapter, the care team communicates to the family that this specific pattern, bilateral and severe basal ganglia-thalamic involvement, carries a high likelihood of significant motor impairment, while acknowledging the genuine uncertainty that remains regarding the precise degree of eventual functional outcome, and a coordinated early-intervention referral is initiated immediately rather than deferred pending further developmental assessment alone.

Case Presentation: Watershed Pattern After Prolonged Labor

A term neonate is born after a prolonged second stage of labor complicated by sustained, category-two fetal heart rate tracing abnormalities over several hours, with a cord pH of 7.05 and moderate encephalopathy by Sarnat staging. Therapeutic hypothermia is initiated, and post-rewarming MRI on day of life five demonstrates bilateral parasagittal cortical and subcortical white matter restricted diffusion with sparing of the deep gray structures, a classic watershed pattern consistent with the sustained, partial nature of the perinatal history. The care team explains to the family that this pattern is more specifically associated with cognitive, language, and visuomotor outcome domains than with the motor-predominant outcome discussed in the prior case, and structures the recommended developmental follow-up specifically around early language and cognitive screening milestones, illustrating how the specific injury pattern identified on imaging directly shapes the individualized follow-up plan rather than a single generic hypoxic-ischemic encephalopathy follow-up protocol applied uniformly to every affected child.

Case Presentation: A Combined Pattern With Multidomain Counseling

A term neonate is born after a labor complicated first by several hours of sustained fetal heart rate abnormalities and then, late in the second stage, by a sudden, severe bradycardia requiring emergent operative delivery; cord pH is 6.9, and Sarnat staging is severe. Post-rewarming MRI on day of life five demonstrates both parasagittal watershed injury and bilateral basal ganglia-thalamic injury, a combined pattern consistent with the two-phase clinical history of sustained partial compromise followed by a superimposed acute, profound event. Applying the reasoning developed in this chapter, the care team explains to the family that this combined pattern places the child at risk across both the motor and cognitive-language domains discussed separately in the two preceding cases, and structures a comprehensive, multidomain early-intervention and follow-up plan accordingly, illustrating that a combined injury pattern requires combined, rather than single-domain, prognostic counseling and follow-up planning.

Synthesis: Matching Mechanism, Pattern, Timing, and Communication

The four sections of this chapter trace a single continuous clinical pathway: a clinical mechanism and severity established through Sarnat staging and its supporting biochemical and physiologic evidence; an imaging pattern shaped jointly by that mechanism and the gestational age of the brain at the time of injury; a cooling-adjusted timeline that determines when the imaging obtained can be interpreted with full confidence; and a set of specific, pattern-dependent prognostic features that must be communicated to the family with honesty about both what is known and what remains uncertain. A reader who holds all four sections together, rather than treating imaging interpretation as a task separable from clinical staging, cooling timing, and family communication, is equipped to manage the full arc of a hypoxic-ischemic encephalopathy case from the delivery room through the long-term developmental follow-up period this chapter has emphasized throughout.

Crossing 1 Recap: Diffusion-weighted imaging obtained between approximately day five and ten of life should never be interpreted in isolation, given the well-documented pseudonormalization phenomenon in this window.

Chapter Anchor: The pattern of hypoxic-ischemic injury, basal ganglia-thalamic versus watershed versus combined, reflects the mechanism and timing of the perinatal insult and carries distinct, specific prognostic implications that should be communicated precisely, not as an undifferentiated single prognosis.

Summary and Key Concepts

Neonatal encephalopathy is a clinical syndrome staged by the Sarnat system and increasingly correlated with continuous electroencephalographic monitoring before imaging is obtained; hypoxic-ischemic injury is the most common but not the only cause, and cord blood gas and multiorgan involvement support the etiologic diagnosis.

The basal ganglia-thalamic (acute profound), watershed (partial prolonged), and combined injury patterns reflect distinct mechanisms and are each associated with distinct clinical histories and distinct prognostic domains; the preterm brain shows a distinct periventricular pattern of vulnerability.

Diffusion-weighted imaging pseudonormalizes between approximately day five and ten of life; conventional T1 and T2 sequences, MR spectroscopy, and clinical severity must be weighted more heavily during this window.

Therapeutic hypothermia is supported by robust randomized trial evidence, slows injury evolution on imaging, and the optimal prognostic MRI is generally obtained after rewarming, around day of life four to seven, rather than during active cooling.

Basal ganglia-thalamic injury is the strongest predictor of motor outcome; watershed injury is more specifically associated with cognitive and language outcome; cerebellar and brainstem injury affects coordination and feeding; prognostic communication should be honest, proportionate, explicit about remaining uncertainty, and framed within an ongoing longitudinal follow-up plan.

CHAPTER 5: PREMATURITY-RELATED BRAIN INJURY

Learning Objectives

1. Grade germinal matrix and intraventricular hemorrhage using the standard severity classification and describe its major complications.
2. Distinguish cystic from diffuse periventricular leukomalacia and correlate each with expected motor and cognitive outcome.
3. Recognize primary and secondary patterns of cerebellar injury in the preterm infant and their distinct detection challenges.
4. Correlate the severity and combination of prematurity-related brain injuries with long-term neurodevelopmental outcome and structure appropriate follow-up.

Germinal Matrix and Intraventricular Hemorrhage

Germinal matrix hemorrhage and its intraventricular extension remain the most common form of significant brain injury identified in the preterm infant, and cranial ultrasound screening for this specific injury, introduced in Chapter 1 and developed fully here, is among the highest-yield routine imaging practices in all of pediatric neuroradiology given its direct, well-established link to both immediate complications and long-term outcome.

Anatomy and Vulnerability of the Germinal Matrix

The germinal matrix, introduced in Chapter 2 as the richly cellular, highly vascularized source of neuronal and glial precursors lining the lateral ventricles, is maximally prominent between approximately twenty-four and thirty-two weeks gestation and is uniquely vulnerable to hemorrhage during this window because its immature capillary bed lacks the structural support of a mature basement membrane and glial investment, making it susceptible to rupture during the fluctuations in cerebral blood flow and venous pressure common in the sick preterm infant. This vulnerability explains why germinal matrix hemorrhage is overwhelmingly a disease of infants born before thirty-two weeks gestation and becomes progressively less common as gestational age at birth increases toward term, mirroring the involutional timeline of the germinal matrix itself described in Chapter 2.

Fluctuations in cerebral blood flow sufficient to precipitate germinal matrix rupture arise from a range of clinical circumstances common in the preterm intensive care setting, including hypoxia, hypercapnia, rapid volume expansion, pneumothorax, and the hemodynamic instability accompanying patent ductus arteriosus, each of which transiently disrupts the preterm brain's limited capacity for cerebral autoregulation; minimizing these precipitating events through careful, gentle handling and hemodynamic management in the first days of life is a central component of neonatal intensive care practice specifically aimed at reducing germinal matrix hemorrhage incidence.

Antenatal corticosteroid administration to the mother when preterm delivery is anticipated has been independently associated with reduced germinal matrix hemorrhage incidence and severity in the resulting preterm infant, reflecting an accelerating effect on both pulmonary and cerebrovascular maturation that extends the neuroprotective benefit of this intervention beyond its better-known respiratory indication; this association is one of several reasons antenatal corticosteroid administration, when clinically feasible given the timeline to delivery, is considered a component of the broader neuroprotective care bundle for the anticipated preterm infant, alongside the postnatal hemodynamic management practices described above.

Grading System for Intraventricular Hemorrhage

The widely used Papile grading system classifies germinal matrix and intraventricular hemorrhage into four grades of increasing severity: grade one, hemorrhage confined to the germinal matrix without ventricular extension; grade two, intraventricular hemorrhage without ventricular dilation; grade three, intraventricular hemorrhage with ventricular dilation; and grade four, historically termed intraventricular hemorrhage with parenchymal extension, though contemporary understanding recognizes this parenchymal component as a distinct venous hemorrhagic infarction rather than a direct extension of the intraventricular blood itself, a distinction developed further below.

This grading system, while imperfect and subject to ongoing refinement in the literature, remains the standard clinical language for communicating hemorrhage severity across neonatology and radiology, and its consistent, correct application, including the important grade three versus four distinction regarding mechanism, is essential for accurate communication with families and for appropriate risk stratification regarding the complications discussed later in this section.

Screening Ultrasound Protocols and Timing

Standard neonatal intensive care practice includes routine cranial ultrasound screening in infants born before approximately thirty-two weeks gestation, typically performed within the first week of life to detect early hemorrhage, given that the great majority of germinal matrix hemorrhage occurs within the first three to four days after birth, with a repeat study performed later, typically around thirty-six to forty weeks corrected age, to assess for the periventricular leukomalacia and cerebellar findings discussed later in this chapter, which characteristically evolve or become fully apparent only after this later time point. A single early screening study alone, without this later follow-up study, therefore risks missing injury patterns that have not yet fully evolved at the time of the first scan.

Complications: Posthemorrhagic Hydrocephalus and Venous Infarction

Posthemorrhagic ventricular dilation, arising from impaired cerebrospinal fluid resorption secondary to blood products within the ventricular system and subarachnoid space, is a common complication of grade three and, less predictably, lower-grade hemorrhage, and is monitored through serial cranial ultrasound measurement of ventricular size, discussed further in Chapter 10 alongside the broader hydrocephalus literature; progressive ventricular dilation exceeding defined thresholds prompts consideration of temporizing or, in some cases, permanent cerebrospinal fluid diversion. Periventricular hemorrhagic venous infarction, the contemporary understanding of what was historically termed grade four hemorrhage, arises from obstruction of the medullary veins draining into the terminal vein by an adjacent large germinal matrix or intraventricular hemorrhage, producing a secondary, typically asymmetric, fan-shaped parenchymal hemorrhagic infarction rather than a direct extension of intraventricular blood, a mechanistic distinction with direct prognostic relevance, since venous infarction carries a substantially worse prognosis than intraventricular hemorrhage alone.

Risk Factors and Prevention Strategies

Beyond gestational age itself, recognized risk factors for germinal matrix hemorrhage include lack of antenatal corticosteroid exposure, vaginal delivery in some studies, early-onset sepsis, and the hemodynamic instability factors named above; antenatal corticosteroid administration to the mother when preterm delivery is anticipated has been consistently associated with reduced hemorrhage incidence and severity in the resulting infant, reflecting accelerated maturation of multiple organ systems including, plausibly, the germinal matrix vasculature itself, and is a cornerstone of modern perinatal care specifically aimed at mitigating this and other complications of prematurity.

Coagulation Status and Platelet Function in the Preterm Infant

The preterm infant's coagulation system is developmentally immature, with reduced levels of several coagulation factors and, in the sickest infants, an increased likelihood of acquired coagulopathy from sepsis, disseminated intravascular coagulation, or severe hepatic dysfunction, each of which compounds the underlying vascular fragility of the germinal matrix described above; correcting a significant coagulopathy or severe thrombocytopenia identified in a preterm infant at elevated hemorrhage risk, when clinically feasible and indicated, is accordingly incorporated into hemorrhage-prevention practice at many neonatal intensive care units, alongside the hemodynamic stabilization measures already discussed, reflecting the recognition that vascular fragility and coagulation status act as compounding, rather than independent, risk factors.

Timing of Hemorrhage Relative to Delivery

While the great majority of germinal matrix hemorrhage occurs within the first several days after birth, a meaningful minority of cases arise antenatally, before delivery, or represent a later, delayed extension of an initially smaller antenatal hemorrhage; a germinal matrix hemorrhage identified on the very first cranial ultrasound obtained shortly after birth, particularly one already showing chronic-appearing features such as porencephalic change or established gliosis rather than the acute appearance typically expected of a peripartum event, should prompt consideration of an antenatal onset, with implications for antenatal counseling and evaluation analogous to the antenatal-onset hypoxic-ischemic injury pattern discussed in Chapter 4.

Multiple Births and Twin-Specific Considerations

Preterm multiple gestation pregnancies, particularly monochorionic twin pregnancies complicated by twin-to-twin transfusion syndrome, carry a distinct set of germinal matrix hemorrhage risk considerations beyond gestational age alone, since the donor and recipient twins in a transfusion syndrome pregnancy experience distinct hemodynamic profiles, hypovolemic and hypervolemic respectively, that can each independently predispose to hemorrhage through different mechanisms; a clinician managing a preterm infant from a complicated multiple gestation pregnancy should incorporate this specific antenatal history into the overall hemorrhage risk assessment, rather than applying only the generic gestational-age-based risk framework developed earlier in this section.

Ventricular Access and Temporizing Measures in Detail

When posthemorrhagic ventricular dilation progresses beyond the intervention threshold discussed above, several temporizing cerebrospinal fluid diversion techniques are available before a decision is made regarding permanent shunt placement, including serial lumbar or ventricular taps, a ventricular access device allowing repeated percutaneous aspiration without a new procedure for each intervention, and a ventriculosubgaleal shunt providing continuous drainage into a subgaleal reservoir; the choice among these temporizing approaches depends on the infant's specific clinical trajectory, the anticipated duration of temporizing management needed before the infant is large enough and stable enough for definitive shunt placement, and institutional expertise and preference, and is developed in full alongside the broader hydrocephalus management literature in Chapter 10.

Long-Term Ventricular Outcome After Temporizing Intervention

A subset of infants who undergo temporizing cerebrospinal fluid diversion for posthemorrhagic ventricular dilation subsequently stabilize without requiring conversion to a permanent shunt, as spontaneous cerebrospinal fluid resorption capacity recovers over the following weeks to months; conversely, a substantial proportion do progress to permanent shunt dependence, and distinguishing which infants will follow which trajectory in advance remains an area of ongoing clinical uncertainty, meaning serial ventricular monitoring continues well beyond the initial temporizing intervention itself, with the decision to proceed to permanent shunting made based on the infant's demonstrated trajectory over time rather than predicted definitively at the time of the initial temporizing procedure.

Interpreting Serial Ultrasound Trends Rather Than Single Measurements

The clinical value of the serial ventricular measurement protocol described throughout this section lies substantially in the trend across sequential studies rather than in any single measurement viewed in isolation, since normal measurement variability between studies, differences in technologist positioning technique, and the inherent limitations of a two-dimensional ultrasound measurement of a three-dimensional structure all introduce a degree of measurement noise that a single time point cannot distinguish from genuine, clinically meaningful progression; plotting sequential measurements against the gestational-age-specific normative curve referenced earlier in this section, rather than comparing only the two most recent values, gives the clearest picture of whether true progression is occurring and helps avoid an intervention decision driven by measurement noise rather than genuine clinical change.

Family Communication During the Acute Hemorrhage Period

The initial identification of germinal matrix or intraventricular hemorrhage on routine screening ultrasound frequently occurs before the family has had time to process the broader reality of a preterm birth, and communicating this finding requires the same honest, proportionate approach developed throughout this book, explicitly distinguishing the generally favorable prognosis associated with lower-grade, uncomplicated hemorrhage from the more guarded prognosis associated with higher-grade hemorrhage or venous infarction, while acknowledging that the fullest prognostic picture will not be available until the term-equivalent MRI discussed in the final section of this chapter; providing this initial finding without either false reassurance or premature worst-case framing, and explicitly previewing the more complete assessment still to come, helps the family engage with the extended prematurity course ahead with realistic, appropriately calibrated expectations.

Figure 5.1: Germinal Matrix Hemorrhage Grading on Cranial Ultrasound

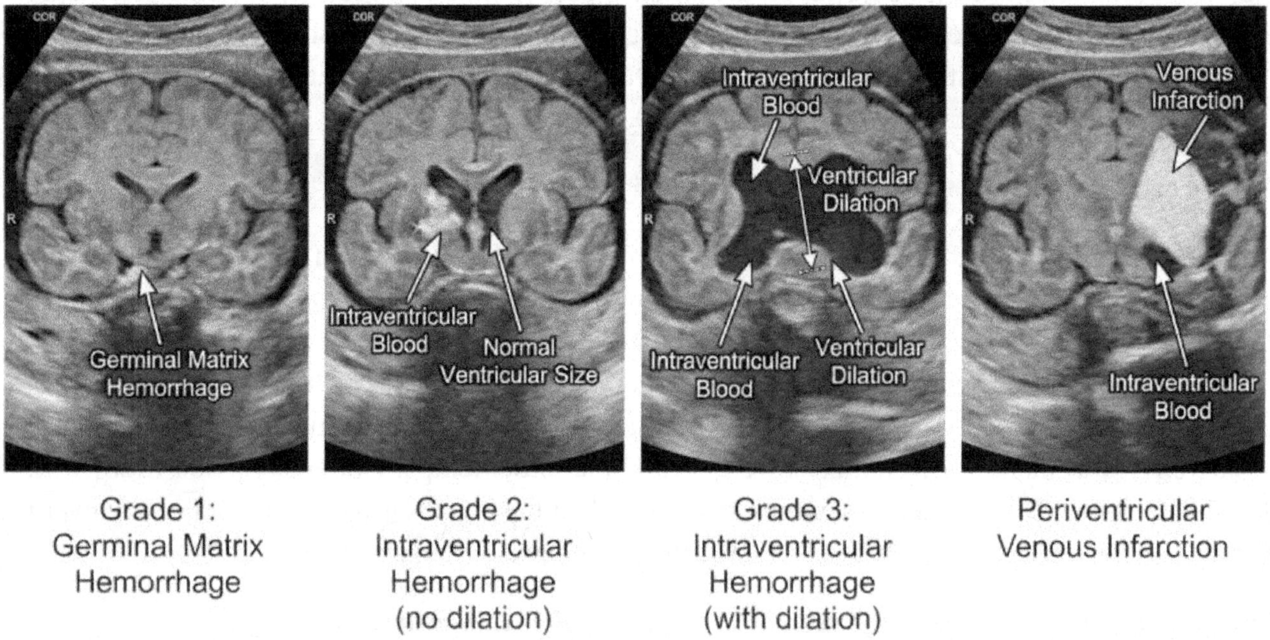

THE CLINICAL-IMAGING CROSSWALK SYSTEM — Grade 4 Hemorrhage Is a Venous Infarction, Not Simple Extension

The Crossing: A preterm infant with a grade three intraventricular hemorrhage develops a new, asymmetric, fan-shaped area of increased echogenicity in the adjacent periventricular white matter on follow-up ultrasound, prompting the referring team to describe it simply as progression to grade four hemorrhage.

Presentation Signature: A preterm infant with an established, graded intraventricular hemorrhage who develops a new, typically asymmetric, wedge- or fan-shaped parenchymal echogenic lesion on follow-up imaging.

Imaging Correlate: The asymmetric, fan-shaped distribution radiating from the region of the terminal vein, rather than a symmetric or diffuse parenchymal change, reflects venous obstruction and hemorrhagic infarction of the medullary veins draining into the terminal vein, a distinct secondary mechanism from the intraventricular hemorrhage itself.

Trap Logic: Describing this finding simply as extension or progression of the intraventricular hemorrhage obscures the distinct venous-infarction mechanism and its correspondingly more guarded prognosis; the terminology and the underlying mechanism should be communicated precisely to the family and care team, not conflated with a simple worsening of the intraventricular grade.

Crossing Anchor: A new asymmetric, fan-shaped parenchymal lesion adjacent to a graded intraventricular hemorrhage represents periventricular hemorrhagic venous infarction, a distinct mechanism with a distinct, more guarded prognosis than intraventricular hemorrhage alone, and should be named and explained as such.

Periventricular Leukomalacia and White Matter Injury

Periventricular leukomalacia, injury to the periventricular white matter of the preterm brain, is distinguished from the terminal zones of myelination discussed in Chapter 2 by a specific set of imaging features and clinical context developed throughout this section, and represents, together with germinal matrix hemorrhage, one of the two dominant injury patterns defining prematurity-related brain injury.

Pathophysiology of Periventricular White Matter Vulnerability

Periventricular white matter is selectively vulnerable in the preterm infant because of the combination of a watershed vascular distribution between the long and short penetrating cerebral arteries in this specific region during the preterm period, before the vascular supply matures further toward term, and the presence of a large population of premyelinating oligodendrocyte precursor cells that are, as introduced in Chapter 4, maximally vulnerable to both hypoxic-ischemic and inflammatory injury during this specific developmental window; this combination of vascular and cellular vulnerability, unique to the preterm period, explains why periventricular leukomalacia is characteristically a disease of prematurity rather than of the term infant.

Cystic Versus Diffuse (Noncystic) Periventricular Leukomalacia

Cystic periventricular leukomalacia, the classic, severe form recognized since the earliest descriptions of this condition, features frank cystic necrosis of the periventricular white matter, typically becoming apparent on cranial ultrasound or MRI within two to four weeks after the initial insult and most reliably identified on the later follow-up ultrasound timing established in the previous section; this cystic pattern, while still encountered, has become substantially less common in contemporary neonatal intensive care practice, reflecting improvements in perinatal and neonatal management over recent decades.

Diffuse, or noncystic, periventricular leukomalacia, now the more commonly encountered pattern in contemporary practice, features a subtler combination of diffuse periventricular T2 signal abnormality, reduced periventricular white matter volume, and secondary ventricular enlargement from volume loss rather than frank cystic change, and requires MRI, not cranial ultrasound alone, for reliable detection given the relative insensitivity of ultrasound to this subtler, diffuse pattern; this shift toward the diffuse, MRI-detected pattern as the more common contemporary presentation is itself a significant, well-documented evolution in the epidemiology of prematurity-related white matter injury.

Imaging Timeline and Sequence Selection

The imaging appearance of periventricular leukomalacia evolves over a well-characterized timeline: an acute phase in the first one to two weeks may show increased periventricular echogenicity on ultrasound or subtle diffusion restriction on MRI if imaging is obtained very early, followed by a subacute phase in which cystic change, if present, becomes apparent, and a chronic phase, typically established by term-equivalent age, in which periventricular volume loss, ventricular enlargement with irregular, angular ventricular margins, and thinning of the corpus callosum, particularly the posterior body and splenium, become the dominant, stable findings; MRI at term-equivalent age, incorporating T1, T2, and diffusion sequencing, is the most sensitive and specific approach for full characterization of both cystic and diffuse periventricular leukomalacia.

Diffuse White Matter Injury and Punctate Lesions

Beyond the classic periventricular leukomalacia pattern, punctate white matter lesions, small, discrete foci of T1 hyperintensity or diffusion restriction scattered through the white matter without the confluent periventricular distribution of classic periventricular leukomalacia, are increasingly recognized as a further, distinct pattern of preterm white matter injury, associated with a milder but still clinically meaningful risk of adverse neurodevelopmental outcome relative to the more severe cystic and diffuse patterns described above; distinguishing punctate lesions from the normal, symmetric terminal zones of myelination discussed in Chapter 2 relies on the same discriminating features, asymmetry, irregular margins, and a plausible clinical context of preterm vulnerability, developed throughout this book.

Differentiating True Periventricular Leukomalacia From Normal Variants

The Chapter 2 discussion of terminal zones of myelination as a normal-variant mimic of periventricular leukomalacia applies with particular relevance in this chapter's population, since the preterm infant undergoing term-equivalent MRI is, by the very nature of the comparison, being imaged at an age when terminal zones of myelination are themselves a genuinely expected normal finding; applying the discriminating features developed in Chapter 2, symmetry, smooth margins, and expected resolution with further myelination, against the specific corrected age of the preterm infant rather than chronologic age, is essential to avoid both false-positive overcalling of a normal finding as periventricular leukomalacia and, in the opposite direction, false-negative undercalling of true, asymmetric or irregularly margined injury as normal variation.

Inflammatory and Infectious Contributors to White Matter Injury

Chorioamnionitis and other antenatal or early postnatal infectious and inflammatory exposures are independently associated with periventricular white matter injury risk, acting through fetal and neonatal inflammatory cytokine exposure that directly affects the vulnerable premyelinating oligodendrocyte precursor population described earlier in this section, a mechanism distinct from, though frequently additive to, the vascular hypoxic-ischemic mechanism also discussed; a preterm infant with a documented history of chorioamnionitis or early sepsis, even in the absence of a specific hypoxic-ischemic sentinel event, carries independently elevated white matter injury risk and warrants the same rigorous term-equivalent MRI evaluation as an infant with a more classic hypoxic-ischemic risk profile, since the two mechanisms are not mutually exclusive indications for careful white matter assessment.

White Matter Injury and Corpus Callosum Thinning

Because commissural fibers of the corpus callosum traverse the periventricular white matter regions most vulnerable to the injury patterns discussed throughout this section, significant periventricular leukomalacia is frequently accompanied by secondary thinning of the corpus callosum, most pronounced in the posterior body and splenium given the caudal-to-rostral vulnerability gradient of the periventricular white matter itself; corpus callosum thinning identified on term-equivalent MRI should prompt careful, correlated assessment of the adjacent periventricular white matter rather than being reported as an isolated finding, since it frequently serves as a secondary marker pointing toward a primary periventricular white matter injury that itself warrants full characterization and reporting.

Diffusion Tensor Imaging and Quantitative White Matter Assessment

Diffusion tensor imaging, introduced in Chapter 1 and revisited in Chapter 2 as a quantitative correlate of myelination, offers a further, increasingly used adjunct for characterizing periventricular white matter injury in the preterm population, since fractional anisotropy values within specific white matter tracts can be reduced even in regions that appear qualitatively unremarkable on conventional T1 and T2 sequences, capturing a subtler degree of microstructural disruption than conventional imaging alone detects; while not yet a routine component of every term-equivalent MRI protocol at every institution, diffusion tensor imaging is increasingly incorporated at centers with a dedicated preterm neuroimaging research or clinical program, particularly when a more precise, quantitative assessment of white matter integrity is needed to inform an individual child's prognostic counseling or research participation.

Structured Reporting for Periventricular White Matter Injury

Given the multiple distinct patterns and severity gradations discussed throughout this section, a structured report explicitly addressing the presence or absence of cystic change, the extent and distribution of diffuse signal abnormality, the number and distribution of any punctate lesions, and the presence or absence of associated ventricular enlargement or corpus callosum thinning gives the referring clinician and family a substantially clearer, more actionable picture than an unstructured qualitative description alone; adopting the same structured-reporting discipline introduced in Chapter 1 for this specific, complex injury category reduces the risk that a clinically important component of the full injury picture, such as a small number of punctate lesions accompanying a more prominent diffuse signal change, is omitted from the report simply because it seemed secondary to the more visually striking primary finding.

Regional Variation in Periventricular Injury Distribution

Periventricular white matter injury does not distribute uniformly around the ventricular system, and injury adjacent to the trigones and occipital horns, the region most classically involved in both cystic and diffuse periventricular leukomalacia, carries somewhat different functional implications than injury more anteriorly distributed near the frontal horns, given the differing white matter tracts and cortical projection targets traversing each region; documenting the specific regional distribution of injury, not only its overall presence and severity, allows the subsequent developmental follow-up program discussed later in this chapter to anticipate and specifically screen for the functional domains most plausibly linked to the particular region affected in an individual child.

Ex-Utero Growth Restriction and Its Interaction With White Matter Injury

Postnatal growth restriction, in which a preterm infant fails to achieve expected growth velocity across the neonatal intensive care hospitalization despite adequate nutritional support, has been independently associated with reduced brain volume and, in some cohorts, with white matter injury severity, plausibly reflecting shared underlying illness severity or a direct nutritional contribution to ongoing brain development during this critical postnatal growth window; nutritional optimization throughout the neonatal intensive care course, coordinated between neonatology and nutrition specialists, is accordingly understood not merely as a general supportive care measure but as a component of the broader neuroprotective strategy this chapter has emphasized throughout, alongside the more specific hemorrhage- and white-matter-injury-prevention measures already discussed.

Bronchopulmonary Dysplasia and Its Association With White Matter Outcome

Bronchopulmonary dysplasia, chronic lung disease of prematurity requiring prolonged respiratory support, frequently coexists with the white matter injury patterns discussed throughout this section, sharing overlapping risk factors including prolonged mechanical ventilation, recurrent hypoxic episodes, and systemic inflammation, and infants with significant bronchopulmonary dysplasia warrant particular attention to white matter assessment on term-equivalent imaging given this documented association; the coexistence of significant respiratory and neurologic morbidity in the same infant further reinforces the family-wide, multidisciplinary counseling and follow-up coordination emphasized throughout this chapter, since these families are simultaneously navigating respiratory and neurodevelopmental follow-up systems that benefit from coordinated, rather than fragmented, communication between the respective specialist teams, ideally through a single, integrated follow-up visit rather than separate, uncoordinated respiratory and neurodevelopmental appointments scheduled independently.

Feature	Cystic PVL	Diffuse (Noncystic) PVL	Punctate White Matter Lesions
Detection modality	Ultrasound or MRI	MRI (ultrasound insensitive)	MRI
Timing of full evolution	2-4 weeks post-insult	Term-equivalent age	Term-equivalent age
Contemporary frequency	Decreasing	Now most common pattern	Common, often mild
Typical severity association	Severe motor outcome risk	Variable, correlates with extent	Milder but meaningful risk

THE CLINICAL-IMAGING CROSSWALK SYSTEM — Diffuse PVL Requiring MRI When Ultrasound Is Reassuring

The Crossing: A former twenty-six-week preterm infant has a reassuring discharge cranial ultrasound without cystic change, but the family and care team want to know whether a term-equivalent MRI adds meaningful additional information.

Presentation Signature: A preterm infant born below the gestational age threshold associated with meaningful white matter injury risk, with a normal or unremarkable cranial ultrasound that did not show frank cystic periventricular leukomalacia.

Imaging Correlate: Term-equivalent MRI, not the reassuring discharge ultrasound alone, is the appropriate study to detect the diffuse, noncystic periventricular leukomalacia pattern and punctate white matter lesions described in this section, both of which are frequently missed by ultrasound given its relative insensitivity to these subtler patterns.

Trap Logic: A normal cranial ultrasound reassures against the classic cystic pattern but does not exclude the diffuse, noncystic pattern that has become the more common contemporary presentation; treating a normal ultrasound as equivalent to a normal MRI in this population overstates the ultrasound's sensitivity.

Crossing Anchor: A reassuring cranial ultrasound in a very preterm infant does not exclude diffuse periventricular leukomalacia or punctate white matter lesions; term-equivalent MRI is the appropriate study for full white matter injury characterization in this population.

Cerebellar Injury in the Preterm Infant

Cerebellar injury has emerged over the past two decades as an increasingly recognized and increasingly important component of prematurity-related brain injury, historically underappreciated relative to the supratentorial injury patterns discussed above because of the specific detection challenges developed in this section.

Mechanisms of Cerebellar Vulnerability in Prematurity

The cerebellum, as introduced in Chapter 2, undergoes its most rapid growth phase during the third trimester, a developmental timing that places the preterm cerebellum at a particularly vulnerable stage of active growth at precisely the time the infant is removed from the intrauterine environment; this vulnerability is compounded by the cerebellum's external granular layer, a transient proliferative structure present only during this developmental window, which is itself susceptible to both direct hemorrhagic injury and the disruptive effects of the systemic inflammatory and hypoxic-ischemic insults common in the sick preterm infant.

Primary Cerebellar Hemorrhage

Primary cerebellar hemorrhage, ranging from small, punctate hemorrhagic foci to larger, destructive hemorrhage, occurs with a documented, non-negligible incidence in very preterm infants and shares several risk factors with the supratentorial germinal matrix hemorrhage discussed earlier in this chapter, including hemodynamic instability and coagulopathy; larger cerebellar hemorrhages are associated with a substantial risk of subsequent cerebellar volume loss and, correspondingly, with the motor coordination and, in some cases, cognitive and behavioral outcome associations discussed later in this chapter.

Secondary (Remote) Cerebellar Injury and Diaschisis

Beyond primary hemorrhagic injury, the preterm cerebellum can also show secondary, remote volume reduction following a supratentorial injury, most notably severe intraventricular hemorrhage or periventricular leukomalacia, through a mechanism termed crossed cerebellar diaschisis or a related remote trophic effect, in which disruption of cerebro-cerebellar connections following a supratentorial insult impairs subsequent cerebellar growth even in the absence of any direct cerebellar hemorrhage or structural injury; recognizing this secondary growth-impairment pattern, typically apparent only on later, term-equivalent or follow-up imaging rather than in the acute period, is important because it means a preterm infant with a severe supratentorial injury but an unremarkable acute cerebellar appearance may still develop clinically significant cerebellar volume reduction over time, warranting the same long-term surveillance discussed in the final section of this chapter.

Imaging Detection Challenges With Ultrasound Versus MRI

Cranial ultrasound, the primary screening modality for germinal matrix hemorrhage discussed earlier in this chapter, has substantially lower sensitivity for cerebellar hemorrhage than for supratentorial hemorrhage, both because the standard anterior fontanelle acoustic window provides a less favorable viewing angle to the posterior fossa and because smaller cerebellar hemorrhages in particular are more easily missed on ultrasound than on MRI; this detection gap is a principal reason cerebellar injury was historically underrecognized before term-equivalent MRI became standard practice in many preterm follow-up protocols, and it reinforces, from a distinct anatomic angle, the same broader point developed throughout this chapter that ultrasound and MRI are complementary rather than interchangeable tools in the preterm brain injury evaluation.

Cerebellar Growth Trajectory and Outcome Correlation

Quantitative cerebellar volume measurement, whether from primary hemorrhagic injury or secondary remote growth impairment, correlates with subsequent motor, and in some published cohorts cognitive and behavioral, outcome in a dose-dependent fashion, reinforcing the specific clinical value of dedicated posterior fossa assessment as a routine, explicit component of every preterm term-equivalent MRI, rather than a supplementary or secondary consideration addressed only when a supratentorial finding prompts specific concern.

Distinguishing Cerebellar Hemorrhage From Normal Neonatal Cerebellar Appearance

The rapidly evolving, actively foliating preterm cerebellum can present interpretive challenges distinct from those affecting the supratentorial brain, since the immature, incompletely foliated cerebellar surface and the transient external granular layer itself can produce a signal appearance on early imaging that is unfamiliar to a reader trained primarily on term or older pediatric cerebellar anatomy; distinguishing this normal, actively maturing preterm cerebellar appearance from true, subtle hemorrhagic injury requires the same age-specific interpretive discipline established in Chapter 2, applied with particular care given both the smaller absolute size of the structures involved and the genuine unfamiliarity many readers have with the preterm cerebellum's specific developmental appearance relative to the more extensively documented supratentorial developmental timeline.

Interaction Between Cerebellar and Supratentorial Injury Severity

Cerebellar injury and supratentorial injury are not independent risk factors that simply sum arithmetically toward a combined outcome estimate; published outcome data suggest that the combination of significant cerebellar and significant supratentorial injury carries a disproportionately elevated risk relative to either injury pattern alone, plausibly reflecting the extensive, bidirectional cerebro-cerebellar connectivity through which each region's injury compounds the functional impact of injury in the other; this interaction is a further reason the combined-injury case presented later in this chapter warrants a more intensive follow-up recommendation than would be generated by considering either the supratentorial or cerebellar findings in isolation.

Brainstem Involvement Alongside Cerebellar Injury

Severe cerebellar hemorrhage or the extreme end of the secondary volume-loss spectrum discussed above can, less commonly, extend to or coexist with brainstem signal abnormality, given the close anatomic proximity and shared vascular supply of these posterior fossa structures; brainstem involvement carries additional clinical significance for early feeding, oromotor, and respiratory function beyond the motor coordination and cognitive-behavioral associations already discussed for isolated cerebellar injury, and a dedicated, explicit assessment of the brainstem, not only the cerebellar hemispheres and vermis, is warranted whenever significant posterior fossa injury is identified on term-equivalent imaging.

Emerging Postnatal Cerebellar Growth Monitoring Strategies

Given the recognized limitation of standard cranial ultrasound for cerebellar assessment discussed above, some centers have begun incorporating dedicated, protocol-driven mastoid fontanelle ultrasound views into routine preterm screening, alongside quantitative cerebellar biometry compared against published preterm normative growth curves, as a lower-cost, more accessible complement to term-equivalent MRI for serial cerebellar growth monitoring across the neonatal intensive care course, rather than relying solely on a single term-equivalent MRI time point to capture cerebellar injury; this practice remains institution-dependent rather than universal at present, but reflects the broader recognition, developed throughout this section, that cerebellar assessment deserves the same systematic attention historically reserved for supratentorial structures.

Practical Recommendations for Cerebellar Assessment in Clinical Practice

Translating the mechanisms and detection challenges developed throughout this section into practical guidance, this book recommends explicit, documented cerebellar assessment, including qualitative appearance and, where institutional capacity allows, quantitative volume or biometric measurement, as a standard, non-optional component of every preterm term-equivalent MRI report, regardless of whether the supratentorial findings alone would otherwise have prompted specific cerebellar concern; given the secondary, remote injury mechanism discussed earlier in this section, a preterm infant with severe supratentorial injury has, if anything, a heightened rather than diminished need for careful cerebellar assessment, the inverse of an intuitive assumption that cerebellar assessment matters most only when a primary cerebellar abnormality is already suspected.

Historical Underrecognition and Its Ongoing Clinical Implications

Because reliable, routine cerebellar assessment in the preterm population is a relatively recent addition to standard neuroimaging practice compared to the decades-long history of germinal matrix hemorrhage and periventricular leukomalacia recognition, a meaningful proportion of older children and adolescents who were themselves born preterm before this recognition became standard practice may carry undiagnosed cerebellar injury contributing to previously unexplained motor coordination or cognitive-behavioral difficulty; a clinician evaluating an older child or adolescent with a preterm birth history and an otherwise unexplained coordination, attentional, or behavioral concern may reasonably consider whether earlier-generation neuroimaging, if available for review, adequately assessed the posterior fossa, or whether updated imaging is warranted to complete a historically incomplete evaluation.

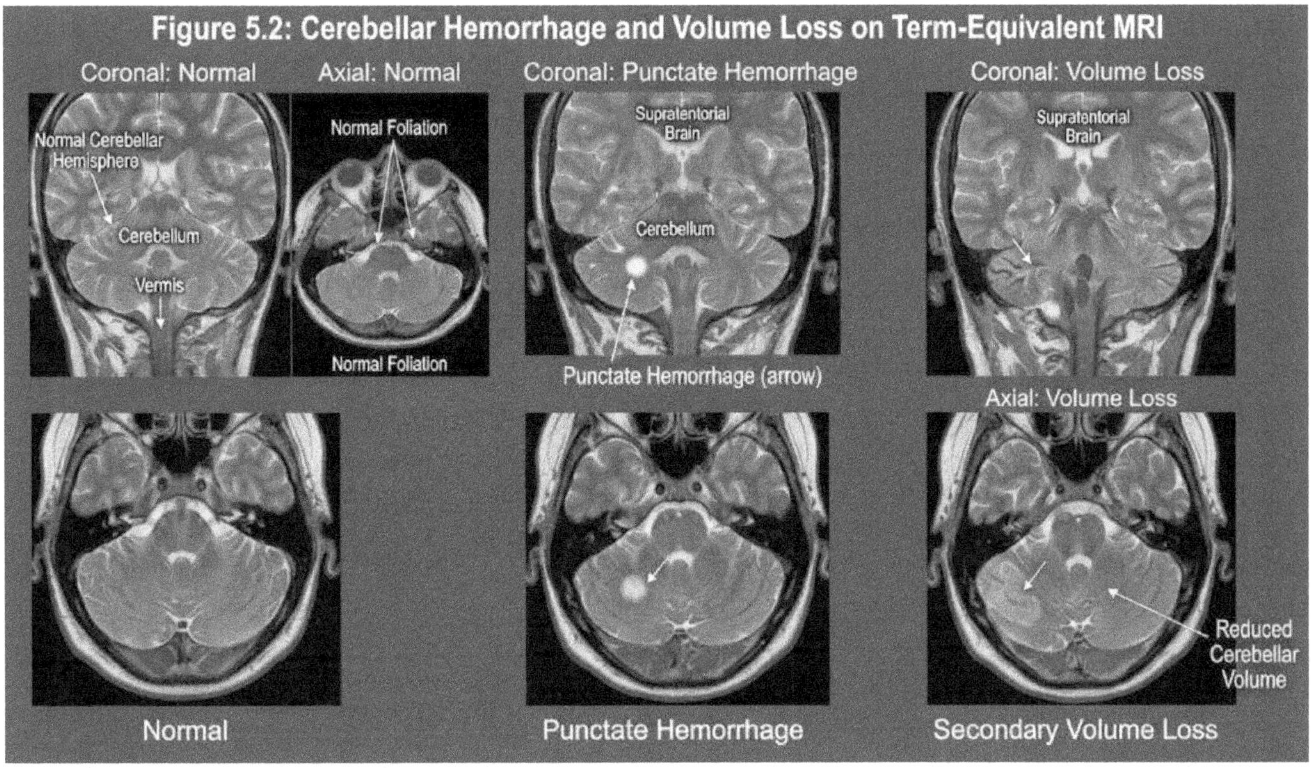

Long-Term Neurodevelopmental Correlates

The ultimate clinical significance of the injury patterns catalogued throughout this chapter lies in their correlation with long-term neurodevelopmental outcome, and this final section synthesizes that correlation while establishing the structured follow-up framework that translates newborn-period imaging into meaningful, ongoing clinical care.

Motor Outcome and Cerebral Palsy Risk by Injury Severity

Cerebral palsy risk rises in a well-documented, graded fashion with increasing severity of periventricular white matter injury, with cystic periventricular leukomalacia carrying the highest documented risk among survivors, severe grade three or four intraventricular hemorrhage carrying substantial additional risk, particularly when periventricular hemorrhagic venous infarction is present, and diffuse, noncystic white matter injury carrying a more variable, generally lower but still clinically meaningful risk that correlates with the extent of white matter volume affected; this graded relationship allows a structured, evidence-based prognostic discussion tailored to the specific severity and pattern of injury identified in an individual infant, rather than a single undifferentiated prematurity-related outcome discussion applied uniformly regardless of the specific imaging findings.

Cognitive and Behavioral Outcome

Beyond motor outcome, periventricular white matter injury, diffuse supratentorial volume reduction, and cerebellar injury are each independently associated with cognitive, language, attentional, and behavioral outcome domains in published longitudinal cohorts, associations that frequently become clinically apparent only well beyond infancy, at school age or later, when the cognitive and academic demands placed on the child exceed what earlier developmental screening was designed to detect; this delayed manifestation is a central rationale for the extended, structured follow-up programs discussed below, rather than a brief follow-up period ending in early childhood.

The Role of Serial Imaging in Outcome Prediction

While the term-equivalent MRI discussed throughout this chapter provides the most comprehensive newborn-period prognostic imaging assessment, serial imaging, when clinically indicated, whether to monitor evolving ventricular size, to assess an initially indeterminate finding, or to investigate a new clinical concern arising later in infancy, adds incremental prognostic value beyond a single time-point study; the general principle from Chapter 4, that imaging is one component of an integrated prognostic assessment alongside clinical trajectory rather than a single definitive verdict, applies with equal force to prematurity-related brain injury.

Socioeconomic and Environmental Modifiers of Outcome

Published outcome data increasingly recognize that the relationship between newborn brain injury severity and eventual developmental outcome is modified, sometimes substantially, by postnatal environmental factors, including socioeconomic circumstances, access to early intervention services, and the quality and consistency of the child's early caregiving environment; two infants with imaging findings of similar severity can experience meaningfully different developmental trajectories depending on these postnatal factors, a reality that argues against treating the newborn imaging severity as a fixed, deterministic outcome predictor and in favor of the structured follow-up and early-intervention connection emphasized throughout this section, since these postnatal factors are, unlike the injury itself, ones the care team and family can actively influence going forward.

Transitioning From Neonatal Intensive Care to Outpatient Follow-Up

The transition from the neonatal intensive care unit to outpatient structured follow-up represents a vulnerable point in a preterm infant's care continuum, at which families, often exhausted from a prolonged hospitalization, must independently coordinate a series of outpatient appointments and assessments that were previously managed for them within the structured hospital environment; a formal, structured discharge process that directly schedules the first structured follow-up appointment before hospital discharge, rather than leaving the family to independently arrange it afterward, measurably improves follow-up program engagement and reduces the number of families lost to follow-up during this specific transition period.

Sibling and Family-Wide Considerations in Counseling

Prognostic counseling following significant prematurity-related brain injury frequently occurs within a family context that includes other children, sometimes a surviving co-twin from the same complicated pregnancy, and family-wide considerations, including how to communicate the affected child's needs to siblings in age-appropriate terms and how to support parental capacity to engage with a medically complex child alongside other family responsibilities, meaningfully shape the practical, sustainable follow-up plan a family can actually carry out; a follow-up plan that is clinically ideal in isolation but does not account for the family's full practical circumstances is less likely to be successfully sustained than one developed collaboratively with explicit attention to these family-wide realities.

Synthesis: Integrating the Three Injury Categories Into One Prognostic Picture

A complete term-equivalent MRI assessment integrates the germinal matrix and intraventricular hemorrhage findings, the periventricular white matter findings, and the cerebellar findings discussed across the three preceding sections of this chapter into a single, coherent injury summary, since, as the interaction discussion earlier in this section established, these three injury categories interact rather than simply coexist independently; a structured, comprehensive reporting template addressing all three categories explicitly, rather than three separate, disconnected findings buried within a longer report, best supports the kind of integrated, honest, and appropriately individualized family counseling this chapter has emphasized throughout, and is the reporting standard this book recommends for every preterm term-equivalent MRI.

Anticipating and Preparing Families for the Term-Equivalent MRI Conversation

Because the term-equivalent MRI discussed throughout this chapter often represents the single most comprehensive prognostic data point a family will receive during the neonatal intensive care hospitalization, preparing the family in advance for both the logistics of the study, including whether sedation will be required per the framework developed in Chapter 1, and the general nature of the results conversation that will follow, reduces acute anxiety around the study itself and allows the family to arrive at the results discussion already oriented to receive complex, nuanced information rather than encountering both the fact of the study and its results simultaneously and without warning; scheduling a dedicated, unhurried time for the results conversation, separate from routine daily rounding, further supports the depth of discussion this complex, multidomain prognostic information genuinely requires.

Research Participation and Its Role in Advancing This Field

Much of the evolving evidence base referenced throughout this chapter, including the outcome correlations for cerebellar injury, diffusion tensor imaging findings, and the socioeconomic and environmental modifiers discussed above, derives from longitudinal research cohorts that depend on sustained family participation across years of structured follow-up assessment; a clinician discussing structured follow-up with a family is well positioned to mention, where a relevant research program exists at the treating institution, that continued participation not only benefits the individual child through more frequent, structured monitoring but also contributes directly to the evidence base that will refine prognostic counseling for future families, a framing that some families find meaningfully motivating for sustained, longitudinal engagement with what can otherwise feel like an open-ended follow-up commitment.

Structured Follow-Up Programs for Preterm Infants

Dedicated preterm follow-up programs, typically incorporating structured developmental assessment at defined intervals through early childhood and, at many centers, extending to school-age assessment given the delayed manifestation of cognitive and behavioral outcomes discussed above, represent the standard of care for infants born at the gestational ages and injury severities discussed throughout this chapter; imaging findings from the newborn period are used within these programs to risk-stratify the intensity and focus of ongoing surveillance, with infants carrying the most severe injury patterns receiving the most intensive, longest-duration follow-up, while infants with milder or no identified injury still benefit from at least baseline structured developmental screening given the imperfect sensitivity of even comprehensive newborn imaging for predicting every domain of eventual outcome.

Case Presentation: Severe Combined Injury and Comprehensive Counseling

An infant born at twenty-four weeks gestation develops a grade three intraventricular hemorrhage with periventricular hemorrhagic venous infarction identified on first-week cranial ultrasound. Term-equivalent MRI subsequently demonstrates diffuse periventricular white matter volume loss, a small punctate cerebellar hemorrhage with associated mild cerebellar volume reduction, and posthemorrhagic ventricular enlargement stabilized after a temporizing cerebrospinal fluid diversion procedure. Applying the graded, pattern-specific reasoning developed throughout this chapter, the care team explains to the family that this combination of findings, venous infarction, diffuse white matter injury, and cerebellar involvement, places the child at meaningfully elevated risk across the motor, cognitive, and behavioral domains discussed in this section, while emphasizing the genuine individual variability in outcome even among infants with similar imaging findings, and enrolls the infant in the institution's structured, extended preterm follow-up program with planned assessments through school age.

Case Presentation: Mild Isolated Finding and Calibrated Reassurance

An infant born at thirty weeks gestation has a grade one germinal matrix hemorrhage on first-week ultrasound without ventricular extension, and term-equivalent MRI demonstrates a small number of punctate white matter lesions without confluent periventricular signal change, normal cerebellar volume, and no ventricular enlargement. Applying the same graded framework, the care team explains that this pattern is associated with a comparatively favorable, though not entirely risk-free, prognosis, distinguishing it explicitly from the more severe combined-injury pattern of the preceding case, and recommends standard, rather than intensive, structured follow-up, illustrating how the specific severity and pattern of findings, not a single generic prematurity diagnosis, calibrates both the content of family counseling and the intensity of the follow-up plan.

Retinopathy of Prematurity as a Parallel Screening Paradigm

Retinopathy of prematurity, a distinct but conceptually parallel complication of prematurity affecting the developing retinal vasculature, is screened through a similarly structured, protocol-driven examination timeline coordinated by ophthalmology, and infants undergoing structured neuroimaging screening per the protocols developed throughout this chapter frequently undergo retinopathy screening concurrently during the same hospitalization; a shared awareness across the neonatal intensive care team of both screening timelines, and coordination between neurology, radiology, and ophthalmology teams evaluating the same medically complex infant, exemplifies the multidisciplinary care model this chapter has emphasized as essential to the comprehensive management of prematurity-related morbidity, of which brain injury is the single most extensively developed example in this book, but by no means the only complication requiring this kind of structured, protocol-driven surveillance.

Documenting Hemorrhage Grade Changes Across Serial Studies

When serial cranial ultrasound demonstrates a change in apparent hemorrhage grade between studies, most often an increase from a lower to a higher grade as evolving hemorrhage or new bleeding is identified, the report should explicitly state both the current and the prior grade and characterize whether the change reflects genuine interval progression, resolution of an earlier overestimate as blood products clear and become easier to characterize precisely, or a technical difference in image quality or acquisition angle between the two studies; this explicit, comparative documentation prevents a family or referring clinician from being confused by an apparent change in severity that may, on closer review, reflect improved characterization rather than a true worsening of the underlying process.

Synthesis: A Continuum, Not a Single Diagnosis

The reader closing this chapter should carry forward one integrating idea above the many specific findings, mechanisms, and grading systems catalogued throughout: prematurity-related brain injury is not a single diagnosis but a continuum spanning three interacting anatomic categories, germinal matrix and intraventricular hemorrhage, periventricular white matter injury, and cerebellar injury, each evolving over a distinct, well-characterized imaging timeline, each carrying distinct but interacting outcome associations, and each requiring the specific, age- and modality-appropriate detection strategy developed section by section in this chapter. Holding this continuum framework in mind, rather than treating any single ultrasound or MRI finding as a final, isolated verdict, is what allows a clinician to counsel families accurately, structure follow-up appropriately, and recognize evolving injury or reassuring stability as the child's clinical course unfolds over the months and years following a preterm birth.

THE CLINICAL-IMAGING CROSSWALK SYSTEM — Prematurity-Related Injury Grading and Detection

---

Crossing 1 Recap: A new asymmetric, fan-shaped parenchymal lesion adjacent to a graded intraventricular hemorrhage represents periventricular hemorrhagic venous infarction, a distinct mechanism from simple hemorrhage extension.

Crossing 2 Recap: A reassuring cranial ultrasound in a very preterm infant does not exclude diffuse periventricular leukomalacia or punctate white matter lesions; term-equivalent MRI is required for full characterization.

Chapter Anchor: Prematurity-related brain injury spans germinal matrix hemorrhage, periventricular white matter injury, and cerebellar injury, each with distinct mechanisms, distinct optimal detection modalities and timing, and distinct, gradable contributions to long-term motor, cognitive, and behavioral outcome.

Summary and Key Concepts

Germinal matrix hemorrhage is graded by the Papile system; grade four hemorrhage is mechanistically a periventricular hemorrhagic venous infarction, not simple intraventricular extension, and carries a distinctly worse prognosis.

Cystic periventricular leukomalacia has become less common as diffuse, noncystic white matter injury and punctate white matter lesions, both requiring MRI rather than ultrasound for reliable detection, have become the more common contemporary patterns.

The preterm cerebellum is vulnerable to both primary hemorrhage and secondary, remote volume reduction following supratentorial injury; ultrasound has substantially lower sensitivity than MRI for cerebellar injury.

Cerebral palsy risk rises in a graded fashion with white matter injury severity; cognitive and behavioral outcomes, associated with white matter, diffuse volume, and cerebellar injury, frequently manifest only at school age or later.

Structured, extended preterm follow-up programs, risk-stratified by newborn imaging severity, are the standard of care given the delayed manifestation of important outcome domains and the imperfect predictive sensitivity of any single newborn-period study.

CHAPTER 6: NEONATAL AND INFANT INTRACRANIAL HEMORRHAGE AND STROKE

Learning Objectives

1. Recognize the clinical presentation and characteristic vascular distribution of perinatal arterial ischemic stroke and apply correct imaging timing.
2. Identify cerebral sinovenous thrombosis on imaging and distinguish it from normal dural venous variants.
3. Generate an appropriate differential diagnosis for nontraumatic neonatal intracranial hemorrhage beyond germinal matrix hemorrhage.
4. Distinguish expected birth-related extra-axial hemorrhage from hemorrhage requiring further evaluation for a pathologic or abusive etiology, applying distribution, timing, and clinical correlation as the guiding reasoning structure throughout.

Arterial Ischemic Stroke in the Neonate and Infant

Perinatal arterial ischemic stroke is among the more common causes of significant, focal, permanent brain injury in the term infant, and its distinctive clinical presentation, characteristic vascular distribution, and specific imaging timing considerations distinguish it clearly from both the diffuse hypoxic-ischemic injury discussed in Chapter 4 and the venous processes discussed later in this chapter.

Epidemiology and Risk Factors

Perinatal arterial ischemic stroke occurs at a well-documented incidence among term live births, making it one of the more common causes of unilateral cerebral palsy in children who do not have a hypoxic-ischemic encephalopathy history; recognized risk factors include maternal and placental factors such as preeclampsia, chorioamnionitis, and placental thrombotic pathology, perinatal factors including a difficult or instrumented delivery, and, in a subset of cases, an underlying prothrombotic tendency in either the mother or the infant, though a specific identifiable risk factor is absent in a meaningful proportion of cases, a pattern that has driven considerable research interest into the placenta itself as an underrecognized source of embolic material in this population.

Clinical Presentation: Seizures as the Dominant Sign

In striking contrast to stroke presentation at any other stage of life, perinatal arterial ischemic stroke does not typically present with an obvious focal deficit, since the profound plasticity and incomplete corticospinal tract myelination of the neonatal brain, developed in Chapter 2, mean that even a substantial unilateral infarct frequently produces a subtle or entirely absent focal motor asymmetry in the newborn period; the dominant, and often the only, presenting clinical sign is a focal or apparently generalized seizure, typically occurring on day one or two of life in an otherwise well-appearing term infant, a presentation pattern distinct enough that perinatal arterial ischemic stroke should be an active differential consideration in any term neonate presenting with new seizures and no other clear explanation.

Vascular Territory and the Middle Cerebral Artery Predilection

Perinatal arterial ischemic stroke shows a marked predilection for the left middle cerebral artery territory, and specifically its lenticulostriate and cortical branches, a distribution pattern whose exact mechanism remains incompletely understood but is thought to relate to the specific hemodynamics of the fetal and perinatal cerebral circulation, including the geometry of flow from the fetal circulation through the region; recognizing this characteristic distribution helps the reader anticipate the expected imaging appearance and also informs the counseling conversation regarding the specific functional domains, most often affecting the contralateral upper extremity motor function given the classic middle cerebral artery distribution, that are most likely to be affected.

Imaging Timing and Diffusion-Weighted Imaging Sensitivity

Diffusion-weighted imaging, applying the same principles developed in Chapter 1 and Chapter 4, is highly sensitive for acute perinatal arterial ischemic stroke and is typically markedly abnormal within the vascular territory affected by the time a symptomatic neonate is imaged, generally within the first several days of life when seizures prompt urgent evaluation; because the diagnosis frequently is not suspected until seizures develop, which may occur somewhat after the presumed timing of the ischemic event itself, the diffusion abnormality identified may already be evolving toward the pseudonormalization phenomenon discussed in Chapter 4 if imaging is delayed, underscoring the same age- and timing-aware interpretive discipline emphasized throughout this book.

Distinguishing Perinatal Stroke From Later-Presenting Childhood Stroke

A distinct entity, presumed perinatal ischemic stroke, refers to a stroke with imaging features consistent with a perinatal-timing injury, including established encephalomalacia and gliosis rather than acute signal change, identified later in infancy or childhood, typically because the child presents with an asymmetric hand preference or early hemiparesis rather than through the acute neonatal seizure presentation described above; recognizing the established, chronic-appearing imaging signature of presumed perinatal stroke, and distinguishing it from a genuinely new, acute childhood arterial ischemic stroke discussed fully in Chapter 18, depends on the same signal-timing reasoning introduced in Chapter 4, applied here to a presentation that by definition lacks a documented acute neonatal history to anchor the timing directly.

Thrombophilia Workup and the Role of Placental Pathology

A limited, targeted thrombophilia evaluation, rather than an exhaustive panel applied indiscriminately, is generally pursued following perinatal arterial ischemic stroke, particularly when there is a family history of thrombotic disease or when the clinical picture suggests an underlying prothrombotic contribution; placental pathology examination, when the placenta has been retained and is available for review, has emerged as an increasingly important complementary diagnostic step, since placental findings including chorionic vessel thrombosis and fetal vascular malperfusion are identified in a meaningful proportion of perinatal arterial ischemic stroke cases and can provide an etiologic explanation that a purely infant-focused hematologic workup would miss entirely.

Cardioembolic Sources in the Neonate

Congenital heart disease, particularly lesions involving intracardiac shunting or requiring early catheter-based or surgical intervention, represents an important cardioembolic risk factor for perinatal and early infantile arterial ischemic stroke, and a neonate with known structural heart disease presenting with new seizures or a stroke-consistent imaging finding warrants echocardiographic review specifically for a potential embolic source, including a patent foramen ovale with paradoxical embolism, alongside the placental and thrombophilia evaluation discussed above; the presence of a cardiac risk factor does not exclude a concurrent placental contribution, and the two evaluations are pursued in parallel rather than sequentially when both are clinically indicated.

Multifocal and Bilateral Presentations

While perinatal arterial ischemic stroke is classically unilateral and confined to a single vascular territory, a bilateral or multifocal presentation, though less common, should prompt heightened consideration of a systemic embolic or prothrombotic process, including disseminated intravascular coagulation, sepsis-associated coagulopathy, or a significant inherited thrombophilia, rather than the more typical isolated placental or perinatal mechanical mechanism; the distribution pattern itself, unifocal versus multifocal, therefore carries direct diagnostic weight and should inform the scope of the subsequent hematologic evaluation.

Neuroimaging Follow-Up and Volume Loss Assessment

Follow-up imaging beyond the acute period, typically obtained months later once the acute and subacute injury evolution has fully resolved into its chronic, established appearance, characterizes the final extent of encephalomalacia and volume loss within the affected territory and provides the more definitive anatomic basis for the long-term motor outcome counseling discussed throughout this book; this follow-up study is also the point at which the diagnosis of presumed perinatal ischemic stroke, discussed above for infants who present later in infancy, is most directly comparable in appearance to a documented acute perinatal stroke imaged at a comparable chronic interval, reinforcing the value of the signal-evolution timeline developed in Chapter 4 as a unifying interpretive framework across this entire category of injury.

Early Recognition of Hand Preference as a Later Clinical Clue

For the presumed perinatal stroke population who did not present acutely with neonatal seizures, an early, consistent hand preference emerging well before the typical age at which hand dominance is expected to develop, generally not before approximately one year of age in a typically developing infant, is a recognized and clinically useful early clue prompting imaging evaluation; a family or pediatrician who notes this early asymmetric hand use pattern and refers for neurologic evaluation is applying, whether explicitly or not, the same territory-specific functional reasoning developed in this chapter, since early hand preference reflects exactly the corticospinal and upper extremity motor pathway involvement characteristic of the classic middle cerebral artery distribution.

Counseling Framework for Presumed Perinatal Stroke

Because presumed perinatal stroke is identified without the benefit of an acute-phase clinical history to anchor the injury timeline directly, family counseling in this circumstance carries a distinct emphasis relative to the acutely diagnosed case: the family is counseled honestly that the precise timing and inciting cause of the injury cannot be established with certainty from a single later study, that the finding nonetheless explains the observed early hand preference or other presenting concern, and that the same territory-specific outcome counseling and developmental surveillance framework developed throughout this chapter applies regardless of whether the diagnosis was made acutely in the newborn period or later through this presumed, retrospective pathway.

Arterial Imaging and the Role of Vessel Wall Assessment

Dedicated intracranial arterial imaging, most commonly MR angiography obtained as part of the acute stroke protocol, is performed to assess for an underlying arteriopathy that might have contributed to the stroke or that might predict recurrence risk, though a demonstrable arteriopathy is identified in only a minority of perinatal arterial ischemic stroke cases relative to the childhood arterial ischemic stroke population discussed in Chapter 18, where arteriopathy is a substantially more common contributing factor; when arterial imaging does demonstrate a focal irregularity or narrowing, correlating this finding with the clinical and placental evaluation discussed above, rather than treating the arterial finding as an isolated, sufficient explanation, provides the most complete etiologic picture.

Recurrence Risk and Implications for Future Pregnancies

Recurrence risk for perinatal arterial ischemic stroke in a subsequent pregnancy is generally low in the absence of an identified severe maternal or infant prothrombotic condition, and this reassurance is an important component of family counseling, since parents not uncommonly express significant anxiety regarding future pregnancies following a perinatal stroke diagnosis; when a specific, heritable prothrombotic condition has been identified through the evaluation discussed above, referral to maternal-fetal medicine or genetics for counseling regarding a subsequent pregnancy, including consideration of enhanced antenatal surveillance, is appropriately incorporated into the family's longer-term care plan.

Distinguishing Stroke From Neonatal Seizure Mimics

Before attributing a neonatal seizure to perinatal arterial ischemic stroke, the clinician should actively consider and exclude the broader neonatal seizure differential, including hypoxic-ischemic encephalopathy discussed in Chapter 4, metabolic derangement such as hypoglycemia or electrolyte disturbance, central nervous system infection discussed in Chapter 15, and benign neonatal sleep myoclonus or other nonepileptic movement phenomena that can be mistaken for true seizure activity by an inexperienced observer; imaging findings consistent with a discrete arterial territory infarct provide strong, specific support for the stroke diagnosis once obtained, but the initial clinical evaluation and basic metabolic screening proceed in parallel with, not sequentially after, the imaging evaluation, given the range of readily treatable alternative or coexisting causes this broader differential includes.

Figure 6.1: Perinatal Arterial Ischemic Stroke in the Middle Cerebral Artery Territory

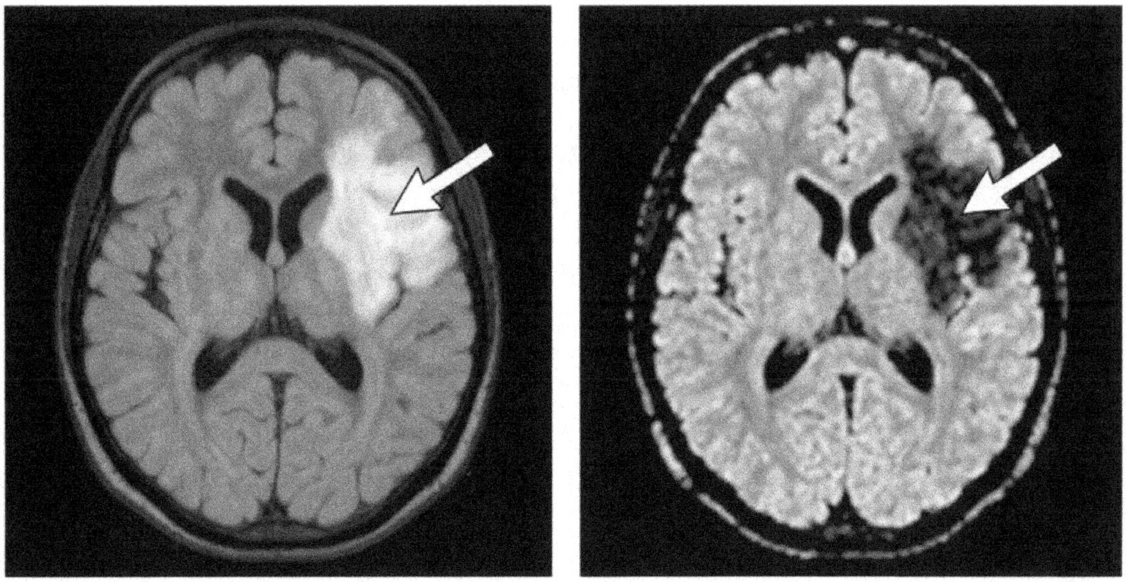

DWI ADC

Cerebral Sinovenous Thrombosis

Cerebral sinovenous thrombosis, a distinct entity from arterial ischemic stroke with its own risk factors, imaging appearance, and management considerations, requires the reader to hold a separate diagnostic framework in mind rather than treating every neonatal vascular brain injury as a variation on the arterial stroke pattern discussed above.

Risk Factors and Clinical Presentation

Cerebral sinovenous thrombosis in the neonate and young infant is associated with a distinct risk factor profile from arterial ischemic stroke, including dehydration, systemic infection and sepsis, underlying prothrombotic conditions, and, in the older infant, local infectious processes such as mastoiditis or sinusitis that can extend to involve the adjacent dural venous sinus directly; clinical presentation is often nonspecific, including seizures, lethargy, and irritability, with the diagnosis frequently made only once dedicated venous imaging is obtained specifically because the initial presentation did not clearly point toward a venous, as opposed to arterial or diffuse, process.

Venous Anatomy and Imaging Technique

Confirming cerebral sinovenous thrombosis requires dedicated venous-phase imaging, either MR venography or CT venography, rather than relying on the venous-phase information incidentally present on a routine, non-venous-optimized study, since a filling defect within a dural venous sinus can be subtle or entirely missed on conventional sequences not specifically optimized for venous flow assessment; the specific technique selected depends on clinical circumstance, with MR venography generally preferred when feasible given its avoidance of radiation and iodinated contrast, consistent with the modality-selection reasoning developed in Chapter 3.

Venous Infarction and Hemorrhagic Transformation

Unlike arterial ischemic stroke, which produces infarction within a discrete arterial territory, cerebral sinovenous thrombosis produces venous congestion and, when severe, venous infarction in a pattern that does not respect arterial territorial boundaries and frequently, unlike the majority of acute arterial infarcts, shows hemorrhagic transformation, reflecting the distinct pathophysiology of venous outflow obstruction and resulting venous hypertension rather than arterial inflow occlusion; recognizing a hemorrhagic parenchymal lesion that does not conform to a recognizable arterial territory should prompt active consideration of an underlying venous thrombosis as the primary process, rather than a purely hemorrhagic diagnosis considered in isolation.

Distinguishing True Thrombosis From Normal Venous Variants

Building directly on the normal dural venous variant discussion in Chapter 2, distinguishing a filling defect representing true thrombosis from a normal variant such as asymmetric transverse sinus hypoplasia or a prominent arachnoid granulation requires careful attention to the specific imaging features that discriminate the two: true thrombosis shows an expansile, space-occupying filling defect with absence of normal flow-related signal and often an abnormal signal characteristic on the thrombus itself, while a normal variant shows a congenitally small or absent sinus segment without expansile change and, critically, without an accompanying clinical picture suggestive of a new, acute venous process.

Treatment Considerations and Follow-Up Imaging

Anticoagulation is considered for cerebral sinovenous thrombosis in selected cases, balancing the thrombotic extension and venous infarction risk against the hemorrhage risk in an already frequently hemorrhagic lesion, a risk-benefit calculation generally made in conjunction with a pediatric hematology consultation; follow-up venous imaging to assess for recanalization, typically obtained some weeks to months after the acute presentation depending on institutional protocol and clinical trajectory, informs both the duration of any anticoagulation therapy and the long-term prognostic counseling regarding persistent venous outflow impairment.

Underlying Prothrombotic and Infectious Workup

Once cerebral sinovenous thrombosis is confirmed, a evaluation for an underlying contributing cause is pursued in parallel with acute management, including assessment for dehydration and its correction, evaluation for a systemic or local infectious source such as mastoiditis or meningitis, discussed further in Chapter 15, and, particularly when the presentation is severe or recurrent, a thrombophilia evaluation analogous to that discussed for arterial ischemic stroke earlier in this chapter; identifying and correcting a modifiable contributing factor, such as dehydration, is itself an important component of preventing extension or recurrence, distinct from but complementary to the anticoagulation decision itself.

Sinus Involvement Patterns and Their Clinical Significance

The specific dural venous sinus or combination of sinuses involved carries clinical significance beyond simple anatomic description: superior sagittal sinus thrombosis is most classically associated with bilateral parasagittal venous infarction and hemorrhage, transverse and sigmoid sinus involvement is more frequently associated with an adjacent infectious source such as mastoiditis in the older infant, and deep venous system thrombosis, involving the internal cerebral veins and vein of Galen, though less common, carries a particularly severe prognosis given the deep gray and thalamic structures drained by this system; documenting the full extent of sinus involvement, rather than noting only the most prominent finding, therefore directly informs both the severity assessment and the anticipated injury pattern.

Long-Term Outcome and Recurrence Risk

Long-term neurodevelopmental outcome following cerebral sinovenous thrombosis correlates most strongly with the extent of associated venous infarction and hemorrhage rather than with the thrombosis itself, consistent with the general principle developed throughout this book that the resulting parenchymal injury, not the vascular event alone, determines functional prognosis; recurrence risk, while overall low in infants without an identified severe underlying prothrombotic condition, is a further consideration incorporated into the family counseling conversation, particularly when a specific, persistent risk factor such as a significant inherited thrombophilia has been identified through the workup discussed above.

Distinguishing Cerebral Sinovenous Thrombosis From Benign Intracranial Hypertension

Cerebral sinovenous thrombosis and idiopathic intracranial hypertension, discussed further in Chapter 10, can present with overlapping clinical features, including headache and papilledema in the older infant or child capable of manifesting these signs, and transverse sinus stenosis is itself a recognized, usually secondary, finding in idiopathic intracranial hypertension, occasionally raising diagnostic ambiguity as to whether a venous narrowing represents thrombosis or a flow-related stenosis secondary to elevated intracranial pressure; dedicated venous imaging demonstrating a true filling defect with expansile change, rather than simple luminal narrowing without an intraluminal filling defect, distinguishes true thrombosis from this alternative, non-thrombotic explanation.

Multidisciplinary Coordination in Cerebral Sinovenous Thrombosis Management

Management of confirmed cerebral sinovenous thrombosis typically involves coordinated input from child neurology, pediatric hematology, and, when a local infectious source is implicated, pediatric infectious disease, reflecting the multiple, overlapping management considerations, anticoagulation risk-benefit assessment, treatment of any underlying infectious or dehydration-related precipitant, and neurologic monitoring for evolving parenchymal injury or seizures, that this diagnosis requires; establishing this multidisciplinary coordination early in the hospitalization, rather than sequentially as each new consideration arises, generally produces a more efficient and better-integrated care plan than a series of independent, uncoordinated specialist consultations.

Seizure Risk and Antiseizure Management

Seizures, whether at presentation or emerging during the acute hospitalization, are common in cerebral sinovenous thrombosis given the frequent parenchymal venous infarction and hemorrhage discussed earlier in this section, and continuous electroencephalographic monitoring, applying the same electroclinical dissociation reasoning developed in Chapter 4, is similarly indicated in this population to capture electrographic seizures that may not manifest clinically; antiseizure medication selection and duration follow general neonatal and infant seizure management principles, with the decision to continue treatment beyond the acute period informed by the presence and severity of the underlying structural injury rather than by the venous thrombosis diagnosis in isolation.

Imaging Follow-Up Beyond Recanalization Assessment

Beyond the recanalization-focused venous follow-up study discussed earlier, a subset of infants with significant venous infarction undergo additional structural follow-up imaging later in infancy to assess the final extent of parenchymal volume loss and to correlate imaging severity with the emerging developmental trajectory, applying the same longitudinal surveillance principle developed in Chapters 4 and 5 for other categories of newborn brain injury; this later structural follow-up is distinguished from the earlier, more narrowly focused venous recanalization study by its broader purpose, characterizing the full anatomic consequence of the injury rather than specifically tracking the vascular finding that initiated the diagnosis.

When to Suspect Cerebral Sinovenous Thrombosis in a Nonspecific Presentation

Because the presenting features of cerebral sinovenous thrombosis, lethargy, poor feeding, and irritability, overlap substantially with numerous more common, benign pediatric presentations, maintaining an appropriate index of suspicion without triggering unnecessary imaging in every irritable infant requires attention to the specific combination of features that should raise concern: a recent history of dehydration, systemic infection, or a known prothrombotic risk factor, combined with a bulging fontanelle, new seizure activity, or a clinical trajectory that fails to improve as expected with treatment of the presumed underlying illness, together shift the presentation from the broad, low-yield category discussed in Chapter 3 into one warranting dedicated venous imaging.

Feature	Arterial Ischemic Stroke	Cerebral Sinovenous Thrombosis
Typical distribution	Discrete arterial territory (often left MCA)	Does not respect arterial territories; follows venous drainage
Hemorrhagic transformation	Less common in acute presentation	Common, reflecting venous hypertension
Key imaging study	Diffusion-weighted MRI	MR or CT venography
Typical risk factors	Placental pathology, perinatal events	Dehydration, infection, prothrombotic states

THE CLINICAL-IMAGING CROSSWALK SYSTEM — A Hemorrhagic Lesion That Does Not Fit an Arterial Territory

The Crossing: A three-week-old with a recent febrile illness and new lethargy undergoes brain MRI, which shows a hemorrhagic parenchymal lesion that does not conform to a single recognizable arterial territory.

Presentation Signature: A young infant with a recent dehydrating or febrile illness, nonspecific neurologic symptoms, and a hemorrhagic lesion on imaging whose distribution does not match a classic arterial vascular territory.

Imaging Correlate: Dedicated venous-phase imaging is obtained and confirms thrombosis of the adjacent dural venous sinus, with the hemorrhagic parenchymal lesion representing venous infarction with hemorrhagic transformation secondary to the venous outflow obstruction, not a primary arterial event.

Trap Logic: Interpreting an atypically distributed hemorrhagic lesion as a primary hemorrhage or an unusual arterial infarct without obtaining dedicated venous imaging risks missing the underlying venous thrombosis, delaying the anticoagulation and hematologic workup discussed in this section.

Crossing Anchor: A hemorrhagic parenchymal lesion that does not conform to a recognizable arterial territory should prompt dedicated venous-phase imaging to evaluate for underlying cerebral sinovenous thrombosis before the finding is attributed to a primary arterial or hemorrhagic process.

Nontraumatic Hemorrhage — Differential Considerations

Beyond germinal matrix hemorrhage, discussed fully in Chapter 5, and the venous and arterial processes discussed above, a further differential of nontraumatic causes of neonatal and infant intracranial hemorrhage must be actively considered whenever a hemorrhagic finding does not fit neatly into either of those two categories.

Coagulopathy-Related Hemorrhage

Systemic coagulopathy, whether from sepsis-associated disseminated intravascular coagulation, severe liver dysfunction, or an inherited coagulation factor deficiency, can produce intracranial hemorrhage in a distribution that may mimic other categories discussed in this chapter but is distinguished by the presence of a systemic bleeding diathesis evident on laboratory evaluation and, frequently, evidence of bleeding at other sites beyond the central nervous system; a coagulation screen is a standard component of the evaluation for any neonate or young infant presenting with unexplained intracranial hemorrhage, applied alongside, not instead of, the imaging-based etiologic reasoning developed throughout this chapter.

Vascular Malformation as a Hemorrhage Source

An underlying vascular malformation, including an arteriovenous malformation or, particularly in the neonate, a vein of Galen malformation, discussed fully in Chapter 18, can present with intracranial hemorrhage as the initial clinical manifestation; a hemorrhage with an atypical location, an associated enlarged or abnormal vessel visible on the initial study, or an unexpectedly severe presentation relative to the apparent hemorrhage volume alone should prompt dedicated vascular imaging to exclude an underlying malformation as the source, rather than attributing the hemorrhage to a presumed primary process without this additional evaluation.

Hemorrhagic Transformation of Ischemic Stroke

Both arterial ischemic stroke and cerebral sinovenous thrombosis, discussed earlier in this chapter, can show secondary hemorrhagic transformation, meaning a hemorrhagic finding identified on imaging may represent a secondary complication of an underlying ischemic process rather than a primary hemorrhagic event; recognizing an accompanying pattern of restricted diffusion or venous filling defect alongside the hemorrhage, rather than evaluating the hemorrhagic component in isolation, is essential to correctly identifying the underlying primary process and therefore the correct management pathway.

Vitamin K Deficiency Bleeding

Vitamin K deficiency bleeding, historically termed hemorrhagic disease of the newborn, remains an important and largely preventable cause of severe, often multifocal intracranial hemorrhage in infants who did not receive standard vitamin K prophylaxis at birth, typically presenting in the classic late form between two and twelve weeks of age; eliciting a specific history regarding vitamin K prophylaxis at birth is a necessary component of the evaluation for any young infant presenting with unexplained intracranial hemorrhage, since this specific, correctable etiology carries distinct implications both for acute management, including vitamin K administration, and for public health counseling regarding future children in the same family.

Exclusively breastfed infants who did not receive vitamin K prophylaxis at birth carry a particularly elevated risk for late vitamin K deficiency bleeding, since breast milk contains comparatively low vitamin K content relative to formula, and this specific risk factor combination, exclusive breastfeeding plus declined or missed prophylaxis, should be actively sought in the history of any infant in the classic two-to-twelve-week presentation window; families who decline vitamin K prophylaxis at birth, for reasons that may include general vaccine or intervention hesitancy, benefit from clear, nonjudgmental counseling regarding this specific, well-documented risk at the time of the initial declination, ideally before a hemorrhagic presentation makes the conversation considerably more difficult.

Alloimmune and Autoimmune Thrombocytopenia

Fetal and neonatal alloimmune thrombocytopenia, in which maternal antibodies directed against a paternally inherited platelet antigen cross the placenta and cause severe fetal or neonatal thrombocytopenia, is a specific and clinically important cause of intracranial hemorrhage, at times occurring antenatally and identified only on the newborn imaging obtained because of a low platelet count discovered at delivery; a severely low platelet count in an otherwise well-appearing term infant, particularly with a hemorrhage pattern not otherwise explained by the categories discussed above, should prompt platelet antigen typing of both parents, since a confirmed diagnosis carries direct implications for the management of future pregnancies in the same family, including antenatal maternal treatment in a subsequent pregnancy.

Structured Approach to the Undifferentiated Hemorrhagic Neonate

Given the breadth of the differential developed across this section, a structured, stepwise approach to the neonate presenting with unexplained intracranial hemorrhage is more reliable than an unstructured search through the full differential simultaneously: gestational age and delivery history first orient the reader toward germinal matrix hemorrhage, discussed in Chapter 5, or birth-related extra-axial hemorrhage, discussed in the next section; the hemorrhage distribution relative to arterial territories and venous drainage patterns then directs consideration toward the arterial and venous processes discussed earlier in this chapter; and only once these more common categories have been actively considered and reasonably excluded does the reader proceed to the less common causes, coagulopathy, vascular malformation, and the specific hematologic entities, discussed in this section, applying the coagulation screen, vascular imaging, and platelet evaluation as targeted next steps rather than as an undirected initial panel.

Genetic Causes of Cerebral Small Vessel Fragility

A small but clinically important subset of nontraumatic neonatal hemorrhage reflects an underlying genetic disorder of cerebral small vessel structural integrity, most notably COL4A1-related disorders, in which a mutation affecting type IV collagen, a key structural component of the cerebral small vessel basement membrane, predisposes to intracranial hemorrhage that can occur antenatally, perinatally, or later in infancy, at times with a recognizable, sometimes bilateral, porencephalic or schizencephalic residual pattern on follow-up imaging; a family history of unexplained stroke, hemorrhage, or antenatal ventriculomegaly in a parent or sibling should prompt consideration of this specific genetic diagnosis, since a confirmed diagnosis carries direct implications for genetic counseling and for surveillance of other organ systems, including renal and ophthalmologic involvement, associated with the same underlying collagen disorder.

Choroid Plexus Hemorrhage as an Isolated Finding

Hemorrhage confined to the choroid plexus, distinct from the germinal matrix hemorrhage discussed in Chapter 5, is an occasionally identified, usually incidental finding on neonatal cranial ultrasound that, in isolation without ventricular extension or associated parenchymal injury, generally carries a favorable prognosis and requires no specific intervention beyond routine follow-up imaging to confirm resolution; distinguishing choroid plexus hemorrhage from the more clinically significant germinal matrix and intraventricular hemorrhage discussed previously depends on correct anatomic localization of the hemorrhage source, a distinction that benefits from careful attention to the specific ultrasound anatomy taught in Chapter 1.

The Value of a Multidisciplinary Hematology-Neurology Case Conference

Given the genuine complexity and breadth of the differential diagnosis developed throughout this section, a case that remains diagnostically unresolved after the initial structured evaluation benefits from formal multidisciplinary case review incorporating child neurology, pediatric hematology, and neuroradiology perspectives together, rather than sequential, siloed consultation; this collaborative review format, increasingly adopted at tertiary centers managing a significant volume of complex neonatal hemorrhage cases, allows each specialty's diagnostic reasoning to inform the others in real time and has been associated, in institutional experience, with more efficient resolution of genuinely ambiguous cases than a purely sequential consultation model.

Maternal Substance Use as a Contributing Factor

Maternal use of certain substances during pregnancy, including cocaine and other vasoactive agents, has been associated with an increased risk of both antenatal and perinatal cerebrovascular events in the infant, including both ischemic and hemorrhagic presentations, through a proposed mechanism involving acute vasoconstriction and resulting vascular injury or rupture; a maternal substance use history, obtained sensitively and nonjudgmentally as part of the standard perinatal history, is a relevant component of the etiologic evaluation for unexplained neonatal hemorrhage or stroke, and its identification does not exclude, and indeed may coexist with, the other etiologic categories discussed throughout this chapter.

Extracorporeal Membrane Oxygenation as a Distinct Risk Context

Infants supported on extracorporeal membrane oxygenation, most commonly for severe cardiac or respiratory failure, carry a substantially elevated risk of both ischemic and hemorrhagic intracranial injury related to the combination of systemic anticoagulation required to maintain the extracorporeal circuit, altered cerebral hemodynamics from the cannulation and flow pattern itself, and the severity of the underlying critical illness necessitating this level of support; neuroimaging surveillance, typically with cranial ultrasound performed at defined intervals throughout the extracorporeal membrane oxygenation course given the impracticality of MRI in this critically supported population, is a standard component of monitoring for this specific, high-risk group, and findings are interpreted with awareness of this distinct risk context rather than applying the general population framework developed elsewhere in this chapter without modification.

Figure 6.2: Differential Considerations in Nontraumatic Neonatal Hemorrhage

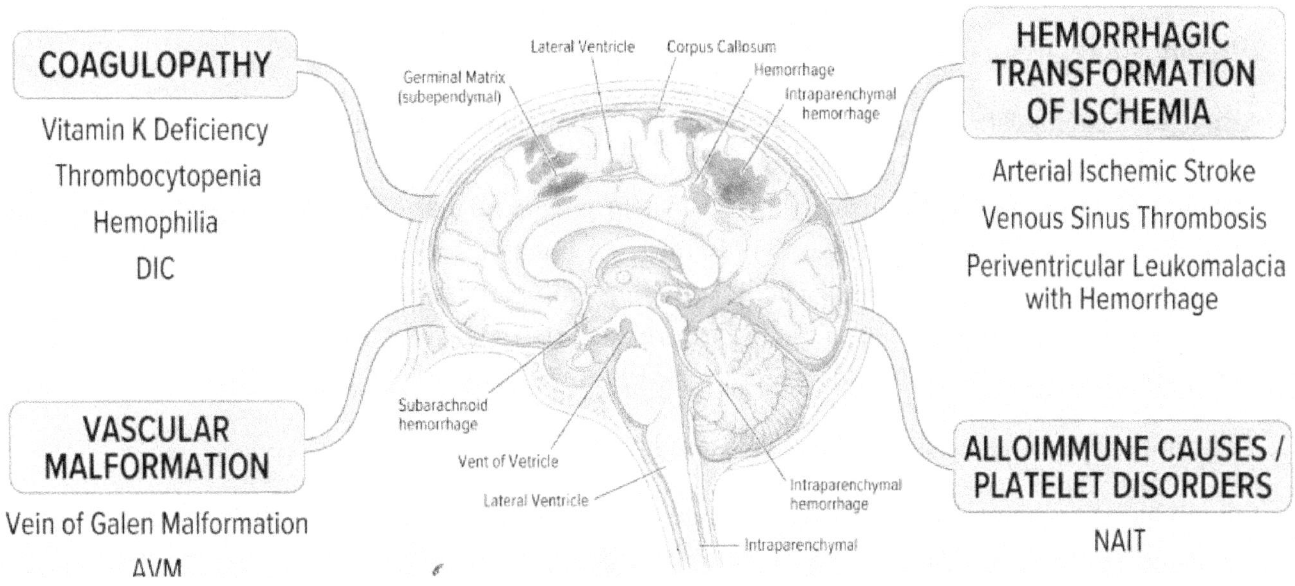

Distinguishing Birth-Related From Pathologic Hemorrhage

A final, clinically and at times legally significant discrimination task addressed in this chapter is distinguishing expected, self-limited hemorrhage related to the normal birth process from hemorrhage that warrants further evaluation for an underlying pathologic or, in specific circumstances, abusive etiology. This discrimination task draws directly on the distribution, timing, and clinical-correlation reasoning structure introduced earlier in this chapter, applied here to a decision with particularly high stakes for the family and, at times, for the broader child protection and legal systems that may become involved.

Extra-Axial Hemorrhage From the Normal Birth Process

Small, thin, layering subdural hemorrhage, most commonly identified over the cerebral convexities or along the tentorium, is a well-documented, common finding on imaging obtained in the first days of life even in entirely asymptomatic, uncomplicated vaginal deliveries, reflecting the normal mechanical forces of transit through the birth canal on the neonatal dural venous structures; this finding, when small, asymptomatic, and without associated parenchymal injury or mass effect, typically resolves spontaneously over the following weeks without specific intervention and should not, by itself, prompt an evaluation for abuse or an underlying bleeding disorder in an otherwise well-appearing, appropriately timed presentation.

Subdural Hemorrhage: Birth-Related Versus Abusive

Distinguishing birth-related subdural hemorrhage from the subdural hemorrhage associated with abusive head trauma, discussed fully in Chapter 19, depends on a constellation of features rather than any single discriminating characteristic: birth-related hemorrhage is typically thin, symmetric or mildly asymmetric, without significant mass effect, identified in the immediate newborn period, and resolving on short-interval follow-up imaging when obtained, while abusive hemorrhage more often presents beyond the immediate newborn period with an inconsistent or absent explanatory history, may be of mixed or varying age suggesting more than one bleeding event, and is more likely to be accompanied by parenchymal injury, retinal hemorrhage, or other suspicious findings developed fully in Chapter 19.

Imaging Features That Discriminate Mechanism

Beyond the clinical timing and history considerations above, specific imaging features assist in this discrimination: susceptibility-weighted or gradient-echo sequences characterizing the specific blood product composition of the hemorrhage can help estimate hemorrhage age, and the identification of hemorrhage of clearly differing ages within the same imaging study, one component appearing acute and another appearing subacute or chronic, is a finding with particular significance for the abuse evaluation discussed in Chapter 19, since a single birth-related bleeding event would not be expected to produce blood products of convincingly different ages on a single study.

Timing and Dating of Hemorrhage on Imaging

Applying the same signal-based hemorrhage-timing framework introduced in Chapter 4 for hypoxic-ischemic injury, hyperacute and acute hemorrhage shows a specific evolving pattern of signal characteristics on T1, T2, and susceptibility-weighted sequences that shifts in a predictable, well-characterized sequence over the following days to weeks as hemoglobin degradation products evolve; while this dating is subject to genuine biological variability and should never be presented to a family or in a legal context as more precise than the underlying science actually supports, a general estimate of hemorrhage age, integrated with the full clinical history, is a legitimate and often clinically important component of the evaluation, developed further in the legal and documentation discussion in Chapter 1 and revisited specifically for trauma in Chapter 19.

Documentation and Communication Considerations

Given the potential legal and child-protection significance of the birth-related-versus-pathologic distinction developed throughout this section, precise, objective, descriptive language in the imaging report, consistent with the documentation discipline established in Chapter 1, is essential whenever this distinction is genuinely at issue; the report should describe the specific imaging findings, including hemorrhage location, extent, and estimated age range, without overstating the certainty of any causal conclusion the imaging alone cannot definitively establish, reserving the integrated causal determination for the multidisciplinary evaluation process rather than a single imaging report acting in isolation.

Instrumented Delivery and Its Specific Hemorrhage Associations

Delivery involving vacuum or forceps assistance carries a somewhat elevated, though still generally low, risk of specific hemorrhage patterns beyond the routine thin subdural collection discussed above, including subgaleal hemorrhage, a potentially serious extracranial collection distinct from the intracranial findings otherwise addressed in this chapter, and, less commonly, a more substantial intracranial hemorrhage associated with a documented difficult extraction; eliciting the specific delivery history, including the type and duration of any instrumentation used, is therefore a necessary component of correctly attributing a hemorrhagic finding identified on early newborn imaging to the birth process itself, and this history should be actively sought rather than assumed absent when not spontaneously offered.

The Role of Repeat Imaging in Resolving Diagnostic Uncertainty

When the initial imaging findings and available clinical history leave genuine uncertainty regarding whether a subdural hemorrhage reflects the normal birth process or warrants further evaluation, short-interval follow-up imaging, typically within one to two weeks, showing the expected resolution or substantial diminution characteristic of birth-related hemorrhage, provides confirmatory reassurance that a single initial study cannot offer; conversely, a hemorrhage that fails to resolve as expected, or that is found to have increased in extent or developed a new component on the follow-up study, shifts the evaluation meaningfully toward the pathologic or abusive categories discussed in Chapter 19, illustrating that the discrimination task addressed in this section is not always fully resolvable from a single time-point study alone.

The Role of Retinal Examination in the Broader Evaluation

Although retinal hemorrhage evaluation itself belongs to the ophthalmologic examination rather than to neuroimaging directly, its presence or absence is frequently discussed alongside the imaging findings when the birth-related-versus-pathologic distinction is genuinely in question, since certain patterns of retinal hemorrhage carry specific associations with abusive trauma developed fully in Chapter 19, while a different, more limited pattern can be seen following even an uncomplicated vaginal delivery; a clinician evaluating a neonate with subdural hemorrhage of uncertain significance should coordinate ophthalmologic examination as a standard, complementary component of the evaluation, understanding that the neuroimaging findings and the retinal findings are interpreted together as part of a single integrated clinical picture, not as independent data points.

Cesarean Delivery and the Expectation of Minimal Extra-Axial Hemorrhage

Because the mechanical forces responsible for the common, benign birth-related subdural hemorrhage discussed throughout this section arise substantially from transit through the vaginal birth canal, an infant delivered by cesarean section, particularly a scheduled cesarean performed before labor has begun, would not be expected to show even the small, thin, physiologic subdural collections seen after vaginal delivery, and the identification of subdural hemorrhage in this specific delivery context accordingly carries somewhat greater diagnostic weight toward an alternative explanation than an identical finding would carry following vaginal delivery; eliciting the specific mode of delivery, and whether labor occurred before a cesarean was performed, is therefore a directly relevant detail the reader should routinely incorporate into the birth-related-versus-pathologic assessment developed in this section.

Practical Guidance for the Ordering Clinician

When a birth-related subdural hemorrhage is identified as an incidental finding on imaging obtained for an unrelated indication in an asymptomatic, appropriately timed newborn, the practical guidance developed throughout this section supports clear, reassuring family communication regarding the expected benign course, explicit documentation of the specific features supporting this determination, and a straightforward, brief follow-up plan rather than an extensive additional evaluation; reserving the more extensive evaluation pathway, including coagulation screening, vascular imaging, and multidisciplinary child protection team involvement, for the cases genuinely departing from the expected birth-related pattern described in this section keeps the response proportionate to the actual clinical concern raised by each specific presentation.

Twin and higher-order multiple pregnancies carry a modestly elevated risk of several of the vascular and hemorrhagic complications discussed throughout this chapter, reflecting factors including a higher rate of preterm delivery, a higher incidence of growth discordance and placental vascular anastomoses in monochorionic pregnancies, and, in the specific setting of twin-twin transfusion syndrome, a recognized risk of both ischemic and hemorrhagic cerebral injury in one or both twins related to the acute hemodynamic shifts this condition produces; a clinician evaluating a twin or higher-order multiple with a vascular or hemorrhagic finding should routinely inquire about chorionicity and any complicated antenatal course specific to the multiple pregnancy, since this history meaningfully informs the etiologic evaluation beyond the singleton-focused risk factors emphasized elsewhere in this chapter.

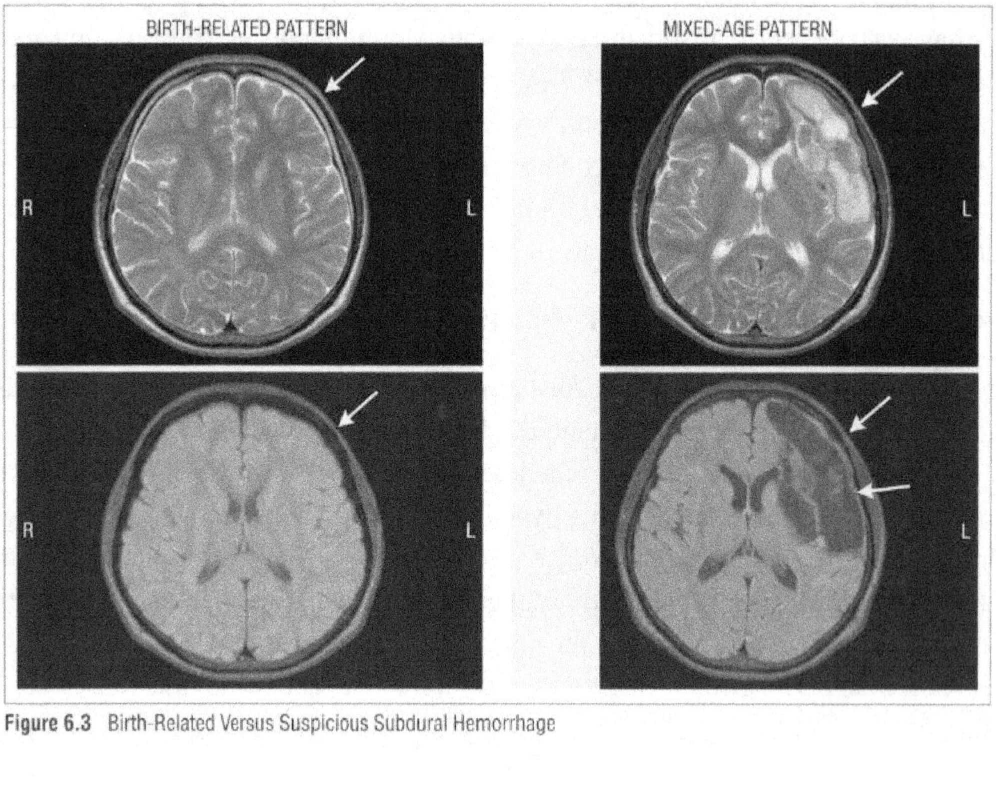

Figure 6.3 Birth-Related Versus Suspicious Subdural Hemorrhage

Case Presentation: Perinatal Stroke Presenting With Seizures

A term neonate develops focal right-sided clonic seizure activity on day two of life, with an otherwise unremarkable delivery history and a normal general neurologic examination between seizures. Applying the reasoning developed in this chapter, perinatal arterial ischemic stroke is considered as a leading diagnosis specifically because of the focal seizure semiology without an accompanying focal examination finding, a pattern this chapter identifies as classic for this diagnosis. Diffusion-weighted MRI confirms restricted diffusion within the left middle cerebral artery cortical and lenticulostriate distribution. Placental pathology, retained and available for review, demonstrates fetal vascular malperfusion, providing a probable etiologic explanation. The family is counseled regarding the expected right-sided motor risk given the specific vascular territory involved, and early motor-focused developmental surveillance is initiated, illustrating how the specific territory identified on imaging directly informs the targeted counseling and follow-up plan.

Case Presentation: Cerebral Sinovenous Thrombosis in a Dehydrated Infant

A six-week-old presents with poor feeding, lethargy, and a bulging fontanelle following several days of viral gastroenteritis with resulting dehydration. Brain MRI demonstrates a hemorrhagic parenchymal lesion in an atypical distribution not matching a recognized arterial territory, prompting the venous-phase imaging discussed in this chapter's rhythm feature, which confirms superior sagittal and transverse sinus thrombosis with associated venous infarction. Pediatric hematology is consulted regarding anticoagulation, and the dehydration, identified as the most likely precipitating risk factor, is corrected. Follow-up venous imaging at six weeks demonstrates partial recanalization, and the family is counseled that ongoing developmental surveillance, rather than the newborn imaging alone, will characterize the eventual functional outcome, consistent with the longitudinal counseling framework developed throughout this book.

Case Presentation: Distinguishing Birth-Related Hemorrhage From a Broader Concern

A term neonate delivered via uncomplicated vaginal delivery undergoes brain MRI on day two of life for evaluation of mild, transient jitteriness, and the study incidentally identifies a thin, symmetric subdural collection layering along the posterior falx and tentorium, without mass effect, parenchymal signal abnormality, or retinal hemorrhage on the coordinated ophthalmologic examination obtained per this chapter's guidance. Applying the reasoning developed in this chapter's final section, the care team recognizes this appearance, timing, and symmetry as fully consistent with the normal birth process rather than a pathologic or abusive etiology, documents this determination explicitly with the specific supporting features noted in the report, and recommends no further evaluation beyond routine well-child follow-up, explaining to the family that this is a common, expected, self-resolving finding rather than a cause for concern. This case illustrates the proportionate, reassuring communication this chapter advocates when the full constellation of findings clearly fits the expected birth-related pattern.

Synthesis: A Shared Reasoning Structure Across Vascular and Hemorrhagic Presentations

The four categories addressed in this chapter, arterial stroke, venous thrombosis, the broader nontraumatic hemorrhage differential, and the birth-related-versus-pathologic distinction, share a common underlying reasoning structure that the reader should carry forward: distribution pattern relative to known arterial territories or venous drainage first orients the diagnosis, timing and evolution on serial or single-timepoint imaging next refines it, and correlation with the full clinical, laboratory, and family history ultimately resolves genuine ambiguity that imaging distribution and timing alone cannot settle. This same three-part reasoning structure, distribution, timing, and clinical correlation, recurs throughout the vascular and hemorrhagic chapters later in this book and is worth recognizing explicitly as a durable, transferable diagnostic habit rather than a set of unrelated facts specific to the neonatal and infant population addressed in this chapter alone.

Beyond the clinical reasoning itself, families navigating a perinatal stroke or hemorrhage diagnosis benefit from connection with condition-specific family support organizations and, where available, hospital-based peer support programs, resources that complement but do not substitute for the direct clinical counseling this chapter has emphasized throughout; providing this information at the time of diagnosis, alongside the specific medical explanation and follow-up plan, acknowledges that a family's need for support extends beyond the purely clinical information this chapter has focused on and into the practical, emotional experience of parenting a child through an uncertain early diagnosis and an extended period of developmental surveillance.

THE CLINICAL-IMAGING CROSSWALK SYSTEM — Vascular and Hemorrhagic Recognition in the Neonate and Infant

---

Crossing 1 Recap: A hemorrhagic parenchymal lesion that does not conform to a recognizable arterial territory should prompt dedicated venous-phase imaging to evaluate for cerebral sinovenous thrombosis before being attributed to a primary arterial or hemorrhagic process.

Chapter Anchor: Neonatal seizures with a normal examination point toward arterial stroke; a nonterritorial hemorrhagic lesion points toward venous thrombosis; and a hemorrhage's timing, distribution, and blood-product age, not its presence alone, determine whether it reflects the normal birth process or warrants further evaluation.

Summary and Key Concepts

Perinatal arterial ischemic stroke classically presents with seizures rather than a focal deficit, shows a marked left middle cerebral artery predilection, and is increasingly linked to placental pathology as an underrecognized etiologic contributor.

Cerebral sinovenous thrombosis requires dedicated venous-phase imaging for diagnosis, produces infarction that does not respect arterial territories, and frequently shows hemorrhagic transformation reflecting venous hypertension.

Nontraumatic hemorrhage beyond germinal matrix hemorrhage includes coagulopathy, underlying vascular malformation, hemorrhagic transformation of ischemic stroke, vitamin K deficiency bleeding, and alloimmune thrombocytopenia, each with a distinct evaluation pathway.

Small, thin, symmetric subdural hemorrhage in the immediate newborn period is a common, usually self-limited finding related to the normal birth process, distinguished from abusive hemorrhage by timing, symmetry, blood-product age uniformity, and the presence or absence of accompanying suspicious findings.

Imaging reports addressing the birth-related-versus-pathologic hemorrhage distinction should use precise, objective, descriptive language, reserving integrated causal determination for the multidisciplinary evaluation process rather than the imaging report in isolation.

CHAPTER 7: MALFORMATIONS OF CORTICAL DEVELOPMENT

Learning Objectives

1. Distinguish neuronal migration disorders from cortical organization disorders based on their distinct embryologic timing and imaging appearance, applying the proliferation-migration-organization framework developed throughout this chapter.
2. Recognize the characteristic imaging features of lissencephaly, subcortical band heterotopia, periventricular nodular heterotopia, polymicrogyria, schizencephaly, and focal cortical dysplasia.
3. Apply an appropriate genetic testing strategy and describe the counseling implications, including recurrence risk and mosaicism, for a confirmed malformation of cortical development.
4. Construct a systematic, imaging-guided differential diagnosis for an abnormal cortical surface, distinguishing malformation from acquired injury.

Neuronal Migration Disorders

Malformations of cortical development arise from disruption at one of several sequential embryologic stages, proliferation, migration, and organization, and this chapter follows that same sequence, beginning with the disorders of neuronal migration, in which cells are generated in appropriate numbers but fail to reach their correct cortical destination. Recognizing which stage of this sequence was disrupted, rather than pattern-matching an imaging appearance against memorized examples alone, is the central diagnostic skill this chapter develops, and it is a skill that transfers directly to the genetic testing strategy and counseling framework addressed later in the chapter.

Normal Neuronal Migration and Its Disruption

Following proliferation within the germinal matrix discussed in Chapter 2, postmitotic neurons migrate outward along radial glial fibers to populate the developing cortex in a characteristic inside-out sequence, in which the earliest-generated neurons occupy the deepest cortical layers and each subsequent wave of migrating neurons passes through the earlier-formed layers to occupy a progressively more superficial position; disruption of this process, whether from a genetic defect in the migration machinery itself, an intercurrent vascular or infectious insult during the migration window, or a defect in the radial glial scaffold the migrating neurons depend upon, produces the spectrum of migration disorders addressed in this section, each reflecting a distinct point and mechanism of disruption within this otherwise tightly choreographed process.

Lissencephaly Spectrum

Lissencephaly, literally smooth brain, represents the most severe end of the migration disorder spectrum, in which neuronal migration arrests early and diffusely, producing a cortex that is either completely smooth, termed agyria, or shows only a few broad, shallow gyri, termed pachygyria, with an abnormally thickened cortical mantle and a smooth gray-white matter junction lacking the normal interdigitating pattern; applying the gyration timeline established in Chapter 2, a cortical surface appearance consistent with lissencephaly is diagnostic only when it persists beyond the gestational age at which normal gyration would be expected to have occurred, underscoring again why gestational or corrected age must accompany every image before a surface finding is characterized as malformation rather than normal immaturity.

Subcortical Band Heterotopia

Subcortical band heterotopia, sometimes termed double cortex syndrome, represents a milder point on the same underlying migration-disorder spectrum as lissencephaly, in which a band of gray-matter-signal neurons becomes arrested partway through their migration, forming a discrete, symmetric or asymmetric band of heterotopic gray matter separated from the overlying, otherwise relatively normal cortex by a thin rim of white matter; this entity is of particular genetic interest because it and classic lissencephaly frequently arise from mutations in the same gene, most notably DCX, with the specific phenotype, band heterotopia versus lissencephaly, differing systematically by sex due to the gene's X-linked inheritance pattern, discussed further in this chapter's genetics section.

Periventricular Nodular Heterotopia

Periventricular nodular heterotopia represents migration arrest at its earliest possible point, in which clusters of neurons fail to leave the periventricular germinal zone at all, forming discrete, gray-matter-signal nodules that line the ventricular margin and remain in continuity with, or immediately adjacent to, the ependymal surface; this entity is frequently bilateral and can be either an isolated finding, at times identified incidentally in an individual presenting with epilepsy in later childhood or even adulthood, discussed further in Chapter 11, or a component of a broader genetic syndrome, most classically FLNA-related periventricular nodular heterotopia, again with an X-linked inheritance pattern carrying specific counseling implications developed later in this chapter.

Cobblestone Malformation and Overmigration

At the opposite mechanistic extreme from the migration-arrest disorders discussed above, cobblestone malformation results from neuronal overmigration, in which a defect in the pial limiting membrane allows migrating neurons to breach the normal cortical boundary and continue migrating past their intended destination into the overlying leptomeninges, producing an irregular, nodular cortical surface with a disorganized, poorly laminated underlying cortex; this malformation is frequently associated with congenital muscular dystrophy syndromes, most notably Walker-Warburg syndrome and related dystroglycanopathies, reflecting the shared molecular pathway connecting the glycosylation defects underlying these muscular dystrophies to the pial basement membrane integrity required for normal migration termination.

Imaging Protocol Considerations for Suspected Migration Disorders

Detecting the subtler migration disorders discussed in this section, particularly periventricular nodular heterotopia and subcortical band heterotopia, requires thin-section, high-resolution T1 and T2 imaging with attention to gray-white matter signal differentiation throughout the full ventricular margin, applying the dedicated, question-specific protocol discipline established in Chapter 1; a standard-resolution, non-dedicated brain protocol can miss subtle nodular heterotopia, particularly small or unilateral nodules, underscoring why a clinical suspicion for a migration disorder, most often arising from a seizure presentation as discussed in Chapter 11, should prompt explicit protocol customization rather than reliance on a routine study.

Tubulinopathies and Other Cytoskeletal Migration Disorders

Beyond the classic lissencephaly and heterotopia genes discussed above, a broader group of disorders affecting the tubulin cytoskeleton and its associated motor proteins, collectively termed tubulinopathies, produce a diverse and often complex combined phenotype incorporating cortical malformation alongside basal ganglia dysmorphism, corpus callosum anomaly, and brainstem or cerebellar hypoplasia, reflecting the broad role these cytoskeletal proteins play in neuronal migration and axon guidance across multiple brain regions simultaneously rather than the cortex in isolation; recognizing this combined, multiregional pattern on imaging, rather than a cortical finding alone, should prompt consideration of a tubulinopathy specifically and inform the choice of a broader gene panel rather than isolated testing of the classic lissencephaly genes alone.

Unilateral and Asymmetric Migration Disorders

While the migration disorders discussed in this section are frequently bilateral, particularly the classic genetic forms, a unilateral or markedly asymmetric presentation should prompt consideration of somatic mosaicism confined to one hemisphere, rather than a germline mutation affecting both hemispheres equally, a distinction addressed further in this chapter's genetics section; a unilateral migration disorder also raises hemimegalencephaly, discussed later in this chapter under organization disorders given its combined migration and organization features, as an important differential consideration, particularly when the affected hemisphere shows associated volume enlargement rather than the normal or reduced volume more typical of an isolated unilateral migration disorder without accompanying overgrowth.

Developmental and Cognitive Outcome by Malformation Severity

Neurodevelopmental outcome across the migration disorder spectrum correlates broadly, though imperfectly, with malformation severity and extent: classic lissencephaly is typically associated with profound, global developmental impairment, subcortical band heterotopia with a wide range of outcome from mild learning difficulty to significant intellectual disability depending on band thickness and location, and isolated, small-volume periventricular nodular heterotopia with outcomes that can range from normal cognitive function with isolated epilepsy to more significant global impairment when the heterotopia is extensive or bilateral; this outcome variability underscores why individualized, imaging-extent-based counseling, rather than a single generic prognosis applied uniformly across the entire migration disorder category, best serves each family.

Eliciting a Structured Family History Before Imaging Review

Before reviewing imaging in a child referred for a suspected migration disorder, obtaining a structured family history spanning at least three generations, specifically screening for a history of epilepsy, intellectual disability, unexplained pregnancy loss, or a known genetic diagnosis in any relative, provides context that can meaningfully change how a subtle imaging finding is interpreted; a family history positive for a similar phenotype in a maternal uncle, for example, immediately raises the X-linked inheritance pattern discussed elsewhere in this chapter as a leading consideration before genetic testing results are even available, allowing more efficient, targeted counseling from the earliest point of contact with the family.

Why CT Has a Minimal Role in Malformation Characterization

Applying the modality-selection reasoning established in Chapters 1 and 3, CT plays only a minimal role in characterizing the malformations of cortical development discussed throughout this chapter, since the gray-white matter contrast resolution CT provides is substantially inferior to MRI for the fine cortical and subcortical detail these malformations require, and the radiation exposure CT entails is difficult to justify for an indication MRI addresses far more effectively; the narrow exception is the specific circumstance in which CT-based detection of periventricular or other calcification, as in the congenital cytomegalovirus pattern discussed earlier in this chapter, adds diagnostically useful information beyond what MRI alone provides, a circumstance addressed with the same targeted, question-specific reasoning applied to every modality decision throughout this book.

Ongoing Research Directions in Migration Disorder Genetics

The genetic landscape underlying neuronal migration disorders continues to expand as sequencing technology and functional genomic studies identify additional causative genes and refine genotype-phenotype correlations for previously identified ones, meaning the specific testing strategies and gene panels described in this chapter should be understood as reflecting current practice rather than a permanently fixed catalog; clinicians managing this population benefit from periodic engagement with updated clinical genetics resources and literature, both to ensure testing strategies remain current and to recognize when a research study or expanded testing program might offer additional diagnostic opportunity for a family whose child's malformation remains genetically unexplained after standard clinical testing.

Microcephaly and Megalencephaly as Associated Findings

Head size, whether abnormally small or abnormally large, frequently accompanies the migration disorders discussed in this section and itself carries diagnostic weight: microcephaly accompanying a migration disorder points toward a primary proliferation defect affecting the total neuronal number generated before migration even begins, a mechanistically distinct process from the migration defects that are this section's primary focus, while macrocephaly or megalencephaly, as seen in hemimegalencephaly discussed later in this chapter, points toward an overgrowth mechanism; documenting head circumference and its growth trajectory alongside the structural imaging findings, rather than treating them as separate, unrelated data points, therefore contributes directly to narrowing the underlying mechanistic category and the corresponding genetic testing strategy.

Figure 7.1: Spectrum of Neuronal Migration Disorders

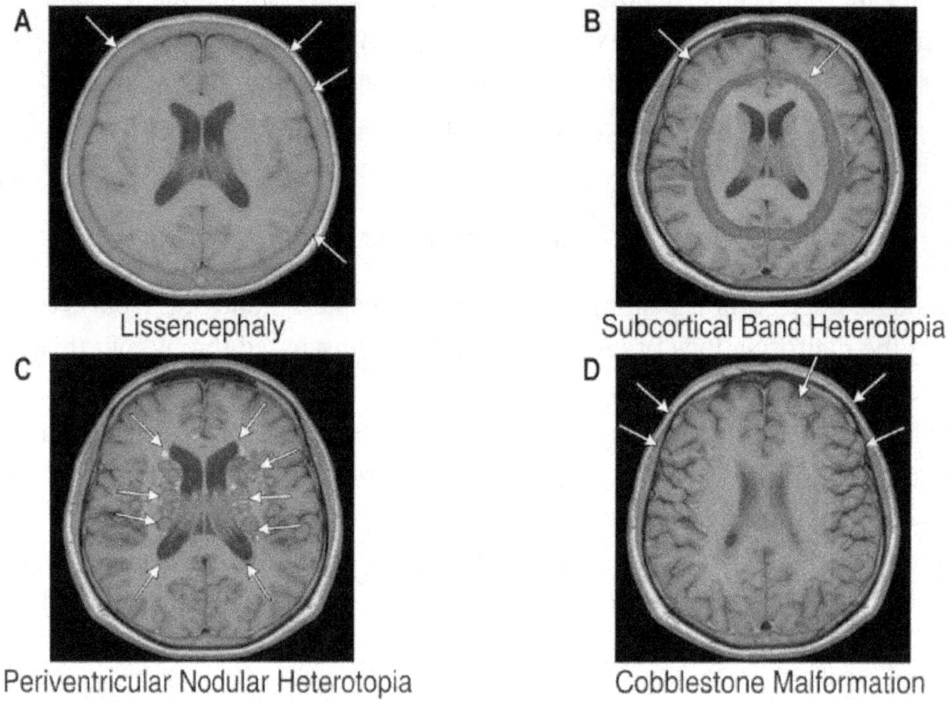

Cortical Organization Disorders

Cortical organization disorders arise from disruption occurring after neurons have reached their correct cortical location, affecting instead the subsequent processes of cortical lamination and synaptic organization, and consequently present with a distinct imaging appearance from the migration disorders discussed above, most often an irregular, abnormally infolded cortical surface rather than the smooth or heterotopic gray matter appearance characteristic of migration arrest.

Polymicrogyria: Pathophysiology and Patterns

Polymicrogyria, characterized by an excessive number of small, abnormally formed gyri separated by shallow, sometimes fused sulci, producing an irregular, bumpy cortical surface with an abnormally thin, poorly laminated cortical mantle, arises from a heterogeneous group of causes acting during the late migration and early organization period, including genetic mutations, intrauterine infection, particularly cytomegalovirus discussed in Chapter 15, and vascular insufficiency; the specific distribution, whether perisylvian, a particularly common and clinically distinctive pattern associated with a recognizable oromotor and language phenotype, bilateral and symmetric, or unilateral, provides diagnostic clues to the underlying cause and is described precisely and consistently in the imaging report given its direct relevance to both the genetic and infectious evaluations this section develops.

Schizencephaly

Schizencephaly, a full-thickness cleft extending from the pial surface to the ventricular ependyma and lined by dysplastic, polymicrogyric gray matter along its margins, is classified as closed-lip, in which the cleft walls are apposed, or open-lip, in which the cleft walls are separated by a cerebrospinal-fluid-filled space communicating between the subarachnoid space and the ventricle; distinguishing schizencephaly from an acquired porencephalic cyst, discussed further in the differential diagnosis section of this chapter, depends critically on the presence of dysplastic, gray-matter-signal, polymicrogyric tissue specifically lining the schizencephalic cleft, a feature absent in a porencephalic cyst, whose margins are instead lined by gliotic white matter reflecting its acquired, destructive rather than malformative origin.

Focal Cortical Dysplasia

Focal cortical dysplasia, a localized region of abnormal cortical lamination frequently associated with an overlying blurred gray-white matter junction, abnormal cortical thickening, and, in the more severe subtypes, a characteristic transmantle signal abnormality extending from the cortical surface toward the ventricle, is among the most common causes of focal, medically refractory epilepsy in children, discussed fully in Chapter 11, and is frequently subtle enough on conventional-resolution imaging to be entirely missed without the dedicated, high-resolution epilepsy protocol discussed in Chapter 1; recognizing this specific detection challenge is essential given the direct surgical implications of an accurately localized, resectable focal cortical dysplasia in an appropriately selected surgical candidate.

Hemimegalencephaly

Hemimegalencephaly, a malformation in which an entire cerebral hemisphere is enlarged and shows a disorganized combination of migration and organization abnormalities, including areas of pachygyria, polymicrogyria, and abnormal white matter signal, typically presents with severe, often medically refractory epilepsy and hemiparesis in the newborn or young infant period, and functional hemispherectomy is considered in appropriately selected, severely affected infants when medical management fails, a decision that depends heavily on the detailed anatomic and functional characterization imaging provides; the marked asymmetry characteristic of this malformation is usually apparent even on a standard, non-dedicated study, distinguishing it from the more subtle focal cortical dysplasia discussed above.

Distinguishing Organization From Migration Disorders on Imaging

Although the migration and organization disorders discussed in this chapter arise from disruption at sequential, related embryologic stages and can coexist within the same malformation spectrum, particularly in the more severe combined presentations, the practical imaging distinction rests on the character of the abnormal cortex itself: migration disorders typically show either a smooth, unmigrated cortical surface (lissencephaly) or discrete, displaced gray-matter-signal heterotopia at an abnormal location, while organization disorders show an irregular, excessively infolded cortical surface (polymicrogyria) or a full-thickness cleft (schizencephaly) with the neurons having reached a location at or near the cortical surface, however disorganized their subsequent lamination. Holding this distinction in mind directly informs both the differential diagnosis and, as developed in the next section, the genetic testing strategy pursued.

Associated Extracranial and Systemic Findings

Several cortical organization disorders, particularly the cobblestone malformation spectrum discussed earlier in this chapter and specific genetic polymicrogyria syndromes, are associated with recognizable extracranial findings, including characteristic facial dysmorphism, ocular abnormalities such as retinal detachment or cataract in the dystroglycanopathies, and systemic muscular involvement; a thorough physical examination, coordinated with genetics and, where indicated, ophthalmology and neuromuscular specialists, complements the imaging findings and can meaningfully narrow the differential diagnosis and guide genetic testing strategy before results are available, consistent with the multidisciplinary evaluation principle emphasized throughout this book.

Perisylvian Polymicrogyria and Its Distinctive Clinical Phenotype

Bilateral perisylvian polymicrogyria, one of the more clinically recognizable polymicrogyria distributions, is associated with a characteristic clinical syndrome of pseudobulbar palsy, including impaired volitional control of facial, tongue, and pharyngeal musculature despite intact or even exaggerated involuntary movement of the same muscles, producing significant feeding and speech difficulty that emerges as a prominent clinical concern independent of, though often accompanying, the seizures more commonly associated with polymicrogyria generally; recognizing this specific oromotor phenotype in a child with an unexplained feeding or speech disorder should prompt consideration of the perisylvian distribution specifically, directing attention to that anatomic region during image review even when the referral indication did not explicitly raise a structural concern.

Polymicrogyria Related to Congenital Cytomegalovirus Infection

Congenital cytomegalovirus infection, discussed fully in Chapter 15, is a well-recognized acquired cause of polymicrogyria, producing a pattern that can closely resemble genetic polymicrogyria on imaging alone but is distinguished by accompanying findings more specific to congenital infection, including periventricular calcification, ventriculomegaly, and, at times, cerebellar hypoplasia; a polymicrogyria finding without a clearly established genetic cause should prompt active consideration of congenital cytomegalovirus testing, since this specific, acquired etiology carries an entirely different recurrence risk and counseling framework than the genetic causes discussed elsewhere in this chapter, illustrating why the imaging-guided differential developed in this chapter's final section explicitly incorporates acquired as well as genetic causes.

Surgical Considerations for Focal Cortical Dysplasia

When focal cortical dysplasia is identified as the likely epileptogenic lesion in a child with medically refractory focal epilepsy, precise anatomic characterization on high-resolution imaging directly informs surgical planning, including the feasibility and expected extent of resection relative to eloquent cortex; postoperative pathologic confirmation and subtyping of the resected tissue, correlated back against the preoperative imaging appearance, both validates the imaging-based localization and refines the reader's ongoing calibration of which imaging features most reliably predict a given pathologic subtype, a feedback loop that exemplifies the case-based, imaging-to-outcome correlation this book's Anchor Section, introduced in Chapter 1, is specifically designed to consolidate across the full range of conditions this book addresses.

Hemispherotomy Versus Hemispherectomy in Hemimegalencephaly

Surgical management of severe, medically refractory hemimegalencephaly has evolved from anatomic hemispherectomy, complete removal of the affected hemisphere, toward functional hemispherotomy techniques that disconnect the affected hemisphere's connections to the rest of the brain while leaving the tissue itself largely in place, an evolution driven by a meaningfully lower complication rate, particularly related to delayed hemosiderosis, with the disconnection-based approach while achieving comparable seizure control; preoperative imaging characterization of the malformation's full anatomic extent, including confirmation that the contralateral hemisphere is genuinely unaffected, remains essential to either surgical approach and is a further example of imaging directly shaping a major, irreversible management decision.

Integrating Structural Imaging With Functional Localization

Beyond the structural characterization emphasized throughout this chapter, functional imaging and mapping techniques, including functional MRI for language and motor localization and, where available, magnetoencephalography, are increasingly incorporated into the presurgical evaluation of a child with a cortical organization disorder being considered for epilepsy surgery, providing complementary information regarding which specific structurally abnormal regions also carry critical functional significance that must be preserved or, conversely, confirming that a structurally abnormal region is functionally silent and can be more safely resected; this multimodal integration, structural malformation characterization paired with functional mapping, exemplifies the broader principle that a single imaging modality, however detailed, rarely provides the complete picture needed for a major surgical decision.

Bilateral Versus Unilateral Distribution and Its Surgical Implications

The distinction between a unilateral and a bilateral organization disorder carries direct surgical significance beyond its diagnostic and genetic implications discussed elsewhere in this chapter: a unilateral malformation, such as unilateral polymicrogyria or hemimegalencephaly, is a substantially more favorable surgical candidate than a bilateral, symmetric malformation, since resective or disconnective surgery targeting one hemisphere is not a viable option when both hemispheres are comparably affected;

this distinction should be explicitly and confidently established on imaging before a family's expectations regarding potential surgical treatment are shaped, since incorrectly characterizing a subtly bilateral malformation as unilateral, or the reverse, can lead to inappropriate surgical counseling in either direction.

Documenting Malformation Extent for Longitudinal Comparison

Given that many children with a cortical organization disorder undergo repeated imaging over years of clinical follow-up, establishing a clear, reproducible baseline description of malformation extent and location at the time of initial diagnosis, ideally referencing standardized anatomic landmarks rather than only qualitative impression, meaningfully improves the reliability of subsequent comparison, particularly when serial studies are interpreted by different readers over time; this documentation discipline, consistent with the structured reporting principles emphasized throughout this book, is especially valuable for the organization disorders discussed in this section given their frequently irregular, less easily quantified anatomic boundaries relative to the more discrete findings characteristic of the migration disorders discussed earlier in this chapter.

Finding	Migration Disorder Example	Organization Disorder Example	Key Distinguishing Feature
Cortical surface	Smooth (lissencephaly)	Irregular, excessively infolded (polymicrogyria)	Surface texture and gyral pattern
Gray matter location	Displaced/heterotopic (PVNH)	At or near normal location, disorganized lamination	Position relative to expected cortical mantle
Full-thickness defect	Not characteristic	Present (schizencephaly)	Cleft lined by dysplastic gray matter vs. gliotic white matter

THE CLINICAL-IMAGING CROSSWALK SYSTEM — Schizencephaly Versus Porencephalic Cyst

The Crossing: A six-month-old with hemiparesis undergoes brain MRI, which shows a full-thickness cleft extending from the cortical surface to the ventricle, and the referring team asks whether this represents a congenital malformation or an acquired injury.

Presentation Signature: An infant or child with a full-thickness cerebral cleft identified on imaging, with a clinical history that may or may not include a documented perinatal vascular event.

Imaging Correlate: The cleft margins are carefully assessed for lining tissue: dysplastic, gray-matter-signal, polymicrogyric tissue lining the cleft confirms schizencephaly, a true malformation, while gliotic, T2-hyperintense white matter lining the cleft, without polymicrogyric gray matter, indicates an acquired porencephalic cyst, most often related to a perinatal vascular insult such as the arterial ischemic stroke discussed in Chapter 6.

Trap Logic: Both entities can appear grossly similar as a cerebrospinal-fluid-containing cleft on a cursory review, and failing to specifically characterize the cleft lining risks conflating a true malformation, with its associated genetic and counseling implications, with an acquired, generally non-heritable vascular injury.

Crossing Anchor: A full-thickness cerebral cleft is characterized as schizencephaly only when its margins are lined by dysplastic, polymicrogyric gray matter; gliotic white matter lining instead indicates an acquired porencephalic cyst, a distinction with direct genetic-counseling and recurrence-risk implications.

Genetic Correlates and Counseling Implications

Confirming a genetic diagnosis underlying a malformation of cortical development carries direct implications for recurrence risk counseling, prognosis, and, at times, targeted management, and this section develops the genetic testing strategy and counseling framework that follows a confirmed or suspected malformation identified using the imaging reasoning developed above.

Genetic Testing Strategies for Malformations of Cortical Development

The specific imaging phenotype identified substantially narrows the genetic testing strategy pursued: lissencephaly and subcortical band heterotopia prompt targeted testing of the well-characterized causative genes, most notably LIS1 and DCX, before proceeding to a broader gene panel or exome sequencing if targeted testing is unrevealing; periventricular nodular heterotopia prompts FLNA testing, particularly in a female proband given the X-linked inheritance pattern discussed below; and polymicrogyria, given its more heterogeneous genetic and acquired etiologic landscape, typically prompts a broader diagnostic approach incorporating both congenital infection screening and a genetic panel or exome sequencing, since a single, universally applicable genetic test does not exist for this more etiologically diverse malformation category.

Inheritance Patterns and Recurrence Risk

Inheritance patterns among malformations of cortical development vary substantially by specific genetic diagnosis and carry direct, differing recurrence risk implications: LIS1-related lissencephaly is most commonly caused by a de novo mutation, carrying a low recurrence risk for future pregnancies except in the specific circumstance of parental germline mosaicism discussed below; DCX-related disorders follow X-linked inheritance, in which an affected male typically presents with the more severe lissencephaly phenotype while a carrier female presents with the milder subcortical band heterotopia phenotype, a sex-differential pattern with direct implications for interpreting a family history and for counseling regarding future pregnancies of each sex; and FLNA-related periventricular nodular heterotopia follows a similar X-linked pattern, in which the condition is typically lethal in affected males in utero, explaining the strong female predominance observed clinically in this specific diagnosis.

Mosaicism and Its Implications for Recurrence Risk Counseling

Somatic and germline mosaicism, in which a causative genetic variant is present in only a subset of an individual's cells, including, critically, a parent's germline cells without being detectable in that parent's standard peripheral blood genetic testing, represents an important and sometimes underappreciated source of recurrence risk that a negative parental blood test does not fully exclude; families counseled regarding recurrence risk should understand this residual, generally low but nonzero risk related to potential parental germline mosaicism, particularly relevant when a second affected pregnancy occurs despite an apparently negative parental genetic evaluation, a scenario that should prompt reconsideration of mosaicism as an explanation rather than an assumption of coincidence or laboratory error.

Prenatal Diagnosis and Its Role in Subsequent Pregnancies

Once a specific causative genetic variant has been identified in an affected child, targeted prenatal testing, whether through chorionic villus sampling, amniocentesis, or, where clinically appropriate and available, preimplantation genetic testing in the context of assisted reproduction, becomes available for a subsequent pregnancy, allowing the family concrete, actionable information rather than the more limited reassurance a general population recurrence risk estimate alone can offer; this option is presented as part of comprehensive genetic counseling, with full acknowledgment that the decision whether to pursue prenatal testing, and what to do with the resulting information, belongs entirely to the family and is never presented as an expectation or obligation.

The Multidisciplinary Genetic Counseling Team

Comprehensive counseling following a confirmed or suspected genetic malformation of cortical development is most effectively delivered through coordinated involvement of child neurology, clinical genetics, and a genetic counselor, each contributing a distinct but complementary perspective: child neurology addresses the functional and prognostic implications of the specific structural finding, clinical genetics interprets the molecular result and its broader syndromic implications, and the genetic counselor addresses inheritance pattern, recurrence risk, and the practical and emotional process of family decision-making; coordinating this team from the point of diagnosis, rather than a series of sequential, uncoordinated referrals, provides the family with a more coherent, less fragmented counseling experience.

Variants of Uncertain Significance and Communicating Genetic Uncertainty

Genetic testing not uncommonly identifies a variant of uncertain significance, a genetic change whose relationship to the child's clinical presentation cannot be confidently established at the time of testing, either because the specific variant has not been previously characterized in the medical literature or because available functional or population data remain insufficient to classify it as clearly pathogenic or clearly benign; communicating this genuine uncertainty honestly to the family, distinguishing it clearly from both a confirmed diagnosis and a fully negative result, while explaining that reclassification may occur as scientific understanding advances and that periodic re-review of the variant's classification is a reasonable component of ongoing care, applies the same honest, proportionate, uncertainty-acknowledging communication principle this book has emphasized throughout, now extended specifically into the genetic counseling context and documented clearly in the chart for any future clinician reviewing the case.

Syndromic Associations Beyond the Isolated Cortical Finding

A malformation of cortical development is, in a meaningful subset of cases, one component of a broader genetic syndrome affecting multiple organ systems rather than an isolated central nervous system finding, and recognizing this possibility shapes the evaluation beyond neuroimaging and targeted neurogenetic testing alone; a dysmorphology evaluation, screening for congenital heart disease, renal anomaly, or skeletal involvement where the specific imaging phenotype or family history raises this possibility, and coordinated genetics involvement from the outset help ensure that a syndromic diagnosis is not missed by a narrowly neurology-focused evaluation that stops once the structural brain finding itself has been characterized.

Psychosocial Support Throughout the Genetic Evaluation Process

The genetic evaluation process for a malformation of cortical development frequently extends over weeks to months, spanning initial testing, results interpretation, and, at times, subsequent reflex or confirmatory testing, and this extended timeline itself represents a source of ongoing family stress distinct from the initial diagnostic imaging finding; proactively offering psychosocial support resources, including social work involvement and connection with condition-specific family support organizations where one exists for the specific diagnosis identified, throughout this extended evaluation period, rather than only at the point of a final confirmed diagnosis, supports the family through the genuine uncertainty this evaluation timeline necessarily involves.

Practical Access Considerations for Genetic Testing

Access to comprehensive genetic testing, including exome sequencing and specialized panels, varies meaningfully by insurance coverage, geographic access to a genetics specialist, and, at an institutional level, by whether a given center has an established clinical genetics program capable of ordering, interpreting, and counseling around these tests; a clinician practicing in a setting with more limited direct genetics access can still initiate the imaging-guided, phenotype-directed testing strategy developed in this chapter through general pediatric or telehealth genetics consultation, and coordinating early referral, rather than deferring the genetics conversation until every other evaluation avenue has been exhausted, reduces the overall time to a diagnosis that, as this chapter has emphasized throughout, carries direct implications for family counseling and future reproductive planning.

Transitioning Genetic Counseling Into Adulthood

As a child with a confirmed malformation of cortical development approaches adulthood, the genetic counseling conversation appropriately shifts to directly engage the young adult, rather than the parents alone, particularly regarding the young adult's own future reproductive decisions and recurrence risk for their own children, a conversation that carries a different character and requires different consent considerations than the counseling initially provided to parents at the time of the child's diagnosis; coordinating this transition with adult genetics services as part of the broader adult care transition process, discussed further in the transition-of-care literature beyond this book's pediatric focus, ensures continuity of this genetic counseling relationship rather than a gap in care at the pediatric-to-adult transition point.

Reanalysis of Prior Negative Genetic Testing

Genetic testing technology and the underlying gene-disease association knowledge base both advance continuously, meaning a comprehensive genetic evaluation that returned negative or inconclusive several years earlier may yield a diagnosis if reanalyzed against current knowledge and current testing technology, since genes newly associated with a given malformation phenotype are regularly added to the medical literature after an individual child's initial evaluation; periodically revisiting a previously unexplained malformation of cortical development for reanalysis or repeat testing, particularly at a meaningful clinical transition point such as entry into adolescence or when family planning becomes an active consideration, reflects the same evolving-evidence principle this book applies broadly and can convert a previously uncertain family into one with the concrete, actionable information a confirmed diagnosis provides.

Supporting Siblings Through the Diagnostic and Counseling Process

Unaffected siblings of a child with a confirmed genetic malformation of cortical development frequently have their own questions and concerns, both regarding their own carrier or recurrence risk status where relevant to the specific inheritance pattern discussed earlier in this chapter, and regarding the family's overall experience of the diagnosis, and age-appropriate inclusion of siblings in at least some portion of the genetic counseling process, calibrated to the sibling's developmental stage and the family's preferences, is increasingly recognized as a valuable component of whole-family support rather than a conversation reserved exclusively for parents and the affected child. A designated family point of contact, most often the genetic counselor introduced earlier in this section, who remains consistent across the multiple specialist visits this evaluation typically requires, further reduces the fragmentation a family might otherwise experience navigating child neurology, clinical genetics, and, where relevant, additional subspecialty involvement across an extended diagnostic timeline.

Figure 7.2: Inheritance Patterns Across Common Migration Disorder Genes

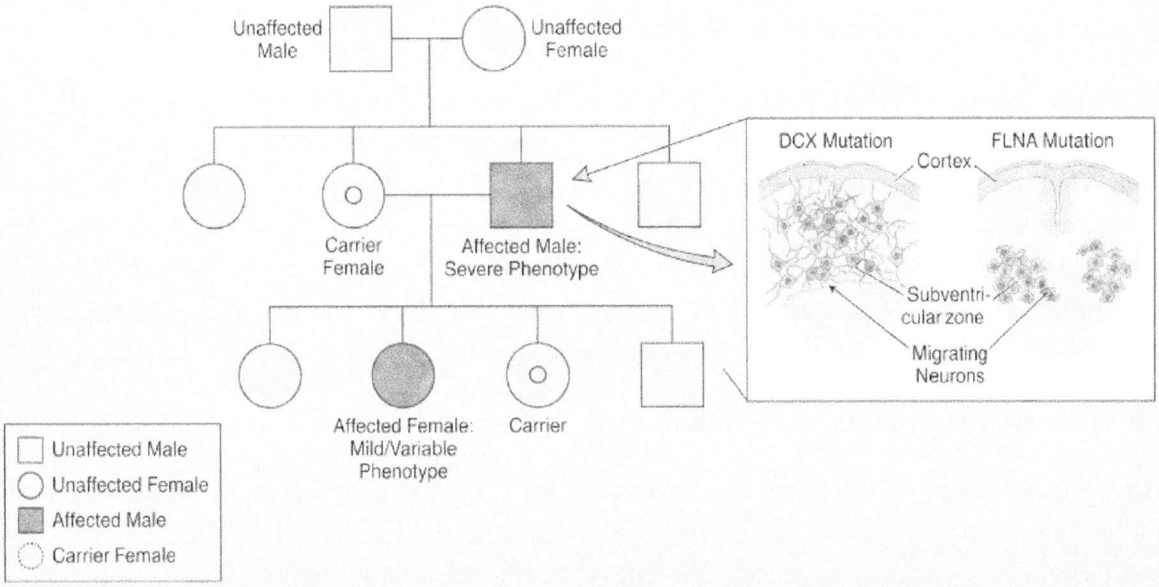

Imaging-Guided Differential Diagnosis

This closing section consolidates the reasoning developed throughout the chapter into a systematic, imaging-guided approach to the child presenting with an abnormal cortical finding, whether identified prenatally, in the setting of new seizures, or as an incidental finding on a study obtained for an unrelated indication.

Systematic Approach to an Abnormal Cortical Surface

Evaluating an abnormal cortical finding systematically begins with characterizing the surface itself, smooth and thickened, irregularly infolded, or interrupted by a full-thickness cleft, then localizing any displaced or heterotopic gray matter, then assessing distribution, diffuse, focal, unilateral, or bilateral, and finally correlating the imaging pattern against the specific gene-phenotype associations developed in the previous section to focus the subsequent genetic evaluation; applying this structured sequence, rather than pattern-matching against memorized examples alone, equips the reader to reason through malformation presentations this chapter has not specifically named.

Differentiating Malformation From Acquired Injury

Beyond the schizencephaly-versus-porencephaly distinction developed in this chapter's Crossing, the broader task of distinguishing a true developmental malformation from acquired, destructive injury, including the hypoxic-ischemic injury discussed in Chapter 4 and the infectious injury discussed in Chapter 15, depends on similar principles: a malformation typically shows dysplastic, abnormally organized but present tissue, while acquired injury shows tissue loss and gliosis, an absence rather than a disorganization of the expected structure; timing also assists this distinction, since a malformation is present from the earliest imaging performed, while acquired injury shows an evolving appearance over serial studies consistent with the injury timeline principles developed in Chapter 4.

Timing of Imaging in a Suspected Malformation

Because the normal cortical surface itself is still actively maturing throughout gestation and into the early postnatal period, as established in Chapter 2, imaging obtained too early in this maturation window can either falsely suggest a malformation that is, in fact, normal immaturity for gestational age, or, conversely, fail to fully characterize a genuine subtle malformation not yet distinguishable from the still-immature normal surface; when clinical suspicion for a malformation exists but early imaging is equivocal, scheduled follow-up imaging once cortical maturation has more fully progressed, rather than a single early determination, provides the more reliable diagnostic answer.

The Role of Fetal MRI in Prenatal Detection

Fetal MRI, introduced in Chapter 1, plays an increasingly important role in the prenatal detection and characterization of malformations of cortical development, particularly the more severe migration disorders discussed earlier in this chapter, allowing earlier family counseling and delivery planning than postnatal detection alone would permit; the same gestational-age-specific interpretive caution developed throughout this chapter and in Chapter 2 applies with particular force to fetal imaging, given the still-evolving normal fetal cortical surface, and a suspected prenatal finding is, per the reasoning developed in Chapter 2, generally confirmed or revised on postnatal imaging once the confounding effect of ongoing fetal cortical maturation and fetal motion has been eliminated.

Structured Reporting for Cortical Malformations

Applying the structured reporting principles established in Chapter 1, a report describing a suspected or confirmed malformation of cortical development should explicitly characterize the surface finding, the specific distribution, and, where relevant, the presence or absence of associated findings such as heterotopic gray matter, ventricular abnormality, or corpus callosum anomaly, using precise, standardized terminology consistent with this chapter rather than informal or ambiguous descriptive language; a precisely worded report both facilitates the genetics referral and testing strategy discussed earlier in this chapter and improves the reliability of comparison should follow-up imaging later be obtained.

Coordinating Imaging Findings With the Epilepsy Evaluation

Because many malformations of cortical development, particularly focal cortical dysplasia and periventricular nodular heterotopia, present clinically through epilepsy rather than through an antenatal or early infancy structural concern, close coordination between the structural imaging interpretation developed throughout this chapter and the electroencephalographic and, where presurgical evaluation is pursued, functional localization discussed in Chapter 11 is essential; a malformation identified on imaging that does not correlate with the electroencephalographic seizure onset zone should prompt reconsideration of whether the imaging finding is truly the epileptogenic lesion or an incidental, non-epileptogenic malformation, a distinction with direct implications for surgical candidacy that neither the imaging nor the electroencephalographic data alone can fully resolve.

Synthesis: A Shared Embryologic Framework

The malformations addressed across this chapter, however diverse their individual imaging appearances and genetic causes, share a single organizing embryologic framework: proliferation determines neuronal number, migration determines neuronal location, and organization determines neuronal lamination and connectivity, and a malformation's imaging phenotype reflects, with reasonable fidelity, which of these sequential processes was disrupted and at what point in gestation that disruption occurred. Holding this embryologic framework in mind, rather than treating each named malformation as an isolated pattern to memorize independently, is the durable diagnostic skill this chapter is built to transmit, equipping the reader to reason through an unfamiliar or atypical cortical finding using the same underlying logic applied throughout this chapter to the specific, named entities discussed. This same framework recurs, adapted to each region's specific embryology, throughout the remaining congenital and developmental chapters of this book.

When to Seek Subspecialty Neuroradiology Consultation

Given the genuine subtlety of several entities discussed in this chapter, particularly focal cortical dysplasia and mild forms of polymicrogyria, a general pediatric radiologist or a clinician reviewing images without dedicated pediatric neuroradiology training should maintain a low threshold for subspecialty neuroradiology consultation whenever a malformation of cortical development is suspected clinically but not clearly confirmed on initial review, or whenever the specific subtype and distribution require precise characterization to guide the genetic testing and, where relevant, epilepsy surgical evaluation discussed throughout this chapter; this consultation threshold reflects the same principle developed in Chapter 1 regarding when advanced or second-opinion imaging expertise meaningfully changes management, applied here specifically to the malformation spectrum this chapter addresses.

The Value of Longitudinal Imaging Review Across a Child's Care

A child with a confirmed malformation of cortical development frequently accumulates multiple imaging studies over years of follow-up, obtained for evolving clinical questions including seizure characterization, presurgical planning, and routine developmental surveillance, and reviewing this full longitudinal imaging history together, rather than evaluating each new study in isolation without reference to prior studies, allows the interpreting clinician to confirm expected stability of the malformation itself, a finding that supports the malformative rather than progressive nature of the process, while also tracking any evolving, superimposed findings such as new epileptogenic changes or treatment-related effects that a single-study review would not reliably capture.

Translating Imaging Findings Into Educational and Developmental Planning

Beyond the medical and genetic implications developed throughout this chapter, the specific malformation identified and its anticipated functional impact should be translated into concrete guidance for educational planning, informing the specific developmental and educational support services a family pursues through early intervention and, later, school-based individualized education programming; a clinician who can describe not only the diagnosis but its anticipated functional implications, expected motor, language, or cognitive impact in terms an educational team can act upon, meaningfully bridges the gap between a precise radiologic and genetic diagnosis and the practical, day-to-day supports that determine a child's actual functional trajectory.

The Anchor Section at the close of this book indexes every Crossing introduced across this chapter and every other chapter in this book, dual-indexed by presenting complaint and by imaging pattern, allowing a reader who encounters an unfamiliar cortical finding to navigate directly to the relevant reasoning developed here regardless of whether their starting point is a clinical presentation, such as new seizures, or an imaging finding, such as an unexpected cortical surface irregularity noted on a study obtained for an unrelated indication.

Taken together, the four sections of this chapter model a complete diagnostic arc for malformations of cortical development: recognizing the specific migration or organization pattern on imaging, correlating that pattern with an embryologically grounded mechanism, pursuing a phenotype-directed genetic evaluation with honest counseling regarding inheritance and uncertainty, and distinguishing malformation confidently from its acquired mimics. A reader who internalizes this arc, rather than a fixed catalog of named entities, is equipped to manage the full range of cortical malformation presentations this specialty encounters, including those this chapter has not had space to name individually.

Case Presentation: Lissencephaly Identified on Fetal MRI

A fetal MRI obtained at thirty weeks gestation for evaluation of ventriculomegaly identified on routine obstetric ultrasound demonstrates a smooth cortical surface without the expected secondary sulcation pattern for gestational age, applying the timeline established in Chapter 2, raising concern for lissencephaly. Postnatal MRI at term confirms diffuse agyria with a markedly thickened cortical mantle, consistent with classic lissencephaly. Targeted LIS1 genetic testing identifies a de novo pathogenic variant. The multidisciplinary genetic counseling team, applying the reasoning developed in this chapter, explains to the family both the anticipated severe neurodevelopmental prognosis associated with this diagnosis and the low recurrence risk for future pregnancies given the de novo, non-inherited nature of the identified variant, while acknowledging the small residual possibility of parental germline mosaicism, and offers referral for prenatal testing should the family pursue a future pregnancy.

Case Presentation: Perisylvian Polymicrogyria With Congenital Cytomegalovirus

A newborn with microcephaly and a failed newborn hearing screen undergoes brain MRI demonstrating bilateral perisylvian polymicrogyria alongside scattered periventricular calcification and mild ventriculomegaly. Applying the reasoning developed in this chapter, the combination of polymicrogyria with periventricular calcification prompts congenital cytomegalovirus testing rather than proceeding directly to a genetic malformation panel, and urine cytomegalovirus polymerase chain reaction testing, obtained within the first three weeks of life to distinguish congenital from perinatally acquired infection, confirms the diagnosis. The family is counseled that this specific, acquired etiology carries a low recurrence risk for future pregnancies, in contrast to the genetic malformations discussed elsewhere in this chapter, and antiviral treatment and hearing surveillance are coordinated with pediatric infectious disease and audiology, illustrating how correctly distinguishing an acquired from a genetic cause fundamentally redirects both the counseling conversation and the broader management pathway.

Case Presentation: Incidental Periventricular Nodular Heterotopia in a Teenager With New Seizures

A fifteen-year-old girl with a new-onset focal seizure undergoes the dedicated epilepsy protocol MRI discussed in Chapter 1, which identifies bilateral periventricular nodules along the lateral ventricular margins, consistent with periventricular nodular heterotopia, an incidental long-standing malformation now presenting clinically for the first time in adolescence. Applying the reasoning developed in this chapter, the care team pursues targeted FLNA genetic testing given the classic imaging appearance and the patient's sex, and a pathogenic variant is identified. The family is counseled regarding the X-linked inheritance pattern, including the specific implication that a future male sibling carrying the same variant would face a substantially more severe, often prenatally lethal presentation, information that directly shapes the family's subsequent reproductive counseling discussion, illustrating how a malformation identified in adolescence still carries the same genetic and family-planning implications developed throughout this chapter for a malformation identified in infancy. This case, together with the two preceding it, spans the full range of clinical entry points this chapter has addressed: prenatal detection, newborn presentation, and delayed adolescent recognition, each converging on the same structured, embryology-anchored reasoning process this chapter has developed throughout.

THE CLINICAL-IMAGING CROSSWALK SYSTEM — Cortical Malformation Recognition and Genetic Correlation

---

Crossing 1 Recap: A full-thickness cerebral cleft is characterized as schizencephaly only when lined by dysplastic, polymicrogyric gray matter; gliotic white matter lining instead indicates an acquired porencephalic cyst.

Chapter Anchor: Malformations of cortical development are distinguished by the embryologic stage disrupted, migration versus organization, and the specific imaging phenotype directly narrows the genetic testing strategy and the recurrence-risk counseling that follows.

Summary and Key Concepts

Neuronal migration disorders span a spectrum from lissencephaly (early, diffuse arrest) through subcortical band heterotopia and periventricular nodular heterotopia (partial or minimal migration) to cobblestone malformation (overmigration through a defective pial membrane), with tubulinopathies producing a distinct, multiregional combined phenotype.

Cortical organization disorders, including polymicrogyria, schizencephaly, focal cortical dysplasia, and hemimegalencephaly, arise after neurons reach the cortex and are distinguished from migration disorders by an irregular rather than smooth or heterotopic cortical appearance.

Genetic testing strategy is guided directly by imaging phenotype; DCX and FLNA-related disorders follow X-linked inheritance with sex-differential phenotypes, and parental germline mosaicism can produce recurrence despite negative parental blood testing.

A systematic, stepwise approach, characterizing surface appearance, gray matter location, distribution, and correlation with gene-phenotype associations, distinguishes malformation from acquired injury and equips the reader to reason through presentations beyond those specifically named in this chapter.

Fetal MRI increasingly enables prenatal detection but requires the same gestational-age-specific interpretive caution as postnatal imaging; structured, precise reporting terminology facilitates both genetic testing strategy and future comparison imaging, and counseling appropriately extends from parents through sibling support and, eventually, transition to adult genetic services.

CHAPTER 8: CONGENITAL MALFORMATIONS OF THE BRAIN, SKULL, AND POSTERIOR FOSSA

Learning Objectives

1. Classify holoprosencephaly by severity and recognize its associated midline, facial, and endocrine anomalies, and describe the related septo-optic dysplasia spectrum.
2. Distinguish true posterior fossa malformation from the benign variants introduced in Chapter 2, and recognize the molar tooth sign of Joubert syndrome.
3. Differentiate single-suture from syndromic craniosynostosis and describe the corresponding surgical planning and multidisciplinary team implications.
4. Distinguish complete from partial corpus callosum agenesis and identify the associated findings that shift a case from isolated to syndromic.

Holoprosencephaly and Midline Malformations

Holoprosencephaly, a failure of the forebrain to cleave into distinct cerebral hemispheres, represents one of the earliest and most severe disruptions of normal brain development addressed in this book, arising from a defect in prosencephalic cleavage occurring between approximately the fourth and sixth gestational week; its recognition and classification anchor this chapter's broader discussion of midline malformation. The reasoning developed across this section, severity grading, genetic evaluation, associated facial and endocrine findings, and coordinated multidisciplinary counseling, establishes the template this chapter applies again, adapted to each region's specific anatomy, in the posterior fossa, craniosynostosis, and corpus callosum sections that follow.

Holoprosencephaly Spectrum and Classification

Holoprosencephaly is classified into four grades of decreasing severity based on the degree of hemispheric cleavage achieved: alobar holoprosencephaly, the most severe form, shows a single, undivided monoventricular cavity with fused thalami and absent interhemispheric fissure and falx; semilobar holoprosencephaly shows partial posterior hemispheric separation with fusion persisting anteriorly; lobar holoprosencephaly shows nearly complete hemispheric separation with more subtle fusion typically confined to the frontal horns and a variably absent septum pellucidum; and middle interhemispheric variant, a distinct pattern rather than a simple continuation of this severity gradient, shows fusion confined to the posterior frontal and parietal regions with relative sparing of the frontal and occipital poles.

This grading carries direct prognostic weight, since severity of hemispheric cleavage failure correlates broadly with severity of subsequent neurodevelopmental impairment, though even the mildest, lobar form carries a substantial burden of developmental and endocrine morbidity, discussed further below, meaning no point on this spectrum should be characterized to a family as a mild or reassuring finding in absolute terms. The middle interhemispheric variant in particular is worth distinguishing explicitly from the graded alobar-to-lobar continuum, since its posterior-predominant fusion pattern reflects a distinct embryologic mechanism rather than simply an intermediate point of severity between semilobar and lobar forms.

Genetic and Teratogenic Causes

Holoprosencephaly arises from a heterogeneous group of causes including chromosomal abnormality, most classically trisomy 13, single-gene mutations affecting the sonic hedgehog signaling pathway central to normal prosencephalic cleavage, and teratogenic exposure, most notably maternal diabetes and, less commonly encountered in contemporary practice, certain maternal medication or toxin exposures during the critical early gestational window; a comprehensive genetic evaluation, including chromosomal microarray and, where indicated, targeted sequencing of the sonic hedgehog pathway genes, is pursued for essentially every confirmed case, since the specific genetic or chromosomal cause directly shapes both prognosis and recurrence risk counseling. Maternal diabetes screening, specifically, is worth eliciting explicitly as part of the etiologic evaluation even when a genetic cause is ultimately identified, since a teratogenic and a genetic contributor are not mutually exclusive and both may warrant distinct counseling and, for maternal diabetes, distinct implications for the management of a future pregnancy.

Associated Facial Anomalies

Holoprosencephaly is frequently, though not universally, accompanied by a recognizable spectrum of midline facial anomalies whose severity correlates broadly with the severity of the underlying brain malformation, reflecting the shared embryologic signaling pathways governing both forebrain cleavage and midline facial development; these findings range from cyclopia and proboscis in the most severe alobar cases to a single central incisor or mild hypotelorism in the mildest lobar cases, and the presence of any of these facial findings on prenatal ultrasound should prompt dedicated fetal brain MRI specifically to evaluate for an underlying holoprosencephaly, applying the same fetal MRI indication reasoning developed in Chapter 1.

Septo-Optic Dysplasia

Septo-optic dysplasia, classically defined by the combination of optic nerve hypoplasia, absence of the septum pellucidum, and pituitary hypoplasia with associated hormonal deficiency, occupies a related but mechanistically distinct position from the holoprosencephaly spectrum discussed above, and the two entities show sufficient imaging and clinical overlap, particularly regarding septal absence and pituitary dysfunction, that septo-optic dysplasia is sometimes conceptualized as occupying the milder end of a broader midline malformation continuum rather than as an entirely separate entity; only a minority of children with septo-optic dysplasia demonstrate all three classic components, and a diagnosis is confirmed when at least two of the three are present.

Absence of the Septum Pellucidum as a Diagnostic Clue

Absence of the septum pellucidum, a finding shared across lobar holoprosencephaly, septo-optic dysplasia, and, less commonly, isolated as an incidental finding without other associated malformation, should prompt a systematic evaluation for each of these possibilities rather than being dismissed as a nonspecific finding; this evaluation includes dedicated assessment of the optic nerves and chiasm, careful pituitary gland characterization, and close attention to the degree of hemispheric cleavage, since the presence or absence of accompanying hemispheric fusion is the key feature distinguishing lobar holoprosencephaly from isolated septal absence or septo-optic dysplasia without hemispheric involvement.

Pituitary and Hypothalamic Involvement

Pituitary and hypothalamic dysfunction, ranging from an ectopic posterior pituitary bright spot to frank pituitary hypoplasia and panhypopituitarism, accompanies the midline malformation spectrum discussed throughout this section with sufficient frequency that endocrinology evaluation, including assessment for growth hormone, thyroid, adrenal, and, in the newborn period specifically, diabetes insipidus risk, is a standard, coordinated component of the initial evaluation for any confirmed holoprosencephaly or septo-optic dysplasia diagnosis, applied proactively rather than reactively once a specific endocrine symptom has already emerged clinically.

Imaging Protocol for Suspected Midline Malformation

Evaluating suspected holoprosencephaly or a related midline malformation requires dedicated attention to midline structures on thin-section imaging, including the septum pellucidum, corpus callosum, optic apparatus, and pituitary gland, applying the same protocol-customization principle developed in Chapter 1; dedicated, thin-section pituitary imaging with and without contrast is specifically added to the standard brain protocol whenever septo-optic dysplasia or a related midline malformation is a leading consideration, since the standard brain protocol alone frequently provides insufficient detail to fully characterize the pituitary gland and optic apparatus.

Ocular and Visual Evaluation in Septo-Optic Dysplasia

Because optic nerve hypoplasia is a defining component of septo-optic dysplasia and can range from subtle to profound, coordinated ophthalmologic evaluation, including formal visual acuity assessment and direct funduscopic examination of the optic discs for the characteristic small, pale appearance of a hypoplastic nerve, is a necessary complement to the neuroimaging findings discussed in this section; a normal-appearing optic nerve on imaging does not fully exclude clinically significant hypoplasia, since the imaging assessment of nerve caliber, while useful, is less sensitive than direct ophthalmologic examination for detecting the full range of severity this finding can present with.

Prenatal Counseling for a Suspected Diagnosis of Holoprosencephaly

When holoprosencephaly is suspected on prenatal ultrasound and confirmed on fetal MRI, prenatal counseling led jointly by maternal-fetal medicine and pediatric neurology addresses the specific severity classification identified, its associated facial and endocrine implications, and the full range of options available to the family, including continuation of the pregnancy with coordinated postnatal care planning or, where legally and personally applicable, pregnancy termination, presented without directive pressure toward either path and with explicit acknowledgment of the genuine severity spectrum this diagnosis spans, from a stillbirth-associated alobar presentation to a lobar presentation compatible with longer-term survival and variable functional outcome.

Seizure Risk and Management Across the Holoprosencephaly Spectrum

Seizures occur with substantial frequency across the holoprosencephaly severity spectrum, related both to the underlying cortical malformation itself and, in the more severe alobar and semilobar forms, to the markedly abnormal overall brain architecture, and antiseizure medication selection in this population requires particular attention to the atypical anatomy when interpreting electroencephalographic localization, since the fused, malformed hemispheres do not permit the standard lateralization assumptions applied in a structurally normal brain; coordinated epilepsy management, applying the electroencephalographic correlation principles introduced in Chapter 4 and developed fully in Chapter 11, is a standard component of ongoing neurologic care for this population.

Temperature Dysregulation and Autonomic Involvement

Beyond the endocrine dysfunction discussed earlier in this section, hypothalamic involvement in the more severe forms of holoprosencephaly can produce autonomic dysregulation, including impaired temperature control and altered sleep-wake regulation, findings that carry direct practical implications for caregivers managing an affected child at home and are worth explicitly anticipating and discussing during the initial multidisciplinary counseling conversation rather than allowing a family to discover them without warning as the child grows; coordinated guidance from neurology and endocrinology regarding practical home management of these autonomic features, including environmental temperature control strategies, supports the family's day-to-day caregiving in a way that a purely diagnostic, imaging-focused conversation alone would not address.

Feeding and Growth Considerations Across the Spectrum

Feeding difficulty, related both to oromotor dysfunction common across the holoprosencephaly severity spectrum and to the hypothalamic-pituitary dysfunction discussed earlier in this section, is a near-universal management consideration for the more severely affected infant, and coordinated feeding evaluation incorporating speech-language pathology and, where growth hormone or other endocrine deficiency is identified, endocrinology-directed growth monitoring, is integrated into the same multidisciplinary care structure this chapter has emphasized throughout rather than addressed as an isolated, separate referral disconnected from the broader neurologic and endocrine picture.

The imaging, genetic, and endocrine reasoning developed across this section applies with equal force to the milder end of the midline malformation spectrum discussed earlier, including isolated septo-optic dysplasia without frank hemispheric fusion, underscoring that severity classification, not the mere presence or absence of a midline malformation label, should govern the intensity and specific focus of the multidisciplinary evaluation each child receives.

Long-Term Multidisciplinary Follow-Up for Midline Malformation

Children with a confirmed midline malformation from the holoprosencephaly or septo-optic dysplasia spectrum require sustained, coordinated multidisciplinary follow-up spanning endocrinology, ophthalmology, and developmental pediatrics well beyond the initial newborn evaluation, since pituitary dysfunction can evolve or newly manifest over years of growth and pubertal development rather than presenting fully at birth; establishing this long-term follow-up structure explicitly at the time of initial diagnosis, rather than leaving the family to coordinate an evolving set of specialist needs independently, reflects the same structured, longitudinal surveillance principle emphasized throughout this book for other categories of significant early brain injury or malformation.

Figure 8.1: Holoprosencephaly Severity Spectrum

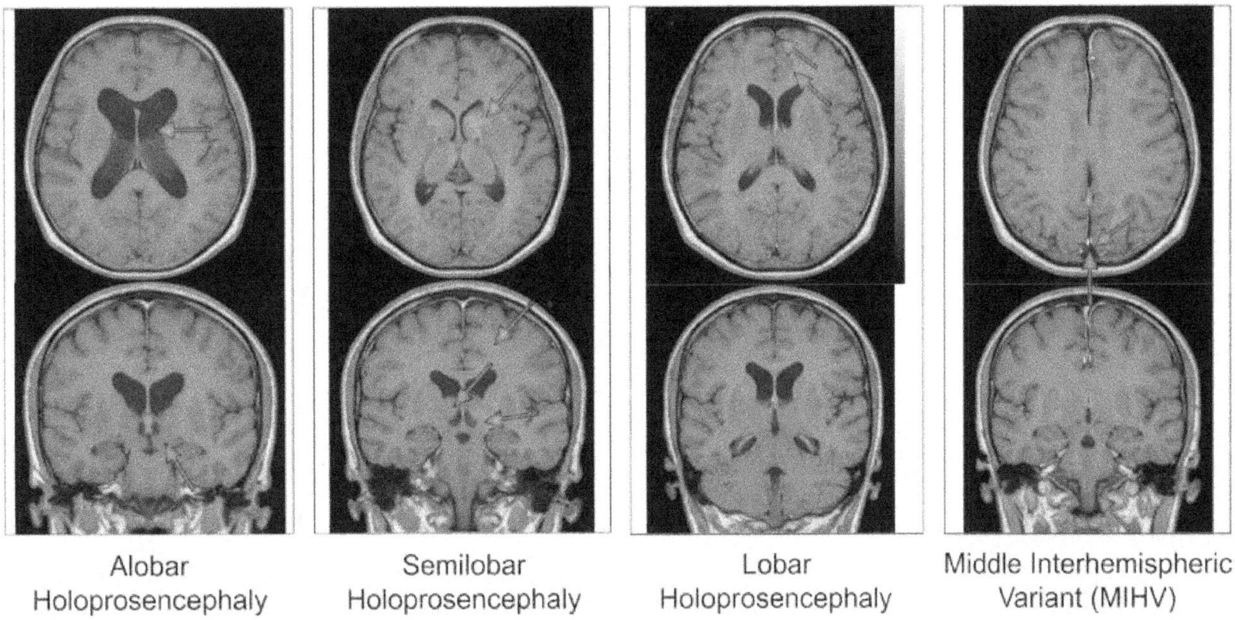

Posterior Fossa Malformations

Building directly on the benign posterior fossa variant discussion in Chapter 2, this section addresses the true posterior fossa malformations that must be actively distinguished from those variants, a distinction with major prognostic and counseling implications given the markedly more severe outcome profile of true malformation. The reader is encouraged to revisit the Chapter 2 discussion of mega cisterna magna and Blake pouch cyst before proceeding, since the vermian-integrity criterion introduced there is the same criterion applied throughout this section to distinguish true malformation from its benign mimics.

Dandy-Walker Malformation

Dandy-Walker malformation, introduced through its Crossing in Chapter 2, is characterized by complete or partial agenesis of the cerebellar vermis, cystic dilatation of the fourth ventricle communicating directly with an enlarged posterior fossa, and elevation of the torcular and tentorium, a constellation collectively termed torcular-lambdoid inversion; this full triad, rather than any single component in isolation, confirms the diagnosis and distinguishes it definitively from the benign mega cisterna magna and Blake pouch cyst variants discussed in Chapter 2, in which the vermis remains fully formed and normally positioned.

Vermian Hypoplasia Spectrum

Between the complete vermian agenesis of classic Dandy-Walker malformation and the fully normal vermis of the benign variants sits a spectrum of partial vermian hypoplasia, in which the vermis is present but reduced in size and, at times, abnormally rotated, a pattern requiring careful distinction from the milder end of true malformation from the mild vermian rotation variant discussed in Chapter 2; volumetric assessment of vermian size relative to age-matched normative data, rather than qualitative visual impression alone, improves the reliability of this distinction in genuinely borderline cases.

Joubert Syndrome and the Molar Tooth Sign

Joubert syndrome, a genetically heterogeneous ciliopathy, produces a highly specific and readily recognizable imaging finding termed the molar tooth sign, in which elongated, thickened, and abnormally horizontally oriented superior cerebellar peduncles combine with a deepened interpeduncular fossa and vermian hypoplasia to produce an axial appearance resembling a molar tooth; this pathognomonic imaging sign, once recognized, should prompt evaluation for the multisystem features characteristic of this ciliopathy spectrum, including retinal dystrophy, renal cystic disease, and hepatic fibrosis, reflecting the broad tissue distribution of the ciliary proteins these genes encode, and genetic testing targeting the growing list of genes associated with Joubert syndrome and related ciliopathies is pursued once this imaging sign is identified.

Rhombencephalosynapsis

Rhombencephalosynapsis, a rarer posterior fossa malformation characterized by fusion of the cerebellar hemispheres across the midline with absence of the vermis, producing a characteristic transverse, horizontally oriented folial pattern rather than the normal vertically oriented vermian folia, is frequently associated with supratentorial anomalies including ventriculomegaly and, at times, holoprosencephaly-spectrum findings discussed earlier in this chapter, reflecting shared disruption of midline patterning signals across both the anterior and posterior neural tube; recognizing the specific transverse folial pattern, rather than simply noting vermian absence, distinguishes this entity from the vermian agenesis of Dandy-Walker malformation, which does not show this fused, transverse hemispheric pattern.

Chiari Malformations I and II

Chiari I malformation, characterized by caudal displacement of the cerebellar tonsils below the foramen magnum, typically identified incidentally or in the evaluation of headache or a syrinx discussed below, is mechanistically and clinically distinct from Chiari II malformation, a more severe malformation characterized by caudal displacement of the cerebellar vermis, brainstem, and fourth ventricle, essentially always associated with a myelomeningocele and the specific supratentorial findings, including a beaked tectum and callosal dysgenesis, that accompany this more severe, syndromic presentation; distinguishing these two entities by their distinct anatomic components and their near-universal association, in the case of Chiari II, with open spinal dysraphism, discussed fully in Chapter 9, prevents the clinically significant error of conflating two malformations with substantially different severity and management implications.

Associated Syringomyelia

Both Chiari I and Chiari II malformation carry an associated risk of syringomyelia, a fluid-filled cavity within the spinal cord parenchyma believed to arise from disrupted cerebrospinal fluid flow dynamics at the crowded craniocervical junction these malformations produce; whenever a Chiari malformation of either type is identified, extending the imaging field of view to include the full spinal cord, applying the field-of-view extension principle established in Chapter 1, is standard practice specifically to evaluate for this association, since an unrecognized syrinx can itself produce a distinct, progressive neurologic deficit requiring its own management consideration independent of the Chiari malformation itself.

Cerebrospinal Fluid Flow Studies in Chiari Evaluation

Beyond static anatomic characterization, dedicated cerebrospinal fluid flow imaging, most commonly a phase-contrast MRI sequence assessing flow velocity and direction across the foramen magnum, is obtained in the evaluation of a symptomatic Chiari I malformation being considered for surgical decompression, providing physiologic information regarding the degree of flow obstruction that static anatomic measurement of tonsillar descent alone cannot capture; a child with borderline tonsillar descent but demonstrably abnormal flow dynamics may be a more appropriate surgical candidate than a child with more pronounced descent but preserved, normal flow, illustrating why this functional assessment complements rather than duplicates the anatomic evaluation.

Genetic Testing in Posterior Fossa Malformation

Beyond the ciliopathy gene panel specifically indicated by a molar tooth sign, discussed earlier in this section, a broader posterior fossa malformation panel or exome sequencing is increasingly pursued for Dandy-Walker malformation, rhombencephalosynapsis, and vermian hypoplasia without a more specific pathognomonic imaging sign directing testing toward a narrower gene set; recognizing that a substantial proportion of posterior fossa malformations remain genetically unexplained even after comprehensive contemporary testing is itself an important, honestly communicated component of family counseling, consistent with the uncertainty-acknowledging communication principle developed throughout this book.

Ventriculomegaly and Hydrocephalus as a Complication of Posterior Fossa Malformation

Several of the posterior fossa malformations discussed in this section, most notably Dandy-Walker malformation, carry a substantial risk of associated hydrocephalus, whether from direct fourth ventricular outflow obstruction or from disrupted cerebrospinal fluid dynamics more broadly across the malformed posterior fossa; serial monitoring of ventricular size using the same standardized measurement approach introduced in Chapter 5 for posthemorrhagic ventricular dilatation, applied here to a congenital rather than acquired hydrocephalus mechanism, guides the timing of any neurosurgical intervention, discussed fully in Chapter 10, that becomes necessary as the malformation and its associated hydrocephalus evolve.

Cognitive and Motor Outcome Across the Posterior Fossa Malformation Spectrum

Neurodevelopmental outcome across the posterior fossa malformations discussed in this section varies considerably by specific diagnosis and severity, ranging from predominantly motor and coordination difficulty in an isolated, mild vermian hypoplasia to the severe, multisystem impairment characteristic of Joubert syndrome with significant ciliopathy-related comorbidity, or the profound impairment frequently accompanying Chiari II malformation and its associated myelomeningocele; the increasing recognition that the cerebellum contributes meaningfully to cognitive and language function, not solely to motor coordination, discussed briefly in Chapter 5, means developmental surveillance for this population should incorporate cognitive and language assessment alongside the motor assessment more traditionally emphasized for cerebellar pathology.

Screening for Multisystem Ciliopathy Involvement

Once the molar tooth sign identifies a likely ciliopathy diagnosis, coordinated screening for the multisystem features these disorders can involve, including baseline and periodic renal ultrasound for cystic disease, liver function testing and imaging for hepatic fibrosis, and ophthalmologic evaluation for retinal dystrophy, is initiated proactively rather than reactively, since these systemic manifestations can emerge gradually over years and are more effectively managed when identified through planned surveillance than when they first present as an acute clinical problem; this proactive, systems-based screening approach exemplifies the broader principle that a pathognomonic imaging sign, once recognized, should trigger a structured, anticipatory evaluation extending well beyond the nervous system alone.

The posterior fossa malformation spectrum addressed throughout this section, from the benign variants of Chapter 2 through true vermian agenesis, pathognomonic ciliopathy signs, and the Chiari malformations, exemplifies this book's broader Clinical-Imaging Crosswalk approach particularly clearly: a single anatomic region, the posterior fossa, generates presentations ranging from entirely reassuring incidental findings to severe, multisystem disease, and confident, precise anatomic characterization is what separates one from the other.

Posterior Fossa Decompression Surgery and Postoperative Imaging

Surgical decompression for a symptomatic Chiari I malformation, typically involving suboccipital craniectomy with or without dural expansion, aims to relieve the crowding at the craniocervical junction responsible for the abnormal cerebrospinal fluid dynamics discussed above, and postoperative imaging assessing for adequate decompression, resolution or stabilization of any associated syrinx, and exclusion of a surgical complication is a standard component of postoperative surveillance; documenting the specific preoperative measurements discussed in this section allows direct, quantitative postoperative comparison rather than a purely qualitative postoperative impression.

Figure 8.2 Molar Tooth Sign of Joubert Syndrome

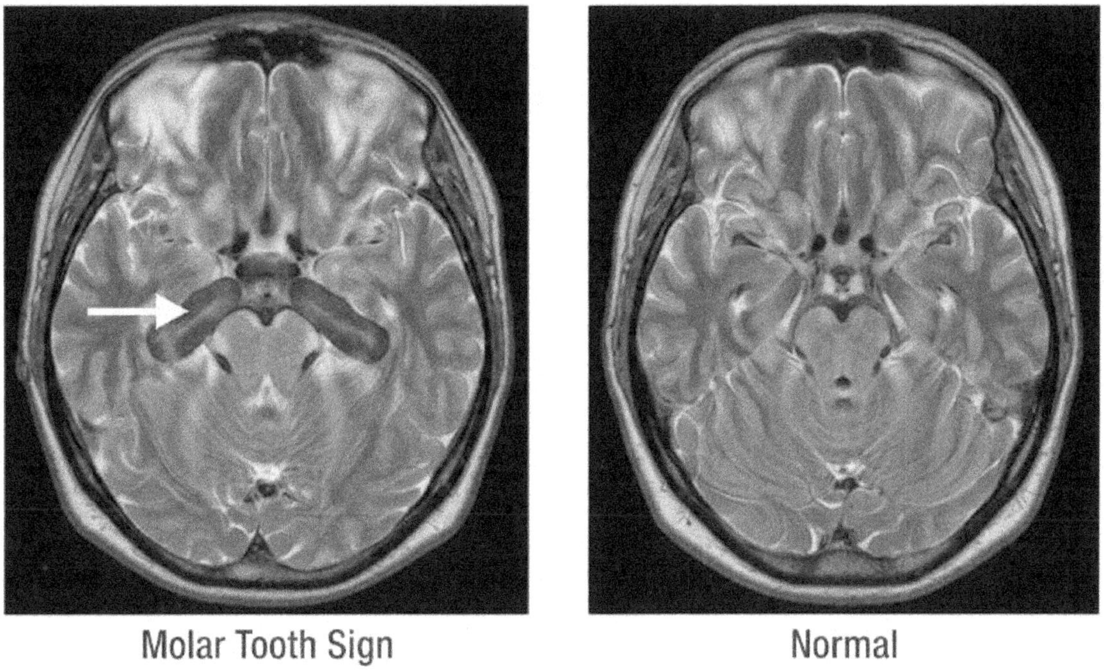

THE CLINICAL-IMAGING CROSSWALK SYSTEM — Chiari I Malformation Discovered Incidentally

---

The Crossing: A twelve-year-old undergoes brain MRI for evaluation of headache, discussed in Chapter 20, and the study incidentally identifies cerebellar tonsillar descent of six millimeters below the foramen magnum.

Presentation Signature: A child with headache as the presenting complaint, no other neurologic symptoms, and incidental tonsillar ectopia identified on a study obtained for an unrelated indication.

Imaging Correlate: The full craniocervical junction and spinal cord are assessed specifically for an associated syrinx, applying the field-of-view extension principle from Chapter 1, and the degree of tonsillar descent, presence or absence of crowding at the foramen magnum, and cerebrospinal fluid flow characteristics are documented.

Trap Logic: Mild, asymptomatic tonsillar ectopia below the classically cited five-millimeter threshold is a common incidental finding that does not, by itself, establish a causal relationship to the presenting headache, and reflexively attributing the headache to an incidentally discovered Chiari I finding without evaluating for red-flag features specific to Chiari-related headache, such as cough- or Valsalva-triggered occipital pain, risks both mismanaging the actual headache etiology and generating unwarranted anxiety about an incidental finding.

Crossing Anchor: Incidental tonsillar ectopia should be evaluated for an associated syrinx and correlated against Chiari-specific red-flag symptoms before being presumed causally related to a presenting headache; asymptomatic, isolated findings without a syrinx are generally managed conservatively rather than surgically.

Craniosynostosis and Skull Base Anomalies

Premature fusion of one or more cranial sutures produces a predictable, named pattern of skull deformity that reflects the specific suture or combination of sutures involved, and correctly characterizing this pattern on imaging directly shapes both the surgical planning discussed in this section and the broader genetic evaluation for syndromic craniosynostosis. This section moves from the underlying growth mechanism through the specific single-suture and syndromic patterns to the imaging technique, surgical timing, and long-term surveillance considerations that together define comprehensive craniofacial care.

Normal Suture Anatomy and the Pathophysiologic Basis of Craniosynostosis

Cranial growth normally occurs perpendicular to each open suture, meaning premature fusion of a specific suture halts growth in that perpendicular direction while compensatory growth continues along the remaining open sutures, producing a predictable, named skull shape deformity specific to which suture or sutures are affected; understanding this underlying growth-restriction mechanism, rather than memorizing each resulting skull shape as an isolated pattern, allows the reader to predict the expected deformity from a known pattern of suture involvement and, conversely, to infer the likely affected suture from an observed skull shape.

Single-Suture Craniosynostosis Patterns

Sagittal synostosis, the most common single-suture pattern, restricts lateral growth while compensatory anteroposterior growth continues, producing a long, narrow skull shape termed scaphocephaly; unilateral coronal synostosis produces an asymmetric, oblique skull deformity termed anterior plagiocephaly, with ipsilateral forehead flattening and contralateral compensatory bossing; bilateral coronal synostosis produces a short, broad skull termed brachycephaly; and metopic synostosis produces a triangular forehead deformity termed trigonocephaly, often accompanied by hypotelorism given the metopic suture's location between the developing orbits.

Syndromic Craniosynostosis

Syndromic craniosynostosis, in which multiple sutures are affected, often bilaterally and symmetrically, and accompanied by characteristic limb, facial, and other systemic findings, includes recognizable entities such as Apert, Crouzon, and Pfeiffer syndromes, most commonly caused by mutations in the fibroblast growth factor receptor genes; recognizing multi-suture, particularly bicoronal, involvement together with any accompanying limb anomaly such as syndactyly should prompt genetics referral and targeted testing, since the syndromic diagnosis carries implications extending well beyond the cranial finding alone, including airway, ophthalmologic, and additional skeletal considerations requiring coordinated multidisciplinary management.

CT and Three-Dimensional Reconstruction Technique

Unlike the great majority of pediatric neuroimaging addressed throughout this book, craniosynostosis evaluation represents one of the specific circumstances, introduced in Chapter 1, in which CT retains a clearly preferred first-line role, since direct visualization of suture fusion requires the bone-detail resolution CT provides and MRI does not; low-dose CT protocols specifically optimized for cranial bone detail, combined with three-dimensional surface reconstruction that allows the surgical team to visualize the full skull shape and suture pattern from any angle, are standard components of the preoperative craniosynostosis evaluation, balancing the radiation stewardship principle from Chapter 1 against the genuine diagnostic and surgical-planning necessity of CT-quality bone detail in this specific circumstance.

Surgical Planning and Timing

Surgical correction of craniosynostosis, whether through open cranial vault remodeling or, for appropriately selected, younger infants with single-suture involvement, minimally invasive endoscopic strip craniectomy followed by helmet therapy, is generally most effective when performed within a defined early window, typically the first year of life, reflecting the greater capacity for compensatory skull remodeling in a younger infant's more malleable, actively growing skull; the specific three-dimensional reconstruction imaging discussed above directly informs the surgical approach selected and the specific osteotomy plan, making precise, detailed preoperative imaging characterization a direct determinant of surgical outcome rather than a purely diagnostic exercise preceding a separately determined surgical plan.

Skull Base Anomalies: Basilar Invagination and Platybasia

Basilar invagination, in which the odontoid process and surrounding upper cervical spine are abnormally displaced upward into the foramen magnum, and platybasia, an abnormally flattened skull base angle, represent a distinct category of skull base anomaly that can produce direct brainstem compression and are associated with several of the skeletal dysplasias and connective tissue disorders discussed elsewhere in this book; dedicated skull base and craniocervical junction measurement using standardized radiographic lines and angles, rather than qualitative visual impression, provides the objective, reproducible characterization needed to guide the decision regarding surgical decompression in a symptomatic child.

Distinguishing Craniosynostosis From Positional Plagiocephaly

Building on the benign positional plagiocephaly discussion and figure in Chapter 2, distinguishing true craniosynostosis from the far more common benign positional skull flattening depends on the specific pattern of deformity, symmetric parallelogram-shaped flattening with ipsilateral ear displacement anteriorly for positional plagiocephaly, versus the suture-specific patterns described in this section for true craniosynostosis, together with the physical examination finding of a palpable bony ridge along the affected suture, present in true craniosynostosis and absent in positional molding; imaging is reserved for cases in which this clinical distinction remains genuinely ambiguous after careful physical examination, rather than obtained reflexively for every infant with an asymmetric head shape.

Airway Considerations in Syndromic Craniosynostosis

Beyond the cranial vault findings emphasized throughout this section, syndromic craniosynostosis frequently carries associated midface hypoplasia that can produce significant upper airway obstruction, and coordinated evaluation with otolaryngology and, where indicated, formal sleep study assessment is a necessary component of the comprehensive management plan for a child with confirmed syndromic craniosynostosis, since this airway risk carries independent morbidity distinct from, though related to, the cranial vault and intracranial pressure considerations that are this chapter's primary imaging focus.

Radiation Dose Optimization in Pediatric Craniofacial CT

Given that craniosynostosis evaluation and surgical planning frequently require more than one CT study across an affected child's care, spanning initial diagnosis, surgical planning, and, at times, postoperative assessment, dose-optimized, pediatric-specific craniofacial CT protocols, applying the radiation stewardship principle established in Chapter 1 with particular rigor given this population's above-average cumulative CT exposure risk, are essential; close collaboration between the ordering surgical team and the imaging department to avoid redundant imaging, reusing existing three-dimensional reconstructions whenever a repeat full CT is not genuinely necessary for the specific surgical planning question at hand, further reduces this population's cumulative radiation burden.

Multidisciplinary Craniofacial Team Coordination

Comprehensive management of craniosynostosis, particularly the syndromic forms discussed in this section, is best delivered through a dedicated, coordinated craniofacial team incorporating neurosurgery, plastic and craniofacial surgery, otolaryngology, ophthalmology, genetics, and developmental pediatrics, meeting collaboratively to review imaging and coordinate the timing and sequencing of the multiple interventions a severely affected child may require across infancy and early childhood; this team-based model, increasingly the standard of care at dedicated craniofacial centers, reduces the fragmentation and redundant evaluation a family might otherwise experience navigating each specialty independently, echoing the multidisciplinary coordination principle emphasized throughout this book for other complex, multisystem presentations.

Ophthalmologic Surveillance in Craniosynostosis

Beyond the airway considerations discussed above, syndromic craniosynostosis carries meaningful risk to the visual system, including exposure keratopathy related to shallow orbits and proptosis, strabismus, and, in severe multi-suture involvement, optic nerve compromise related to the elevated intracranial pressure risk discussed earlier in this section; regular, coordinated ophthalmologic surveillance, distinct from but complementary to the periodic papilledema screening discussed for intracranial pressure monitoring, is therefore a standard, ongoing component of comprehensive craniofacial team follow-up rather than a consultation reserved only for a child with an already-apparent visual symptom.

Psychosocial Considerations in Visible Craniofacial Difference

Beyond the medical and surgical considerations emphasized throughout this section, a child with a visible craniofacial difference, whether from craniosynostosis itself or its surgical correction, may experience social and psychological challenges related to appearance and peer perception as they grow, and proactive psychosocial support, including connection with craniofacial-specific family support resources and, where indicated, referral for psychological support around appearance-related concerns, is an appropriate and increasingly standard component of comprehensive craniofacial team care, extending this chapter's medical and surgical focus into the lived, day-to-day experience of the child and family.

Applying the suture-anatomy-to-deformity reasoning developed at the start of this section to skull base anomalies as well, basilar invagination and platybasia can be understood as a further consequence of abnormal growth restriction, in this instance at the skull base rather than the cranial vault, reinforcing the value of the underlying growth-mechanism framework this section has developed across the full range of skull and skull base anomalies it addresses.

Monitoring for Elevated Intracranial Pressure After Multi-Suture Involvement

Multi-suture craniosynostosis, particularly the syndromic forms discussed above, carries a meaningful risk of chronically elevated intracranial pressure related to restricted overall cranial vault growth relative to ongoing brain growth, a risk that persists even after surgical correction of the visible skull shape deformity and requires its own dedicated, longitudinal monitoring; papilledema screening through serial ophthalmologic examination and, where clinically indicated, direct intracranial pressure monitoring or repeat imaging assessing for signs of chronic pressure elevation such as copper-beaten skull appearance, are incorporated into long-term follow-up specifically because visibly adequate cranial vault reshaping does not, by itself, guarantee normalized intracranial pressure.

Suture Involved	Resulting Skull Shape	Common Term
Sagittal	Long, narrow	Scaphocephaly
Unilateral coronal	Asymmetric, oblique	Anterior plagiocephaly
Bilateral coronal	Short, broad	Brachycephaly
Metopic	Triangular forehead	Trigonocephaly

Corpus Callosum Anomalies

The corpus callosum, introduced in its normal developmental sequence in Chapter 2, is subject to a range of congenital anomalies from complete agenesis through partial, segment-specific absence, each carrying distinct associations and prognostic implications this closing section addresses. As the final section of this chapter, it also draws together several threads developed earlier, the anterior-to-posterior developmental timing established for malformation dating, the isolated-versus-syndromic distinction shaping counseling, and the phenotype-directed genetic testing strategy applied consistently throughout this chapter.

Complete Versus Partial Agenesis

Complete agenesis of the corpus callosum, the total absence of this commissural structure, is distinguished from partial agenesis, in which one or more callosal segments are present while others are absent, by applying the anterior-to-posterior developmental sequence established in Chapter 2: because the genu forms first and the splenium and rostrum form last, partial agenesis characteristically spares the genu and body while the posterior segments are absent, a pattern that both confirms the diagnosis of a true developmental anomaly, as opposed to an acquired callosal injury which would not respect this specific developmental sequence, and helps date the approximate gestational timing of the underlying disruption. This same anterior-sparing logic, once internalized, gives the reader a reliable, mechanism-based check to apply whenever a callosal finding's developmental versus acquired origin is genuinely in question.

Associated Interhemispheric Cysts and Lipomas

Corpus callosum agenesis is frequently accompanied by an interhemispheric cyst, ranging from a small, simple cyst to a large, communicating cyst that can produce mass effect and hydrocephalus, and by an interhemispheric lipoma, a fat-signal mass along the expected callosal course believed to arise from abnormal persistence and differentiation of the embryonic meninx primitiva; recognizing these specific, characteristic associated findings, an interhemispheric cyst or lipoma in the setting of callosal agenesis, rather than treating them as separate, unrelated incidental findings, reinforces the correct primary diagnosis and, in the case of a large or symptomatic interhemispheric cyst, directly informs the need for neurosurgical evaluation.

Isolated Versus Syndromic Corpus Callosum Agenesis

Corpus callosum agenesis identified as an isolated finding, without accompanying malformation elsewhere in the brain and without an associated dysmorphic or multisystem syndrome, carries a substantially more favorable neurodevelopmental prognosis than callosal agenesis occurring as one component of a broader malformation complex or genetic syndrome, underscoring why a thorough search for additional intracranial findings, applying the systematic differential diagnosis approach from Chapter 7, and a coordinated dysmorphology and genetics evaluation are essential before a family is counseled regarding expected prognosis; a substantial minority of apparently isolated cases are ultimately found, on comprehensive genetic testing, to carry an identifiable genetic cause even without an obvious accompanying syndromic feature on examination.

Neurodevelopmental Outcome

Neurodevelopmental outcome in isolated corpus callosum agenesis ranges widely, from normal cognitive function identified only incidentally in adulthood to significant learning and social-cognitive impairment, reflecting the corpus callosum's role in interhemispheric communication and integration; a specific pattern of social cognition and pragmatic language difficulty, sometimes termed the nonverbal learning disability profile, has been particularly associated with this diagnosis even in children with preserved general intellectual function, informing targeted developmental surveillance that extends beyond general cognitive screening alone into these more specific social-cognitive and pragmatic language domains.

Prenatal Diagnosis Challenges

Prenatal diagnosis of corpus callosum agenesis, whether by ultrasound or fetal MRI, carries specific interpretive challenges given the corpus callosum's ongoing, incomplete development throughout gestation, discussed in Chapter 2, meaning a prenatal study performed before the callosum has substantially completed its normal developmental sequence can be genuinely difficult to distinguish from a truly absent structure; when prenatal imaging raises this concern, postnatal confirmation once the callosum's normal developmental window has closed, alongside the comprehensive search for additional findings and the genetic evaluation discussed above, provides the family with more complete, reliable information than the prenatal finding alone can offer.

Genetic Evaluation

Corpus callosum agenesis is associated with a broad and continually expanding range of genetic causes, including chromosomal abnormalities, single-gene disorders, and specific metabolic conditions, and the genetic testing strategy pursued is informed by the presence or absence of associated findings identified through the comprehensive evaluation discussed above, applying the same phenotype-directed testing principle developed in Chapter 7 for the malformations of cortical development; a syndromic presentation with distinctive additional features directs testing toward the specific associated syndrome, while an apparently isolated presentation more often proceeds to broader chromosomal microarray and exome-based testing given the absence of a single, narrowing clinical clue.

Probst Bundles and Colpocephaly as Secondary Imaging Findings

Beyond the primary absence of the callosum itself, corpus callosum agenesis produces characteristic secondary findings that support the diagnosis and reflect the underlying altered white matter tract organization: Probst bundles, longitudinally oriented white matter tracts that would normally have crossed the midline via the callosum but instead run parallel to the interhemispheric fissure along the medial hemispheric wall, and colpocephaly, disproportionate enlargement of the occipital horns of the lateral ventricles relative to the frontal horns, reflecting the altered white matter architecture posteriorly;

recognizing these secondary findings reinforces the primary diagnosis and, particularly for colpocephaly, should not be mistaken for the ventriculomegaly discussed in Chapter 10, since the underlying mechanism and management implications differ substantially between these two entities.

Diffusion Tensor Tractography in Callosal Anomaly Evaluation

Diffusion tensor imaging with tractography, introduced as an advanced technique in Chapter 1, offers a further, complementary tool for characterizing corpus callosum anomalies, directly visualizing the Probst bundles and any residual, atypically coursing callosal fibers that conventional sequences alone may only infer indirectly; this technique is applied selectively, most often in the presurgical evaluation of an associated epilepsy or when the conventional imaging appearance leaves genuine ambiguity regarding whether a thin, residual callosal remnant is truly present or truly absent, consistent with the adjunct-sequence discipline, adding a technique only when it will change the answer to a specific question, established in Chapter 1.

Interhemispheric Transfer Deficits and Targeted Educational Support

The specific pattern of interhemispheric transfer deficit associated with corpus callosum agenesis, in which information processed in one hemisphere is not efficiently shared with the other, can produce subtle but functionally meaningful difficulties with bimanual coordination, rapid cross-modal integration, and the pragmatic, social-inferential language skills discussed earlier in this section, deficits that may not be apparent on general cognitive testing alone; neuropsychological evaluation specifically incorporating tasks sensitive to interhemispheric transfer and social cognition, rather than general intelligence testing alone, provides the more clinically useful basis for targeted educational accommodation planning in this specific population.

Distinguishing Corpus Callosum Agenesis From Acquired Callosal Thinning

Beyond the developmental anomalies emphasized throughout this section, the corpus callosum can also show acquired thinning secondary to a range of processes elsewhere in this book, including significant hydrocephalus discussed in Chapter 10, extensive white matter injury discussed in Chapter 5, and certain metabolic and neurodegenerative conditions discussed in Chapter 17; distinguishing developmental agenesis or hypogenesis from acquired thinning depends on the same principles introduced in Chapter 7 for the broader malformation-versus-injury distinction, namely the presence of the anterior-sparing segmental pattern and associated Probst bundles and colpocephaly characteristic of a true developmental process, against a uniformly thin but structurally complete callosum with all segments present in acquired thinning.

Case Presentation: Isolated Corpus Callosum Agenesis With Favorable Outcome

A prenatal ultrasound at twenty weeks raises concern for absent corpus callosum, and fetal MRI at twenty-eight weeks, timed appropriately per the developmental window discussed in this section, confirms complete agenesis without an associated interhemispheric cyst, additional cortical malformation, or other structural anomaly. Postnatal MRI confirms the isolated finding, with the characteristic Probst bundles and mild colpocephaly discussed in this section but no additional abnormality identified on comprehensive review. Chromosomal microarray is normal. Applying the reasoning developed in this chapter, the family is counseled regarding the genuinely favorable prognostic implications of a truly isolated finding while being honestly informed of the still-meaningful, if reduced, risk of the specific social-cognitive and pragmatic language difficulties discussed in this section, and structured developmental surveillance incorporating targeted neuropsychological assessment, rather than general cognitive screening alone, is scheduled beginning in early childhood. This case, considered alongside the syndromic and combined presentations discussed elsewhere in this chapter, illustrates why the same anatomic finding, callosal absence, requires an individualized rather than uniform counseling approach based on the full context in which it occurs.

Counseling Families Through Genuine Prognostic Uncertainty

The wide neurodevelopmental outcome range characteristic of isolated corpus callosum agenesis, discussed earlier in this section, presents a particular counseling challenge distinct from the more narrowly predictable outcome patterns associated with several other malformations discussed throughout this book; applying the honest, proportionate, uncertainty-acknowledging communication framework developed throughout this book, families are counseled that the isolated nature of the finding is genuinely reassuring relative to a syndromic presentation, while being equally honest that this reassurance does not translate into a confident prediction of normal outcome for their specific child, and that the structured, longitudinal developmental surveillance discussed in Chapter 5 remains the appropriate path to actual, individualized prognostic clarity over time.

Figure 8.3 Complete Versus Partial Corpus Callosum Agenesis

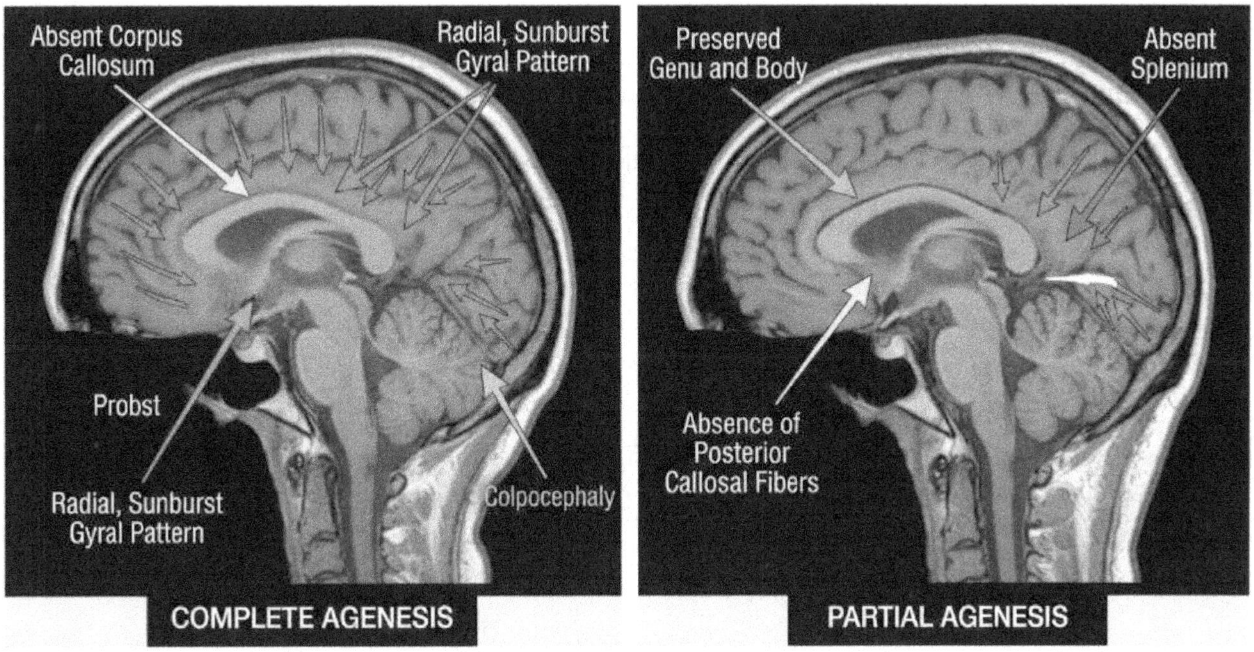

Case Presentation: Semilobar Holoprosencephaly With Endocrine Involvement

A newborn with mild hypotelorism and a single central maxillary incisor identified on newborn examination undergoes brain MRI, which demonstrates semilobar holoprosencephaly with posterior hemispheric separation and anterior fusion, fused thalami, and an absent septum pellucidum. Applying the reasoning developed in this chapter, endocrinology is consulted proactively for pituitary function assessment given the well-documented association between midline malformation and hypothalamic-pituitary dysfunction, identifying subclinical central hypothyroidism on screening labs before any clinical symptom had emerged. Chromosomal microarray and sonic hedgehog pathway gene testing are pursued in parallel, and the family is counseled regarding the anticipated developmental impact of the semilobar classification alongside the specific, proactively identified and now treated endocrine finding, illustrating how the midline malformation framework developed in this chapter directs a coordinated, anticipatory evaluation rather than a purely reactive one.

Case Presentation: Sagittal Synostosis Identified in Infancy

A four-month-old is referred for evaluation of a progressively long, narrow head shape noted by the family and confirmed on examination, including a palpable ridge along the sagittal suture. Applying the reasoning developed in this chapter, the clinical examination findings, ridging along a specific suture rather than the symmetric parallelogram flattening of positional plagiocephaly, support a diagnosis of true craniosynostosis, and low-dose CT with three-dimensional reconstruction confirms isolated sagittal synostosis without involvement of any other suture. Given the infant's young age and isolated single-suture involvement, the craniofacial team recommends endoscopic strip craniectomy followed by helmet therapy rather than open cranial vault remodeling, applying the age-and-severity-based surgical planning framework developed in this section, and the family is counseled that this minimally invasive approach, appropriately timed within the early surgical window discussed in this chapter, offers a favorable expected outcome with a shorter recovery than the open surgical alternative.

Case Presentation: Chiari II Malformation Identified on Prenatal Imaging

A fetal MRI obtained for evaluation of a lumbosacral myelomeningocele identified on prenatal ultrasound, discussed further in Chapter 9, demonstrates the characteristic beaked tectum, caudally displaced cerebellar vermis and fourth ventricle, and moderate ventriculomegaly consistent with Chiari II malformation. Applying the reasoning developed in this chapter, the care team explains to the family that this specific constellation of findings, distinct from the isolated Chiari I pattern discussed in this chapter's Crossing, is essentially always associated with the open spinal dysraphism already identified, and coordinates multidisciplinary counseling incorporating maternal-fetal medicine, pediatric neurosurgery, and pediatric neurology to discuss delivery planning and the postnatal management pathway, including close postnatal monitoring for hydrocephalus given the ventriculomegaly already apparent on the prenatal study, illustrating the close, near-obligate anatomic and counseling linkage between this specific posterior fossa malformation and its associated spinal anomaly. The family's questions regarding fetal surgery, an option for selected myelomeningocele cases discussed further in Chapter 9, are addressed within this same coordinated prenatal counseling conversation rather than deferred to a separate, later visit.

THE CLINICAL-IMAGING CROSSWALK SYSTEM — Congenital Malformation Recognition Across the Brain, Skull, and Posterior Fossa

---

Crossing 1 Recap: Incidental tonsillar ectopia should be evaluated for an associated syrinx and correlated against Chiari-specific red-flag symptoms before being presumed causally related to a presenting headache.

Chapter Anchor: Midline and posterior fossa malformations are distinguished from their benign variant mimics by specific, named anatomic criteria, vermian integrity, degree of hemispheric cleavage, suture-specific skull deformity pattern, and callosal segment involvement, each directly shaping the genetic evaluation, multidisciplinary team composition, and prognostic counseling that follows.

Summary and Key Concepts

Holoprosencephaly is graded alobar through lobar by degree of hemispheric cleavage, correlates broadly with facial anomaly severity, and warrants proactive endocrine, feeding, and autonomic evaluation given frequent hypothalamic-pituitary involvement.

True posterior fossa malformation, including Dandy-Walker malformation, Joubert syndrome's molar tooth sign, and rhombencephalosynapsis, is distinguished from the benign variants of Chapter 2 by vermian agenesis or a specific pathognomonic pattern; Chiari I and II are mechanistically distinct entities each warranting spinal cord evaluation for syrinx and, where relevant, multisystem ciliopathy screening.

Craniosynostosis produces suture-specific, named skull deformities; CT with three-dimensional reconstruction is the preferred modality given its unique bone-detail requirement, and syndromic, multi-suture involvement warrants genetic evaluation, coordinated craniofacial team management, and ongoing airway, ophthalmologic, and intracranial pressure surveillance.

Corpus callosum agenesis, complete or partial, is distinguished from acquired callosal injury by its characteristic anterior-sparing pattern and associated Probst bundles and colpocephaly; isolated agenesis carries a more favorable prognosis than syndromic agenesis, and comprehensive evaluation for additional findings should precede prognostic counseling.

Across this chapter, each malformation category is defined by specific, named anatomic criteria rather than gestalt impression, and correct classification directly determines the genetic testing strategy, multidisciplinary team composition, and honest, individualized counseling that follow.

CHAPTER 9: SPINAL DYSRAPHISM AND CONGENITAL SPINE ANOMALIES

Learning Objectives

1. Distinguish open from closed spinal dysraphism and describe the specific imaging appearance and clinical implications of each major subtype, including the near-obligate Chiari II association of myelomeningocele.
2. Recognize the imaging features of a tethered spinal cord and describe the age-dependent normal conus position that anchors this diagnosis.
3. Identify vertebral segmentation anomalies and their association with other organ system malformations, including VACTERL association and craniocervical instability syndromes.
4. Recognize the cutaneous markers that should prompt spinal imaging in an otherwise asymptomatic infant, and distinguish them from the low-yield simple sacral dimple.

Open and Closed Spinal Dysraphism

Spinal dysraphism, a broad category encompassing failure of normal neural tube closure or subsequent secondary neurulation, is divided fundamentally into open and closed forms based on whether neural tissue is exposed to the environment, a distinction with immediate delivery-room and surgical urgency implications that makes it the organizing framework for this chapter's opening section.

Myelomeningocele: The Prototypical Open Dysraphism

Myelomeningocele, the most common and clinically significant form of open spinal dysraphism, results from failure of neural tube closure typically between the third and fourth gestational week, producing exposed, dysplastic neural tissue continuous with the surrounding skin defect rather than covered by normal skin; this open neural placode is at risk for infection and further injury from direct environmental exposure both before and after birth, making it a surgical urgency requiring closure, whether through the fetal surgery discussed later in this section or prompt postnatal repair, to reduce this ongoing exposure risk. The specific spinal level of the defect, assessed precisely on imaging, correlates broadly with the anticipated motor level of impairment, giving the family and care team an early, imaging-derived basis for anticipating the child's likely functional trajectory even before birth.

The Chiari II Association

As established in Chapter 8, myelomeningocele is essentially always accompanied by Chiari II malformation, reflecting a shared pathophysiologic mechanism in which chronic cerebrospinal fluid leakage through the open spinal defect reduces intracranial pressure during critical stages of hindbrain development, producing the characteristic caudal displacement of the cerebellum and brainstem; recognizing this near-obligate association means that identifying a myelomeningocele on prenatal or postnatal imaging should immediately prompt dedicated brain imaging for Chiari II malformation and its associated hydrocephalus risk, applying the coordinated evaluation principle developed throughout this book. This mechanistic link between a spinal defect and a distant, cranial finding is a clear illustration of why this book insists on evaluating the full neuraxis, not the presenting anatomic region in isolation, whenever a significant congenital anomaly is identified anywhere along it.

Fetal Surgery for Myelomeningocele

Prenatal, in-utero surgical repair of myelomeningocele, performed at specialized fetal surgery centers typically between approximately nineteen and twenty-six weeks gestation, has been shown in randomized trial data to reduce the need for postnatal shunt placement and improve certain motor outcomes relative to standard postnatal repair, reflecting the hypothesis that earlier closure limits the duration of neural tissue exposure and the associated chronic cerebrospinal fluid leakage responsible for the Chiari II mechanism discussed above; eligibility for fetal surgery depends on specific anatomic and maternal criteria evaluated through dedicated fetal MRI and ultrasound at a specialized center, and family counseling regarding this option, where anatomically and logistically feasible, is an important component of prenatal myelomeningocele care.

Myelocele: A Related Open Dysraphism

Myelocele, a related but distinct open dysraphism in which the neural placode lies flush with the skin surface rather than protruding above it within a meningocele sac, carries a similar exposure risk and surgical urgency to myelomeningocele but is distinguished on imaging by the absence of the sac-like protrusion characteristic of the more common myelomeningocele; correctly distinguishing these two entities, while both require prompt surgical attention, assists in precise preoperative surgical planning regarding the specific technique required for closure. Although less commonly encountered than myelomeningocele, myelocele is worth naming explicitly so the reader does not mistake its flush, non-protuberant appearance for a less urgent, closed dysraphism.

Closed Spinal Dysraphism With a Subcutaneous Mass

Closed spinal dysraphism, in which the neural tissue is covered by intact, though frequently abnormal, skin, encompasses a further spectrum of entities including lipomyelomeningocele, in which a fatty mass is contiguous with the spinal cord and extends through a bony defect to a subcutaneous component, and myelocystocele, a rarer entity in which a cystically dilated terminal central canal herniates through the defect; unlike open dysraphism, closed dysraphism does not carry the same immediate infection risk from environmental exposure, but nonetheless typically requires surgical intervention to address the tethering effect discussed in the next section of this chapter and to prevent progressive neurologic decline over time, making it a scheduled rather than emergent surgical priority in the great majority of cases.

Meningocele Without Neural Element Involvement

A simple meningocele, in which cerebrospinal fluid and meninges herniate through a bony defect without any neural tissue involvement, represents a distinct, generally more favorable entity within the closed dysraphism spectrum, since the absence of neural tissue within the herniated sac substantially reduces the risk of the neurologic tethering and progressive deficit associated with the neural-tissue-containing closed dysraphism entities discussed above; careful imaging characterization confirming the absence of any neural element within the sac is nonetheless essential before this more favorable prognosis is communicated to a family, since a small, easily overlooked neural component can be present even in an otherwise typical-appearing meningocele.

Split Cord Malformation

Split cord malformation, in which the spinal cord is divided into two hemicords, either within a single dural tube (type II) or, more commonly requiring surgical attention, within two separate dural tubes divided by an osseous, cartilaginous, or fibrous septum (type I), frequently coexists with the other dysraphic entities discussed throughout this chapter and carries its own distinct tethering mechanism related to the dividing septum itself; identifying the specific septum composition on imaging, since a bony septum is more readily visualized on CT while a fibrous septum may be more apparent on MRI, directly informs surgical planning for septum resection, a necessary component of split cord malformation repair distinct from the cord detethering addressed elsewhere in this chapter. Recognizing split cord malformation as a distinct entity, rather than folding it into the broader tethered cord discussion, matters because its surgical management specifically requires septum resection in addition to, not instead of, standard detethering technique.

Timing of Postnatal Surgical Closure

For infants born with an open myelomeningocele not eligible for or not pursuing fetal repair, postnatal surgical closure is generally performed within the first 24 to 72 hours of life, reflecting the same infection-risk and exposure-duration reasoning discussed earlier in this section applied to the postnatal rather than prenatal timeline; coordinating rapid postnatal imaging, physical examination, and neurosurgical evaluation within this narrow window requires efficient, well-rehearsed institutional protocols, since delay beyond this window incrementally increases infection risk without a corresponding clinical benefit to waiting.

Latex Allergy and Long-Term Management Considerations

Children with myelomeningocele carry a substantially elevated risk of latex allergy, believed to relate to the repeated early and ongoing latex exposure this population experiences through numerous surgical procedures and catheterizations beginning in infancy, and instituting latex-precaution protocols from the earliest surgical encounters, rather than only after a sensitization reaction has already occurred, is a standard, proactive component of comprehensive care for this population; this consideration, while not itself an imaging finding, is worth incorporating into the multidisciplinary counseling conversation this chapter has emphasized throughout, since it directly shapes practical, lifelong medical management decisions for the family.

Bladder and Bowel Management Across the Lifespan

Neurogenic bladder and bowel dysfunction, near-universal in myelomeningocele given the direct involvement of the sacral neural segments governing these functions, requires coordinated, lifelong urology and gastroenterology management extending from infancy, when a clean intermittent catheterization program is typically initiated, through adolescence and into adult transition; imaging surveillance of the urinary tract, including renal ultrasound to monitor for hydronephrosis and reflux-related upper tract change, is integrated into this same coordinated, multidisciplinary follow-up structure rather than pursued independently of the neurologic and orthopedic surveillance this chapter has emphasized throughout.

Prenatal Counseling Timelines and Family Decision-Making

When myelomeningocele is identified on prenatal ultrasound screening, typically around the standard second-trimester anatomy scan, the family faces a compressed decision-making timeline given the gestational age windows for both fetal surgical repair and, where legally and personally applicable, pregnancy termination, each of which narrows as gestation advances; providing the family with clear, prompt access to the full range of specialist input, maternal-fetal medicine, pediatric neurosurgery, and genetics, without unnecessary scheduling delay, respects both the medical urgency of these timelines and the family's need for complete information before reaching a decision, and coordinated, expedited referral pathways for a newly identified prenatal myelomeningocele diagnosis are an important systems-level component of comprehensive care.

Amniotic Band Sequence and Limb-Body Wall Complex as Differential Considerations

A minority of severe, atypical open spinal and body wall defects identified prenatally reflect amniotic band sequence or the related limb-body wall complex, rather than a primary neural tube closure defect, mechanisms involving disruption of already-formed structures by constricting amniotic bands rather than a failure of initial embryologic formation; distinguishing these disruption-mechanism entities from the malformation-mechanism dysraphism entities that are this chapter's primary focus depends on recognizing the characteristic irregular, asymmetric defect margins and, frequently, associated limb constriction rings or amputation defects that accompany amniotic band-related pathology, a distinction with different recurrence risk implications given the sporadic, non-genetic mechanism generally underlying true amniotic band disruption.

Spinal dysraphism, a broad category encompassing failure of normal neural tube closure or subsequent secondary neurulation, is divided fundamentally into open and closed forms based on whether neural tissue is exposed to the environment, a distinction with immediate delivery-room and surgical urgency implications that makes it the organizing framework for this chapter's opening section. This section, in turn, establishes the anatomic vocabulary and evaluation principles that the tethered cord, vertebral segmentation, and cutaneous marker sections build upon throughout the remainder of this chapter.

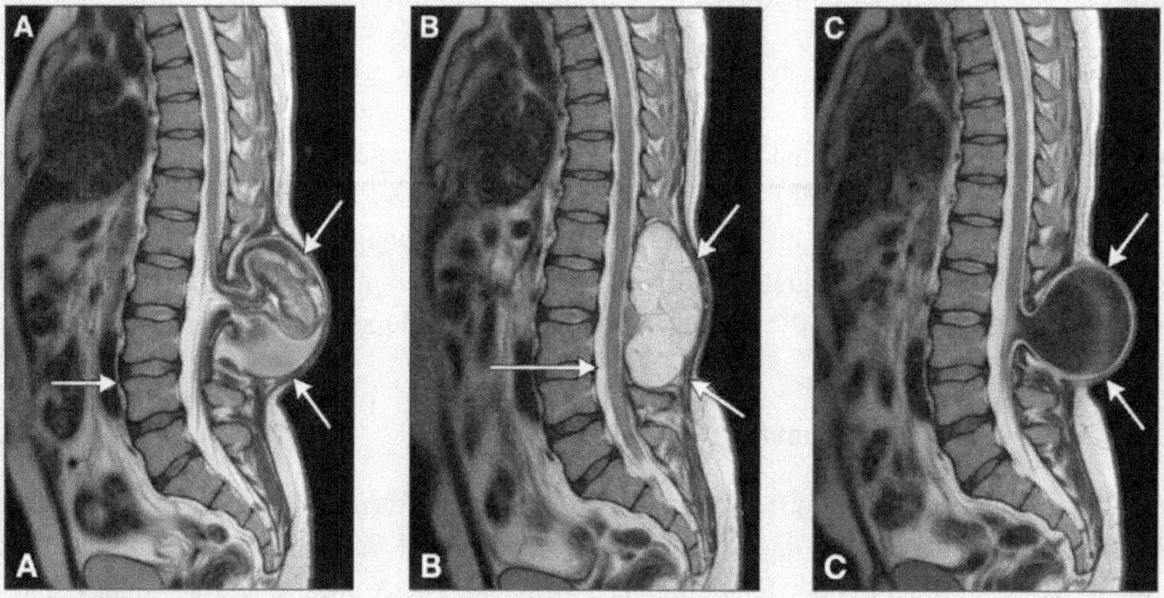

Figure 9.1: Open Versus Closed Spinal Dysraphism

Tethered Cord and Occult Spinal Dysraphism

Tethered spinal cord, a condition in which the spinal cord is abnormally fixed rather than free to ascend normally within the spinal canal during growth, is both a direct complication of the closed dysraphism entities discussed above and a distinct diagnostic consideration in the child with occult, imaging-only evidence of an underlying dysraphic process not apparent on external examination.

Normal Conus Position and Its Age-Dependent Ascent

The spinal cord and vertebral column grow at different rates during fetal development, with the vertebral column growing more rapidly, producing an apparent cephalad migration of the conus medullaris relative to the vertebral bodies as gestation and early postnatal life proceed; by term, the conus normally terminates at or above the L2-L3 disc space, and a conus position below this level, applying the same age-specific interpretive framework established in Chapter 2 for other developmental landmarks, is considered abnormally low and raises concern for tethering, though the precise normal range shows some variation across published normative studies, making mild borderline findings a circumstance warranting careful correlation with the imaging appearance of the filum terminale discussed below rather than conus position in isolation. This differential growth rate is the same underlying embryologic principle, applied here to the spinal axis, that Chapter 2 developed for the cranial structures discussed in that chapter.

The Thickened or Fatty Filum Terminale

A thickened filum terminale, generally defined as exceeding two millimeters in diameter, or a filum containing abnormal fat signal, are each independently associated with tethering even when the conus position itself falls within the normal range discussed above, reflecting the direct mechanical tethering effect this abnormal filum exerts; assessing filum thickness and signal characteristics is therefore a necessary complement to conus position measurement, not a redundant or optional additional step, when the full imaging evaluation for tethered cord is performed.

Clinical Presentation of Tethered Cord

Tethered cord classically presents with a progressive, rather than static, pattern of lower extremity weakness, gait disturbance, bladder and bowel dysfunction, and, in the older child, back or leg pain that worsens with activities involving spinal flexion or growth spurts, reflecting the progressive mechanical stretch injury this condition produces as the child grows while the cord remains abnormally fixed; recognizing this progressive clinical trajectory, rather than a static congenital deficit present from birth, is itself a diagnostic clue supporting tethered cord over an alternative, non-progressive congenital neurologic condition, and any new or worsening lower extremity or urologic symptom in a child with a known risk factor for dysraphism warrants prompt reevaluation rather than routine, unhurried follow-up. This progressive-versus-static distinction is worth stating explicitly to families at the time of an initial, asymptomatic finding, so they understand precisely which future symptoms should prompt them to seek prompt reevaluation rather than waiting for a routinely scheduled visit.

Occult (Skin-Covered) Tethering Without an External Marker

A subset of tethered cord cases present without any of the cutaneous markers discussed in this chapter's final section, identified instead through the urologic or orthopedic evaluation of a presenting symptom such as unexplained bladder dysfunction or a progressive foot deformity, underscoring that the absence of a cutaneous clue does not exclude an underlying dysraphic process; a low threshold for spinal imaging in a child with an otherwise unexplained, progressive neurogenic bladder or progressive lower extremity deformity, even without a cutaneous marker, reflects this chapter's broader theme that imaging-ordering decisions should be driven by the specific clinical presentation and its documented associations, not by the presence or absence of a single, most-commonly-cited clue alone.

Fatty Filum and Terminal Lipoma as a Milder Tethering Spectrum

An isolated fatty filum or a small terminal lipoma without an associated open or closed dysraphism defect elsewhere represents the mildest end of the tethering spectrum discussed in this section, and the decision to pursue prophylactic surgical release in an asymptomatic child with this isolated finding remains an area of genuine practice variation, weighing the risk of progressive tethering symptoms over time against the risks of prophylactic surgery in a currently asymptomatic child; this specific management question is appropriately addressed through shared decision-making between the family and a pediatric neurosurgeon experienced in this condition, applying the same shared decision-making framework developed in Chapter 3 to a surgical, rather than purely imaging, decision.

Imaging Protocol for Suspected Tethered Cord

Evaluating suspected tethered cord requires dedicated, thin-section sagittal and axial imaging of the full lumbosacral spine with attention to precise conus level measurement and filum characterization, applying the protocol-customization principle from Chapter 1; in the young infant with an open posterior fontanelle-equivalent access at the sacrum, spinal ultrasound, introduced in Chapter 1, offers an effective, sedation-free initial screening tool, though MRI remains the definitive study whenever ultrasound is equivocal, the infant is beyond the age at which ultrasound remains reliable, or the specific clinical question requires the more detailed anatomic characterization only MRI provides.

Tethered Cord Syndrome After Prior Myelomeningocele Repair

A child with a history of myelomeningocele repair, whether fetal or postnatal, carries an ongoing, lifelong risk of secondary, re-tethering at the surgical closure site, since the repaired cord, while released from its original open dysraphic attachment, is not restored to a fully normal, freely mobile anatomic configuration; new or progressive symptoms in this population, applying the same progressive-trajectory reasoning developed earlier in this section, should prompt reevaluation for re-tethering rather than being attributed reflexively to the child's baseline, presumed-stable neurologic deficit from the original malformation, a distinction that depends on careful comparison against prior baseline imaging and examination findings whenever available.

Urodynamic Testing as a Complementary Diagnostic Tool

Because bladder dysfunction is frequently among the earliest and most sensitive indicators of tethered cord, particularly in the young child not yet toilet-trained in whom a subtle change in urinary pattern may otherwise go unrecognized, formal urodynamic testing, performed in coordination with pediatric urology, offers a complementary, quantitative assessment of bladder function that can detect early tethering-related change before it becomes apparent on routine clinical history alone; incorporating baseline and, where clinically indicated, serial urodynamic assessment into the structured surveillance plan for a child at risk for tethered cord reflects the same principle of proactive, multidisciplinary monitoring emphasized throughout this book.

Postoperative Imaging After Detethering Surgery

Following surgical detethering, postoperative MRI is generally deferred beyond the immediate postoperative period, since expected postsurgical change, including a degree of persistent low conus position and postoperative scarring at the surgical site, can mimic or obscure the appearance of residual or recurrent tethering if imaging is obtained too early; establishing a documented postoperative baseline once acute surgical change has stabilized, typically several months after surgery, gives the reader a genuine baseline for comparison should re-tethering be suspected later, applying the same baseline-and-serial-comparison principle emphasized throughout this book for other conditions requiring longitudinal imaging surveillance.

Tethered Cord in the Context of Anorectal Malformation

Children with an anorectal malformation, whether isolated or as part of the VACTERL association discussed later in this chapter, carry an increased risk of coexisting occult spinal dysraphism and tethered cord, reflecting shared embryologic disruption of the caudal cell mass from which both the anorectal and distal spinal structures derive; spinal imaging is therefore a standard, proactive component of the newborn evaluation for any infant with an anorectal malformation, applying the same coordinated, association-driven screening approach this chapter applies to VACTERL more broadly, rather than reserved only for an infant who also happens to show one of the cutaneous markers discussed in this chapter's final section.

Anesthetic and Positioning Considerations for Spinal MRI

Obtaining diagnostic-quality spinal MRI in the young infant or child requires attention to positioning that maintains a neutral spinal alignment throughout image acquisition, since flexion or extension artifact can meaningfully distort the conus position measurement central to this section's diagnostic framework; coordinating positioning technique with the sedation and motion-reduction strategies discussed in Chapter 1, and confirming neutral alignment on preliminary localizer images before completing the full diagnostic sequence, protects against the specific, correctable technical pitfall of a falsely low or falsely normal conus measurement caused by positioning artifact rather than true anatomic variation.

Filum Terminale Lipoma Versus Normal Filum Fat

A small amount of fat within an otherwise normal-caliber filum terminale is occasionally identified as an incidental finding and, when the filum thickness itself remains within the normal range discussed earlier in this section, does not necessarily indicate clinically significant tethering, a distinction worth making explicitly since the mere presence of any fat signal within the filum is sometimes over-interpreted as diagnostic of tethering regardless of the accompanying thickness measurement; correlating fat signal with filum caliber, rather than treating fat presence alone as a binary diagnostic criterion, provides the more accurate, nuanced interpretation this section's overall framework depends upon.

Tethered spinal cord, a condition in which the spinal cord is abnormally fixed rather than free to ascend normally within the spinal canal during growth, is both a direct complication of the closed dysraphism entities discussed above and a distinct diagnostic consideration in the child with occult, imaging-only evidence of an underlying dysraphic process not apparent on external examination. The conus-position-plus-filum-characterization framework developed across this section applies consistently whether tethering is suspected because of a cutaneous marker, a progressive neurologic symptom, or an incidental finding on imaging obtained for an unrelated reason.

Feature	Normal	Tethered Cord Concerning Finding
Conus position (at term)	At or above L2-L3	Below L2-L3
Filum thickness	≤2 mm	>2 mm

Filum signal	Normal (no fat)	Fat signal present
Clinical trajectory	Static, non-progressive	Progressive weakness, bladder/bowel change, or pain

THE CLINICAL-IMAGING CROSSWALK SYSTEM — A Borderline Conus Position With a Normal Filum

The Crossing: A two-year-old undergoes spine MRI for evaluation of a sacral dimple, discussed further in this chapter's final section, and the conus terminates at the L2-L3 disc space, a borderline position relative to the normal range discussed in this section.

Presentation Signature: An asymptomatic toddler with a borderline conus level and no progressive neurologic or urologic symptom, referred for a cutaneous marker rather than a specific neurologic complaint.

Imaging Correlate: The filum terminale is carefully assessed and found to be normal in thickness and signal, without fat content, and no other dysraphic finding is identified elsewhere in the spine on the full study.

Trap Logic: A borderline conus position in isolation, without a thickened or fatty filum or another supporting dysraphic finding, does not by itself confirm tethering, and recommending surgical intervention based on conus position alone, without the corroborating filum assessment this section emphasizes, risks an unnecessary surgical referral for a borderline normal variant.

Crossing Anchor: A borderline conus position is interpreted alongside filum thickness and signal, not in isolation; a normal filum and the absence of progressive symptoms support conservative observation rather than surgical referral for an isolated borderline finding.

Vertebral Segmentation Anomalies

Beyond the neural tube and cord anomalies addressed in the preceding sections, disruption of normal vertebral segmentation produces its own distinct spectrum of congenital spine anomalies, frequently coexisting with dysraphism and carrying important associations with malformation elsewhere in the body that this section develops.

Hemivertebrae and Wedge Vertebrae

A hemivertebra, in which only one half of a vertebral body forms, and a wedge vertebra, in which a vertebral body forms asymmetrically without the complete absence of a hemivertebra, each produce focal, angular spinal curvature and are among the most common causes of congenital, as opposed to the more familiar idiopathic, scoliosis; a fully segmented, unilateral hemivertebra with normal disc spaces above and below carries a higher risk of progressive curvature than a partially segmented or incarcerated hemivertebra, making precise segmentation-pattern characterization directly relevant to the surgical decision-making orthopedic spine surgery colleagues undertake for this population. This same segmentation-pattern-to-risk logic recurs throughout the remainder of this section, applied to block vertebrae and the combined patterns discussed next.

Block Vertebrae and Failure of Segmentation

Failure of normal segmentation between adjacent vertebral levels, producing a block vertebra in which two or more vertebral bodies remain fused, is mechanistically distinct from the hemivertebra and wedge vertebra anomalies discussed above, reflecting a failure of the normal segmentation process rather than a failure of formation; a symmetric block vertebra typically produces less curvature than an asymmetric segmentation failure, though a mixed pattern combining both formation and segmentation failure at adjacent levels, sometimes termed a unilateral unsegmented bar, carries a particularly high risk of severe, rapidly progressive curvature given the combined growth-restriction and asymmetric-growth mechanisms acting together.

VACTERL Association

Vertebral segmentation anomalies are a defining component of VACTERL association, a nonrandom co-occurrence of Vertebral anomalies, Anal atresia, Cardiac defects, Tracheoesophageal fistula, Renal anomalies, and Limb abnormalities, and identifying a vertebral segmentation anomaly on spine imaging should prompt systematic screening for the other VACTERL components, including echocardiography, renal ultrasound, and careful examination for anal and limb involvement, since a child meeting criteria for this association requires this specific, coordinated multisystem evaluation rather than a spine-focused evaluation alone; VACTERL is a descriptive association rather than a single genetic syndrome with one identifiable causative gene, and while a subset of cases have an identifiable underlying genetic or chromosomal cause, many do not, a point worth communicating honestly to families seeking a single unifying explanation. The diagnostic threshold conventionally applied requires at least three of the six component findings, a criterion worth stating explicitly so that an isolated vertebral anomaly alone is not mislabeled as VACTERL association without the supporting additional findings this threshold requires.

Klippel-Feil Syndrome

Klippel-Feil syndrome, characterized by congenital fusion of two or more cervical vertebrae, presents with a classic though not universally present clinical triad of a short neck, low posterior hairline, and limited cervical range of motion, and is associated with an increased risk of Sprengel deformity (a congenitally undescended scapula), renal anomaly, and, of particular clinical importance, craniocervical instability that can predispose to serious neurologic injury with relatively minor trauma; recognizing this instability risk and providing the family and any treating clinicians, including sports and physical activity guidance, with clear precautions regarding activities carrying craniocervical injury risk is an important, practical component of the counseling that follows this specific diagnosis.

Imaging Approach to Suspected Segmentation Anomaly

Plain radiography remains a useful, low-cost first-line screening tool for suspected vertebral segmentation anomaly, particularly for longitudinal curvature monitoring over time, while MRI is added specifically to evaluate for an associated intraspinal anomaly, including the dysraphism and tethering entities discussed earlier in this chapter, which coexist with segmentation anomalies frequently enough that MRI evaluation of the full spinal axis is standard practice once a significant segmentation anomaly is identified, applying the same coordinated, question-driven multimodality approach emphasized throughout this book rather than relying on a single modality to answer every relevant question.

Orthopedic Surgical Considerations for Progressive Congenital Curvature

Surgical management of progressive congenital scoliosis related to the segmentation anomalies discussed in this section, including growth-preserving instrumentation techniques in the young child and definitive fusion in the older child approaching skeletal maturity, is coordinated closely between pediatric orthopedic spine surgery and, given the frequent coexisting intraspinal findings discussed above, pediatric neurosurgery, since intraspinal pathology such as a tethered cord or split cord malformation must generally be addressed before or concurrent with orthopedic curvature correction to avoid precipitating an acute neurologic injury during spinal instrumentation and correction.

Sprengel Deformity and Associated Musculoskeletal Findings

Beyond the specific renal, cardiac, and craniocervical associations discussed elsewhere in this section, vertebral segmentation anomalies, particularly in the cervical spine, frequently coexist with additional musculoskeletal findings including Sprengel deformity, an undescended, congenitally malpositioned scapula, and rib anomalies; a coordinated orthopedic evaluation extending beyond the spine itself to the shoulder girdle and chest wall, applying the same principle of active, systematic multisystem examination developed throughout this chapter, ensures these frequently coexisting findings are identified and addressed as part of a comprehensive, rather than spine-only, evaluation.

Genetic Evaluation for Vertebral Segmentation Anomalies

A subset of vertebral segmentation anomalies, particularly those occurring as part of a recognized syndrome such as spondylocostal dysostosis, are associated with identifiable single-gene causes affecting the segmentation clock genes governing normal somite formation during early development, and genetics referral is appropriately pursued when a segmentation anomaly presents alongside a recognizable syndromic pattern rather than as an isolated finding within the broader VACTERL association discussed above, which, as noted, more often lacks a single identifiable genetic cause; distinguishing a syndromic, single-gene segmentation disorder from the more etiologically heterogeneous VACTERL association shapes both the specific genetic testing pursued and the recurrence risk counseling ultimately provided to the family.

Longitudinal Curvature Surveillance Through Growth

Because vertebral segmentation anomalies carry a curvature-progression risk that is highly dependent on the child's growth velocity, serial spine radiographs at intervals timed to the child's growth phase, more frequent during periods of rapid growth such as infancy and puberty and less frequent during the relatively slower mid-childhood growth period, provide the most clinically useful surveillance pattern; a fixed, uniform imaging interval applied without regard to growth phase risks either missing a rapid progression during a high-risk growth period or obtaining unnecessarily frequent imaging during a lower-risk period, reinforcing the value of individualized, growth-informed surveillance planning over a one-size-fits-all interval.

Cervical Spine Considerations in the Skeletal Dysplasia Population

Several skeletal dysplasias beyond Klippel-Feil syndrome, discussed earlier in this section, carry an independently elevated risk of cervical spine instability related to odontoid hypoplasia or other craniocervical junction anomaly, and a child with a known or suspected skeletal dysplasia warrants dedicated cervical spine imaging, including flexion-extension views when clinically tolerated, as part of the baseline evaluation, applying the same proactive screening principle developed throughout this chapter to a population defined by its underlying skeletal, rather than solely spinal, diagnosis; this evaluation carries particular urgency before any procedure requiring neck manipulation or extension, including endotracheal intubation, given the acute injury risk an unrecognized instability poses in that specific clinical circumstance.

Distinguishing Congenital From Idiopathic Scoliosis on Imaging

Congenital scoliosis, arising from the vertebral segmentation anomalies discussed throughout this section and typically apparent from infancy or early childhood, is distinguished from the far more common idiopathic scoliosis of later childhood and adolescence by the presence of a specific, identifiable vertebral anomaly, a hemivertebra, block vertebra, or unsegmented bar, rather than the structurally normal vertebrae characteristic of idiopathic curvature; this distinction carries direct management implications, since congenital scoliosis related to a specific structural anomaly is evaluated and monitored using the anomaly-specific, progression-risk framework developed in this section, while idiopathic scoliosis follows a separate, well-established surveillance and bracing protocol outside this chapter's primary focus.

Beyond the neural tube and cord anomalies addressed in the preceding sections, disruption of normal vertebral segmentation produces its own distinct spectrum of congenital spine anomalies, frequently coexisting with dysraphism and carrying important associations with malformation elsewhere in the body that this section develops. The VACTERL and Klippel-Feil associations discussed in this section exemplify this chapter's recurring theme that a spinal finding is frequently a signal for systematic evaluation well beyond the spine itself.

Figure 9.2: Hemivertebra and Block Vertebra Segmentation Patterns

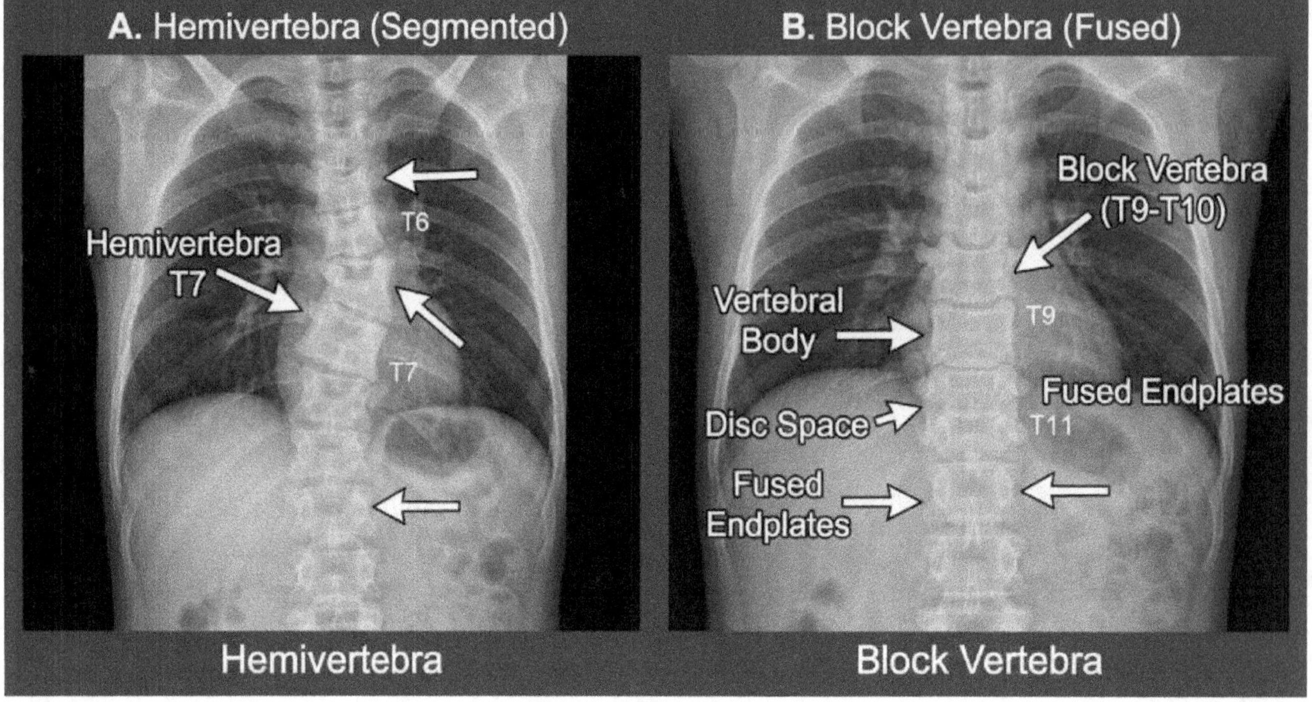

Associated Cutaneous and Clinical Markers

This closing section addresses the specific cutaneous findings that should prompt spinal imaging evaluation in an otherwise asymptomatic infant, translating the anatomic and pathophysiologic reasoning developed throughout this chapter into a practical, bedside screening framework.

The Simple Sacral Dimple: A Low-Risk Finding

A simple sacral dimple, a small, shallow midline pit located within the natal cleft close to the anus, with a visible base and no other associated cutaneous finding, is a common, generally benign finding present in a substantial minority of healthy newborns and does not, by itself, warrant imaging, since published cohort data demonstrate a very low yield of clinically significant underlying dysraphism for this specific, isolated, low-risk pattern; correctly reassuring a family regarding a simple, low-risk sacral dimple, rather than reflexively obtaining imaging for every dimple encountered on newborn examination, is an important application of the low-yield-presentation reasoning developed in Chapter 3 to this specific, high-volume newborn screening context. This same structured, evidence-based approach to distinguishing high-risk from low-risk cutaneous findings extends naturally to the remaining markers discussed throughout the rest of this section.

High-Risk Cutaneous Markers Warranting Imaging

In contrast to the low-risk simple dimple discussed above, a cluster of specific cutaneous findings carries a substantially higher associated risk of underlying dysraphism and warrants spinal imaging: a hairy patch (hypertrichosis) overlying the lower spine, a subcutaneous lipoma, a hemangioma, particularly a large or midline lesion, a dermal sinus tract, especially one located above the natal cleft or with a deep, non-visualizable base, and any dimple that is large, located away from the midline, or associated with an adjacent skin tag or other cutaneous abnormality; the presence of any one of these specific findings, applied as a structured checklist rather than an unstructured gestalt impression, should prompt spinal ultrasound in the young infant or MRI in the older infant, applying the age-based modality selection reasoning developed earlier in this chapter. Each of these findings reflects a distinct embryologic marker of the underlying dysraphic process, whether an ectodermal remnant, a fatty inclusion, or a vascular anomaly, tracing back to the same disrupted neural tube closure or secondary neurulation processes discussed throughout this chapter's earlier sections.

The Dermal Sinus Tract and Infection Risk

A dermal sinus tract, an epithelial-lined tract extending from the skin surface toward or into the spinal canal, carries a distinct and clinically urgent risk beyond the general dysraphism-association discussed above: direct communication between the skin surface and the intradural space creates a pathway for ascending infection, including meningitis and, at times, an intraspinal dermoid or epidermoid abscess, making prompt imaging characterization of tract depth and intraspinal extent a genuine clinical priority rather than a routine, unhurried evaluation, particularly in an infant presenting with fever or signs of meningitis in whom this specific anatomic pathway should be actively considered as a potential infectious source. Surgical excision of the full tract, including any intraspinal component identified on imaging, is generally recommended even in an asymptomatic infant specifically because of this ongoing infection risk, distinguishing the management urgency of this particular finding from several of the other, more conservatively managed cutaneous markers discussed elsewhere in this section.

Combining Multiple Cutaneous Markers

The presence of more than one cutaneous marker in the same infant, such as a hairy patch combined with a subcutaneous lipoma, further increases the associated likelihood of significant underlying dysraphism beyond the risk conferred by either finding in isolation, reinforcing the value of a complete, systematic skin examination of the entire lower back and sacrococcygeal region, rather than stopping evaluation once a single finding has been identified, in every newborn assessment; documenting each specific finding present, rather than a general description such as birthmark noted, gives the interpreting radiologist and the ordering clinician a more precise basis for correlating the specific cutaneous pattern against the specific imaging findings ultimately identified.

Coordinating Newborn Examination Findings With Imaging Referral

Because the cutaneous markers discussed in this section are identified at the newborn examination, typically performed by a pediatrician or nursery clinician rather than a neurologist, clear, structured newborn examination guidance regarding which specific findings warrant referral, incorporating the high-risk-versus-low-risk distinction developed in this section, supports appropriate, timely imaging referral at the point of first contact rather than depending on the finding being recognized as significant only later, at a delayed subspecialty visit; a structured newborn examination checklist or decision aid, distributed to referring pediatric and nursery colleagues, is a practical, systems-level application of the reasoning this chapter has developed at the level of an individual clinical encounter.

Sacrococcygeal Teratoma as a Distinct Midline Mass

A sacrococcygeal teratoma, a germ cell tumor arising at the sacrococcygeal region and among the most common congenital tumors of infancy, must be distinguished from the dysraphism-associated cutaneous markers discussed throughout this section, since although both can present as a midline sacral mass, a teratoma is a distinct oncologic entity requiring its own dedicated imaging characterization, staging, and surgical management pathway rather than the dysraphism-focused evaluation this chapter otherwise emphasizes; a solid or mixed solid-cystic mass with heterogeneous imaging characteristics, as opposed to the simple cystic or fatty appearance typical of the dysraphism-related entities discussed above, should prompt this alternative diagnostic pathway and coordinated oncology involvement.

Family Education on Ongoing Monitoring for Delayed-Presentation Markers

Because some cutaneous markers, particularly a subtle hairy patch or a small dermal sinus tract opening, may not be immediately apparent or may be overlooked at a single newborn examination, particularly if performed briefly or under suboptimal lighting conditions, educating families to continue observing the lower back and sacrococcygeal region during routine care, and to report any newly noticed finding at a subsequent well-child visit, extends this chapter's screening framework beyond the single newborn examination into the ongoing, longitudinal well-child care relationship, applying the same proactive, structured surveillance principle this book emphasizes across many other conditions.

Ultrasound Timing Window and Its Practical Limitations

Spinal ultrasound screening for a cutaneous marker is most reliable before approximately four to six months of age, since progressive ossification of the posterior spinal elements beyond this window increasingly limits the acoustic window available for adequate visualization, applying the same age-dependent imaging-window reasoning developed in Chapter 1 for cranial ultrasound to this related, sacrococcygeal application; an infant referred beyond this window, or one in whom an ultrasound performed within the window yields an equivocal or technically limited result, should proceed directly to MRI rather than a repeat, likely similarly limited ultrasound attempt.

Counseling Families of an Infant With a Reassuring Low-Risk Marker

When a newborn examination identifies only a simple, low-risk sacral dimple without any of the high-risk features discussed in this section, the family is well served by clear, confident reassurance, applying the same evidence-based, honestly communicated reasoning developed in Chapter 3 for other low-yield presentations, rather than a hedged or uncertain response that might inadvertently suggest unresolved concern; explaining specifically why this particular finding does not warrant imaging, referencing the visible base and absence of any of the high-risk features named in this section, gives the family concrete, retainable reasoning rather than a bare reassurance they may not fully trust.

Documentation Standards for Cutaneous Marker Findings

Given the direct clinical significance of the specific cutaneous features discussed throughout this section, precise, structured documentation at the newborn examination, describing the exact location, size, and specific character of any midline lower back finding, using photography where available and consistent with institutional policy, supports both the immediate referral decision and any later comparison should the finding evolve or a new concern emerge; a documentation habit of simply noting dimple present, without the specific descriptive detail this section has developed, provides materially less clinical value to any subsequent clinician relying on that newborn record.

Atypical Presentations Beyond the Classic Newborn Screening Window

Although this section has emphasized newborn examination as the primary point of cutaneous marker identification, a child can occasionally present later in infancy or childhood with a previously unrecognized cutaneous marker, whether because it was genuinely absent or subtle at birth and became more apparent with growth, such as a hairy patch becoming more visible as hair growth progresses, or because it was simply missed on an earlier, less thorough examination; the same high-risk-versus-low-risk evaluation framework developed in this section applies regardless of the child's age at identification, and a delayed identification should prompt the same prompt imaging evaluation this section recommends for the classic newborn presentation, rather than a lower priority response simply because the finding was not identified at birth.

This closing section addresses the specific cutaneous findings that should prompt spinal imaging evaluation in an otherwise asymptomatic infant, translating the anatomic and pathophysiologic reasoning developed throughout this chapter into a practical, bedside screening framework. Applied together with the open-versus-closed dysraphism distinction, the tethered cord evaluation, and the vertebral segmentation reasoning developed earlier in this chapter, this framework equips the reader to move confidently from a newborn examination finding through to a precise, evidence-based imaging and referral decision.

Case Presentation: Fetal Myelomeningocele Repair

A twenty-four-week fetal MRI obtained after prenatal ultrasound identified a lumbosacral myelomeningocele confirms an L4-level defect with Chiari II malformation and moderate ventriculomegaly, and the family meets anatomic and maternal eligibility criteria for fetal surgical repair at a specialized center, discussed earlier in this chapter. Following successful in-utero closure at twenty-five weeks, the family is counseled that fetal repair has been shown to reduce, though not eliminate, the likelihood of postnatal shunt placement, and postnatal MRI after delivery confirms improved, though not fully resolved, hindbrain herniation. Applying the reasoning developed in this chapter, close postnatal surveillance for both hydrocephalus and the tethered cord risk inherent to any myelomeningocele repair, fetal or postnatal, is established as part of the child's long-term, structured neurosurgical follow-up plan, alongside the coordinated urologic and orthopedic surveillance this chapter has emphasized as a necessary companion to the neurosurgical follow-up itself.

Case Presentation: VACTERL Association Identified Through a Vertebral Anomaly

A newborn with imperforate anus identified at delivery undergoes the coordinated multisystem screening this chapter recommends for any infant with an anorectal malformation, including spine radiography, which identifies multiple thoracic hemivertebrae. Applying the VACTERL framework developed in this chapter, echocardiography identifies a small ventricular septal defect, and renal ultrasound identifies a unilateral duplicated collecting system; a tracheoesophageal fistula is excluded on clinical and radiographic evaluation, and limb examination is normal. The family is counseled that this child meets criteria for VACTERL association based on the combination of vertebral, anal, cardiac, and renal findings, that a single unifying genetic cause is often not identifiable despite comprehensive testing, and that ongoing coordinated surveillance across each affected organ system, including the spinal MRI evaluation for occult dysraphism this chapter recommends specifically for anorectal malformation, will structure the child's multidisciplinary care going forward.

Case Presentation: A Newborn With a High-Risk Cutaneous Marker Cluster

A term newborn's routine examination identifies a hairy patch overlying the lower lumbar spine together with an adjacent small subcutaneous lipoma, findings meeting this chapter's high-risk criteria for underlying dysraphism. Spinal ultrasound performed at two weeks of age, applying the sedation-free young-infant imaging approach discussed in this chapter, demonstrates a low-lying conus at L3 with a thickened, fatty filum terminale, confirming an underlying closed dysraphism with tethering. Neurosurgery is consulted, and given the infant's currently normal neurologic examination, elective, rather than emergent, surgical release is planned for early infancy, applying the shared decision-making approach discussed earlier in this chapter to the timing question specifically, while the family is counseled to monitor for any of the progressive symptoms described in this chapter that would prompt more urgent reevaluation in the interim. This case exemplifies the complete diagnostic arc this chapter has developed: a cutaneous marker prompting imaging, imaging confirming tethering through the conus-and-filum framework, and a shared, individualized surgical timing decision informed by the child's current, asymptomatic clinical status.

THE CLINICAL-IMAGING CROSSWALK SYSTEM — Spinal Dysraphism and Segmentation Anomaly Recognition

---

Crossing 1 Recap: A borderline conus position is interpreted alongside filum thickness and signal, not in isolation; a normal filum and absence of progressive symptoms support conservative observation.

Chapter Anchor: Open dysraphism is a surgical urgency from exposed neural tissue; closed dysraphism and vertebral segmentation anomalies are distinguished by their specific anatomic pattern, associated systemic findings, and cutaneous markers, each directly shaping imaging modality, timing, and the multisystem evaluation that follows. The reasoning developed across all four sections converges on a single practical habit: whenever a spinal finding is identified, whether through a cutaneous marker, a progressive symptom, or an incidental imaging finding, the reader should systematically ask what it implies about neural tube closure, cord mobility, vertebral formation, and, where relevant, coexisting organ-system involvement, rather than evaluating the spine in isolation from the rest of the child's development.

Summary and Key Concepts

Open spinal dysraphism, most commonly myelomeningocele, exposes neural tissue and carries surgical urgency and a near-obligate Chiari II association; fetal surgical repair, where anatomically eligible, reduces shunt-placement risk relative to postnatal repair, and lifelong latex precaution, bladder/bowel, and urologic surveillance are standard companion components of care.

Tethered cord is confirmed by a low conus position correlated with filum thickness and signal, not conus position alone, and presents with a progressive, rather than static, clinical trajectory that itself supports the diagnosis; re-tethering risk persists after repair and is assessed against a stable postoperative baseline.

Vertebral segmentation anomalies, including hemivertebrae and block vertebrae, are a defining component of VACTERL association and warrant systematic multisystem screening; Klippel-Feil syndrome and several skeletal dysplasias carry a distinct craniocervical instability risk requiring activity and procedural precautions.

A simple, midline sacral dimple with a visible base is a low-yield finding not warranting imaging; a hairy patch, lipoma, hemangioma, or dermal sinus tract, especially in combination, warrants prompt spinal imaging given the meaningfully higher associated dysraphism risk, applicable regardless of the age at which the marker is first identified.

A dermal sinus tract carries a distinct, urgent infection risk given its direct communication with the intradural space and should be actively considered as a potential source in an infant presenting with fever or meningitis; sacrococcygeal teratoma is a distinct oncologic mimic requiring its own dedicated evaluation pathway.

CHAPTER 10: HYDROCEPHALUS AND DISORDERS OF CSF DYNAMICS

Learning Objectives

1. Classify hydrocephalus as communicating or obstructive and identify the specific imaging pattern associated with each major mechanism, including choroid plexus overproduction as a distinct, less common cause.
2. Recognize the imaging findings of shunt malfunction and describe the appropriate rapid-imaging evaluation pathway, including the specific exceptions posed by slit ventricle syndrome and loculated hydrocephalus.
3. Distinguish idiopathic intracranial hypertension from other causes of papilledema and describe its characteristic, though nonspecific, imaging findings, and from pseudopapilledema mimics such as optic disc drusen.
4. Distinguish an incidental arachnoid cyst from a cyst requiring neurosurgical evaluation, and from its epidermoid, neuroglial, and porencephalic cyst mimics.

Classification and Mechanisms of Hydrocephalus

Hydrocephalus, an excess accumulation of cerebrospinal fluid within the ventricular system producing ventricular enlargement, is classified fundamentally by mechanism into communicating and obstructive forms, a distinction that directly determines both the expected imaging pattern and the surgical approach best suited to each specific case.

Communicating Versus Obstructive Hydrocephalus

Communicating hydrocephalus results from impaired cerebrospinal fluid resorption at the level of the arachnoid granulations, without any obstruction to flow within the ventricular system itself, producing uniform enlargement of all four ventricles; obstructive, or noncommunicating, hydrocephalus results from a mechanical blockage at a specific point along the cerebrospinal fluid pathway, producing enlargement confined to the ventricles proximal to the obstruction while the ventricles distal to the blockage remain normal in size, a distinguishing pattern that itself localizes the level of obstruction before any further evaluation is undertaken, and this pattern-based localization is the single most useful first step in any hydrocephalus workup.

Aqueductal Stenosis as the Prototypical Obstructive Cause

Aqueductal stenosis, narrowing or obstruction of the cerebral aqueduct connecting the third and fourth ventricles, is among the most common causes of congenital obstructive hydrocephalus and produces a characteristic pattern of dilated lateral and third ventricles with a normal-sized fourth ventricle, directly localizing the obstruction to the aqueduct itself; congenital aqueductal stenosis may be idiopathic, genetic, most notably in X-linked hydrocephalus related to L1CAM mutations, or secondary to a prior intraventricular hemorrhage or infection producing aqueductal scarring, each carrying distinct counseling implications the imaging pattern alone cannot fully resolve without correlation to the clinical history. Thin-section, high-resolution sagittal imaging through the aqueduct itself, applying the dedicated-protocol principle from Chapter 1, is often necessary to distinguish a discrete, membranous web from a longer-segment, gliotic stenosis, a distinction that can influence the choice between endoscopic third ventriculostomy and shunt placement discussed later in this chapter.

Posthemorrhagic and Postinfectious Hydrocephalus

Posthemorrhagic hydrocephalus, introduced in Chapter 5 as a complication of germinal matrix and intraventricular hemorrhage, and postinfectious hydrocephalus, arising from inflammatory obliteration of the arachnoid granulations or ventricular pathways following meningitis discussed in Chapter 15, both typically produce a communicating pattern reflecting impaired resorption at the arachnoid granulations, though postinfectious hydrocephalus can additionally produce loculated, obstructive components when inflammatory debris and adhesions partition the ventricular system into isolated, separately pressurized compartments, a more complex pattern requiring correspondingly more complex, multi-catheter surgical management. Distinguishing a purely communicating postinfectious pattern from one already showing early loculation at the time of initial diagnosis, discussed further in the shunt malfunction section of this chapter, allows the surgical team to anticipate and plan for this added complexity from the outset rather than discovering it only after an initial single-catheter shunt has already failed.

Hydrocephalus Associated With Structural Malformation

Several of the congenital malformations discussed in Chapter 8, including Dandy-Walker malformation and the Chiari malformations, carry an independent, malformation-specific hydrocephalus risk operating through mechanisms distinct from the acquired posthemorrhagic and postinfectious causes discussed above, and recognizing the specific underlying malformation, rather than treating hydrocephalus as a generic, undifferentiated finding, directly shapes the anticipated surgical approach, since the obstruction level and the presence of any additional structural abnormality relevant to catheter placement varies by the specific underlying malformation. A shunt catheter trajectory planned without accounting for an associated malformation's distorted ventricular anatomy risks a technically more difficult placement or a suboptimal catheter position, reinforcing why the malformation-specific imaging characterization developed in Chapter 8 remains directly relevant to the surgical planning this chapter addresses.

Choroid Plexus Overproduction Hydrocephalus

A distinct, uncommon mechanism, hydrocephalus from choroid plexus overproduction, most classically associated with choroid plexus papilloma, produces hydrocephalus through cerebrospinal fluid overproduction exceeding normal resorptive capacity rather than through the impaired resorption or mechanical obstruction mechanisms discussed above; identifying an enhancing intraventricular mass, discussed further in Chapter 12, in a child with hydrocephalus should prompt consideration of this overproduction mechanism specifically, since surgical management in this circumstance appropriately targets tumor resection, which frequently resolves the hydrocephalus directly, rather than proceeding immediately to a shunt procedure that would address only the downstream consequence rather than the underlying overproduction source. Distinguishing this overproduction mechanism from the more common obstructive pattern a choroid plexus tumor can also produce through direct mechanical blockage of cerebrospinal fluid pathways requires careful correlation of the tumor's specific location and size against the resulting ventricular pattern, since a single tumor can, in some cases, act through both mechanisms simultaneously.

Ventricular Measurement and Standardized Assessment

Quantifying ventricular size using standardized measurements, including the frontal and occipital horn ratio and, in the neonate, the ventricular index and anterior horn width discussed in Chapter 5, provides a more reproducible, comparable assessment than qualitative visual impression alone, particularly important given the serial imaging surveillance most hydrocephalus diagnoses require over time; applying age-adjusted normative reference ranges to these measurements, consistent with the age-specific interpretive framework established in Chapter 2, avoids both under-recognition of genuinely pathologic enlargement and over-diagnosis of the benign extra-axial fluid patterns and normal ventricular variation discussed elsewhere in this book. Recording these standardized measurements explicitly in every report, rather than only when a value appears subjectively abnormal, builds the consistent longitudinal dataset that later serial comparison depends upon.

Clinical Presentation Across Age Groups

Clinical presentation of hydrocephalus varies substantially by age, reflecting the differing capacity of the skull to accommodate rising intracranial pressure: an infant with open sutures and a patent fontanelle presents with progressive macrocephaly, a bulging fontanelle, and split sutures, allowing some compensatory accommodation before acute decompensation, while an older child with fused sutures presents more acutely with headache, vomiting, and papilledema once compensatory mechanisms are exhausted, since the closed skull cannot expand to accommodate rising pressure in the same way; recognizing this age-dependent presentation pattern directs the urgency and specific findings sought on both examination and imaging.

Endoscopic Third Ventriculostomy as an Alternative to Shunting

For selected cases of obstructive hydrocephalus, particularly aqueductal stenosis, endoscopic third ventriculostomy, in which a surgically created opening in the floor of the third ventricle allows cerebrospinal fluid to bypass the obstruction and flow directly into the subarachnoid space, offers a shunt-independent alternative that avoids the lifelong hardware-related complications discussed later in this chapter; precise preoperative imaging characterization of the third ventricular floor anatomy and the basilar artery position relative to the planned fenestration site is essential to safe surgical planning, and postoperative imaging assessing flow through the newly created stoma, using dedicated cerebrospinal fluid flow sequences, confirms whether the procedure has achieved adequate, durable decompression. Success rates for this procedure vary meaningfully by the child's age and the specific underlying cause of the obstruction, with older children and those with a discrete, focal aqueductal obstruction generally showing more favorable outcomes than very young infants or those with a more diffuse, communicating component to their hydrocephalus.

Fetal and Antenatal Diagnosis of Hydrocephalus

Ventriculomegaly identified on prenatal ultrasound, ranging from mild, isolated enlargement to severe, frank hydrocephalus, prompts fetal MRI evaluation applying the same principles developed in Chapter 1, both to characterize the specific underlying cause where identifiable and to assess for additional structural anomalies elsewhere in the brain that might indicate a broader malformation syndrome rather than isolated hydrocephalus; mild, isolated ventriculomegaly, particularly when stable or only slowly progressive on serial prenatal surveillance, carries a more favorable prognosis than progressive or severe ventriculomegaly accompanied by additional structural findings, information that directly shapes the prenatal counseling conversation this chapter's broader framework consistently emphasizes.

Long-Term Neurodevelopmental Outcome in Treated Hydrocephalus

Neurodevelopmental outcome in treated hydrocephalus depends substantially on the underlying cause and any associated brain injury or malformation rather than on the presence of hydrocephalus or its surgical treatment alone, meaning a child with hydrocephalus secondary to an isolated, successfully treated aqueductal stenosis without other structural abnormality carries a materially different prognosis than a child with hydrocephalus secondary to severe intraventricular hemorrhage with extensive associated parenchymal injury, discussed in Chapter 5; communicating this cause-specific, rather than generic, prognosis is essential to avoid either falsely reassuring or falsely alarming a family based on the hydrocephalus diagnosis alone, independent of its underlying etiology.

Structured Radiology Report Elements for Hydrocephalus

Applying the structured reporting discipline established in Chapter 1, a report characterizing hydrocephalus should explicitly state the specific ventricles involved, the standardized size measurements discussed earlier in this section rather than a purely qualitative descriptor, the presumed level of obstruction where an obstructive pattern is present, and any identified underlying cause or associated malformation; this structured approach gives the referring neurosurgical team the precise, reproducible information needed for surgical planning and gives future readers a genuine, quantitative baseline for the serial comparison this condition typically requires over a child's lifetime.

Hydrocephalus, an excess accumulation of cerebrospinal fluid within the ventricular system producing ventricular enlargement, is classified fundamentally by mechanism into communicating and obstructive forms, a distinction that directly determines both the expected imaging pattern and the surgical approach best suited to each specific case. The mechanistic reasoning developed across this section, applied consistently from congenital through acquired and malformation-associated causes, establishes the diagnostic foundation the remaining three sections of this chapter build upon.

Figure 10.1: Communicating Versus Obstructive Hydrocephalus

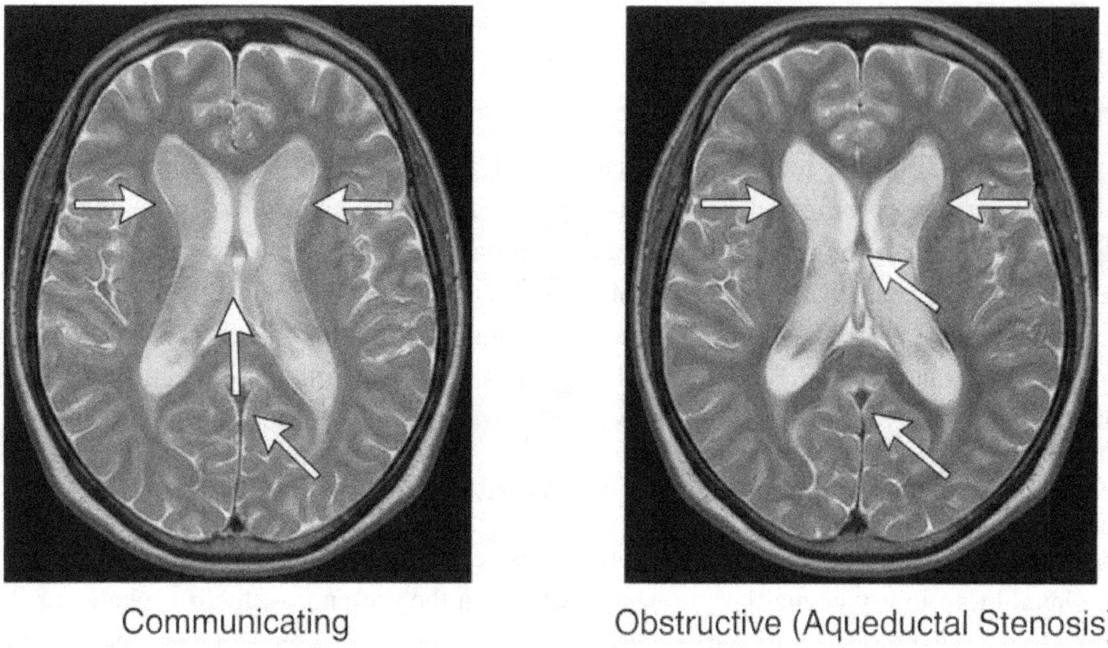

Imaging of Shunt Malfunction and Complications

Ventriculoperitoneal shunting remains the most common surgical treatment for hydrocephalus, and shunt malfunction, a frequent complication over a shunted child's lifetime, represents one of the more common pediatric neurosurgical emergencies a clinician will encounter, making rapid, accurate imaging evaluation for this specific complication a critical skill this section develops.

Clinical Presentation of Shunt Malfunction

Shunt malfunction presents with signs and symptoms of recurrent elevated intracranial pressure, including headache, vomiting, lethargy, and, in the infant with an open fontanelle, a bulging fontanelle and rapidly increasing head circumference, and a family or child with a known shunt is frequently able to recognize these symptoms as consistent with their own or their child's prior malfunction episodes, a history worth eliciting directly and weighting heavily, since a family's pattern recognition from prior episodes is often a highly reliable clinical indicator even before imaging confirmation. In the older child or adolescent, more subtle presentations, including a change in school performance, personality change, or new-onset diplopia from sixth cranial nerve palsy related to elevated pressure, can represent an atypical malfunction presentation that a less experienced clinician might not immediately connect to the underlying shunt, underscoring the value of maintaining a broad symptom index of suspicion in any child with a shunt history presenting with a new, otherwise unexplained neurologic or behavioral change.

Rapid Imaging Protocol for Suspected Malfunction

Evaluating suspected shunt malfunction requires rapid imaging comparing current ventricular size against the child's own established baseline, applying the same baseline-comparison principle emphasized throughout this book, using either fast, motion-robust MRI sequences or CT depending on institutional protocol and the specific urgency of the presentation, consistent with the acute-modality-selection reasoning developed in Chapter 3; a complete shunt series, plain radiographs of the skull, chest, and abdomen tracing the entire catheter course, is obtained alongside the cross-sectional imaging specifically to assess for a mechanical catheter problem, including disconnection, migration, or fracture, that cross-sectional imaging alone may not fully characterize. Many centers have adopted rapid, limited-sequence MRI protocols specifically for this indication, completing acquisition in only a few minutes without sedation in most children, which both reduces radiation exposure relative to CT and reduces the logistical burden that a lengthier, sedated study would impose on an acutely symptomatic child and family.

Ventricular Size Change as the Primary Imaging Indicator

Interval increase in ventricular size compared to the child's established baseline is the primary, most reliable imaging indicator of shunt malfunction, reinforcing why obtaining and clearly documenting a baseline study at a time of known shunt function, rather than relying on a single isolated measurement without a prior comparison, is essential to accurate malfunction assessment; a ventricular size that appears large in absolute terms but is unchanged from the child's own chronic baseline is a fundamentally different, generally reassuring finding compared to a ventricular size that has genuinely increased from that same baseline, a distinction that cannot be made without the comparison study, and this comparison should be explicit and stated directly in the report rather than left for the referring clinician to infer independently.

The Challenge of Slit Ventricle Syndrome

Slit ventricle syndrome, in which chronically over-shunted, small, slit-like ventricles paradoxically fail to enlarge even during a genuine malfunction episode because the ventricular walls have become abnormally noncompliant, presents a specific diagnostic challenge in which the primary imaging indicator discussed above, interval ventricular enlargement, may be absent or minimal despite a genuine, symptomatic malfunction; recognizing this specific scenario in a child with a known history of chronically small ventricles, and correlating imaging findings more heavily with the clinical presentation and, where available, direct intracranial pressure monitoring rather than ventricular size change alone, prevents a falsely reassuring imaging interpretation in this specific subpopulation. Direct intracranial pressure monitoring, whether through a temporary external ventricular or intraparenchymal monitor, is at times the only way to definitively confirm a genuine pressure-related malfunction in this population when the ventricular imaging itself remains ambiguous, underscoring why this chapter treats slit ventricle syndrome as a distinct diagnostic category rather than a simple variant of the standard malfunction evaluation.

Loculated Hydrocephalus as a Complex Malfunction Pattern

Beyond a straightforward single-catheter malfunction, a child with a history of prior infection or multiple prior shunt revisions can develop loculated hydrocephalus, in which the ventricular system becomes partitioned by adhesions into multiple, separately pressurized compartments not effectively decompressed by a single shunt catheter positioned in only one compartment; recognizing this complex pattern on imaging, characterized by asymmetric or compartmentalized ventricular enlargement not uniformly responsive to the existing shunt, directs the surgical team toward a more complex management approach, potentially including multiple catheters or endoscopic fenestration of the separating septations, rather than a straightforward single-catheter revision that would fail to address the compartmentalized anatomy. Careful, systematic review of all ventricular compartments individually, rather than a single global impression of ventricular size, is required to detect this pattern reliably.

Shunt Infection as a Distinct Complication

Shunt infection, a distinct complication from mechanical malfunction though capable of producing overlapping clinical symptoms and, at times, coexisting mechanical obstruction from infected debris, is suspected when fever, marked local erythema or swelling along the shunt tract, or systemic signs of infection accompany the presentation, and evaluation in this circumstance extends beyond the imaging discussed above to include shunt fluid sampling for culture, a component of the evaluation belonging to the neurosurgical and infectious disease literature but worth naming explicitly here, since imaging alone cannot reliably distinguish infected from purely mechanical malfunction, and both possibilities should be actively considered in the presenting child rather than assumed to be mutually exclusive. Infection risk is highest in the weeks following initial placement or revision, a timing pattern worth incorporating into the clinical index of suspicion for a recently shunted or revised child presenting with new symptoms.

Distal Catheter Complications

Beyond the proximal, intracranial catheter complications emphasized throughout this section, the distal catheter, most commonly terminating in the peritoneal cavity, carries its own distinct complication spectrum including catheter migration, abdominal pseudocyst formation around the distal tip, and, rarely, bowel or other visceral perforation, each of which may present with abdominal rather than neurologic symptoms and can be missed if the imaging evaluation focuses exclusively on the cranial portion of the shunt system; the abdominal radiograph and, where a distal complication is specifically suspected, dedicated abdominal ultrasound or CT, are incorporated into the complete shunt evaluation for precisely this reason.

Programmable Valve Considerations

Programmable shunt valves, which allow noninvasive external adjustment of the opening pressure setting, introduce a specific imaging and clinical consideration beyond the fixed-pressure valves discussed implicitly elsewhere in this chapter: because the magnetic field of an MRI scanner can inadvertently alter a programmable valve's setting, applying the MRI safety principle introduced in Chapter 1, a valve setting check is a mandatory component of both pre- and post-MRI care for any child with a programmable shunt, and a family and referring clinicians should be explicitly informed of this requirement so it is not inadvertently overlooked at an outside imaging facility unfamiliar with the child's specific shunt hardware. Some newer valve models incorporate a locking mechanism specifically designed to resist inadvertent reprogramming from an external magnetic field, but confirming the specific valve model and its MRI-conditional status, rather than assuming universal protection, remains the safest, most reliable practice regardless of the specific hardware in place.

The Role of Family and Patient Self-Report

Beyond the objective imaging and radiographic findings emphasized throughout this section, a family's or, in the older child, the patient's own report that current symptoms feel like a prior, confirmed malfunction episode carries substantial diagnostic weight and should be actively elicited and documented, since this pattern-recognition history, developed over a child's own individual shunt history, is a form of clinical data this chapter's imaging-focused discussion does not by itself capture; a clinician dismissing this specific self-reported pattern-match in favor of imaging findings alone risks discounting a genuinely reliable source of diagnostic information unique to each individual shunted child's own established symptom pattern.

Imaging Follow-Up After Shunt Revision

Following surgical shunt revision, postoperative imaging confirming appropriate catheter position and, over subsequent follow-up, stable or decreasing ventricular size relative to the pre-revision study establishes a new, updated baseline for future comparison, applying the same baseline-establishment principle emphasized throughout this section; failing to update the documented baseline after a revision, and instead continuing to compare future studies against an outdated, pre-revision baseline, can produce a misleading interpretation of apparent interval change that in fact reflects the expected, successful outcome of the revision itself rather than a new, developing problem.

Emergency Department Coordination for Suspected Malfunction

Because shunt malfunction frequently presents acutely, often in an emergency department setting rather than a scheduled neurology or neurosurgery clinic visit, establishing clear, institution-specific rapid imaging and neurosurgical notification protocols for any shunted child presenting with symptoms concerning for malfunction reduces the time to definitive evaluation and, where indicated, surgical intervention; a family carrying documentation of their child's specific shunt type, baseline ventricular measurements, and prior malfunction history, whether as a physical card or accessible electronic record, further expedites this evaluation when presenting to an unfamiliar emergency department without immediate access to the child's full prior imaging history.

Ventriculoperitoneal shunting remains the most common surgical treatment for hydrocephalus, and shunt malfunction, a frequent complication over a shunted child's lifetime, represents one of the more common pediatric neurosurgical emergencies a clinician will encounter, making rapid, accurate imaging evaluation for this specific complication a critical skill this section develops. The baseline-comparison, slit-ventricle-awareness, and loculation-recognition principles developed across this section together form the practical toolkit a clinician needs when a shunted child presents acutely, at any hour, with symptoms concerning for malfunction.

Finding	Suggests	Next Step
Ventricles enlarged vs. baseline	Malfunction	Shunt series + neurosurgical evaluation
Ventricles unchanged, chronically small (slit-like)	Possible slit ventricle syndrome	Correlate with clinical exam; consider ICP monitoring
Catheter discontinuity on shunt series	Mechanical disconnection	Surgical revision
Abdominal pseudocyst around distal tip	Distal catheter complication	Abdominal imaging + surgical evaluation

THE CLINICAL-IMAGING CROSSWALK SYSTEM — Unchanged Ventricles in a Symptomatic Shunted Child

The Crossing: A seven-year-old with a shunt placed in infancy for posthemorrhagic hydrocephalus presents with headache and vomiting, and CT shows ventricles that appear essentially unchanged from a prior study obtained one year earlier.

Presentation Signature: A shunted child with symptoms consistent with malfunction but imaging showing no interval ventricular size change compared to a prior baseline.

Imaging Correlate: The child's shunt history is reviewed and reveals chronically small, slit-like ventricles on every prior study, consistent with slit ventricle syndrome; a shunt series is obtained to exclude a mechanical catheter problem, and the clinical presentation is weighted heavily given the recognized limitation of ventricular size assessment in this specific population.

Trap Logic: Assuming unchanged ventricular size excludes malfunction, without recognizing the child's chronic slit ventricle pattern, risks a falsely reassuring interpretation and a missed, genuine malfunction in a population specifically known to not reliably show the primary imaging indicator this chapter otherwise relies upon.

Crossing Anchor: In a child with known chronically small, slit-like ventricles, unchanged ventricular size does not exclude shunt malfunction; clinical presentation and shunt series findings are weighted more heavily than ventricular size change alone in this specific population.

Idiopathic Intracranial Hypertension in Children

Idiopathic intracranial hypertension, elevated intracranial pressure without a demonstrable structural cause on imaging, presents a distinct diagnostic and imaging challenge from the structural hydrocephalus discussed in the preceding sections, since the diagnosis depends substantially on excluding a structural cause rather than confirming a specific positive imaging finding.

Diagnostic Criteria and the Role of Imaging

Diagnosis of idiopathic intracranial hypertension requires papilledema or another sign of elevated intracranial pressure, elevated cerebrospinal fluid opening pressure on lumbar puncture, normal cerebrospinal fluid composition, and, critically for this chapter's focus, neuroimaging that excludes a structural cause of elevated pressure, including hydrocephalus, a mass lesion, or the cerebral sinovenous thrombosis discussed in Chapter 6; imaging in this context therefore serves primarily an exclusionary function, and a normal or near-normal structural study, rather than a specific positive finding, supports rather than refutes this diagnosis once the other clinical and cerebrospinal fluid criteria are met. Because lumbar puncture opening pressure is itself position- and, in a young or anxious child, cooperation-dependent, coordinating puncture technique with appropriately calibrated sedation or positioning support, where needed, protects against a falsely low or falsely elevated pressure reading that could otherwise confound the diagnostic process this section describes.

Characteristic Though Nonspecific Imaging Findings

Despite its exclusionary diagnostic role, idiopathic intracranial hypertension is associated with a cluster of characteristic, though individually nonspecific, secondary imaging findings including an empty or partially empty sella from chronic pressure-related remodeling, flattening of the posterior globes, distension of the optic nerve sheath, and transverse venous sinus stenosis, addressed further below; recognizing this characteristic constellation, while not required to establish the diagnosis given its clinical and cerebrospinal-fluid-pressure basis, supports the diagnosis when present and should not be mistaken for evidence of an alternative structural process.

Transverse Sinus Stenosis: Cause or Consequence

Transverse venous sinus stenosis, frequently identified on dedicated venous imaging in children with idiopathic intracranial hypertension, presents a genuine ongoing question in the field regarding causal direction, whether the stenosis is a primary contributor to the elevated pressure through impaired venous outflow, or whether it is instead a secondary consequence of the elevated pressure itself compressing the pliable venous sinus walls; this bidirectional relationship, an area of active research rather than settled consensus, is relevant to venous sinus stenting, an emerging but not yet universally established treatment approach for selected, medically refractory cases, and the current uncertainty regarding causal direction is worth communicating honestly to a family considering this intervention. This same normal-variant-versus-pathologic-stenosis distinction connects directly back to the dural venous sinus variant discussion in Chapter 2, underscoring why a stenosis identified incidentally in a child without any signs of elevated pressure should not, by itself, be equated with the pathologic stenosis pattern this section describes in the context of confirmed idiopathic intracranial hypertension.

Risk Factors in the Pediatric Population

Idiopathic intracranial hypertension in children shows a different risk factor and demographic profile than the adult population, in which obesity and female sex are dominant, more strongly associated, risk factors; prepubertal children show a more even sex distribution and a weaker obesity association than the postpubertal adolescent population, whose risk factor profile increasingly resembles the adult pattern as puberty progresses, a distinction worth holding in mind when evaluating a prepubertal child, in whom the diagnosis should not be discounted simply because the child does not fit the more classic obesity-associated adult or adolescent presentation. This age-dependent shift in risk factor profile is itself a further instance of the age-specific interpretive discipline this book has emphasized throughout, applied here to epidemiologic risk assessment rather than to imaging signal interpretation directly.

Medication-Associated Idiopathic Intracranial Hypertension

Several medications, most notably tetracycline-class antibiotics, growth hormone therapy, and, less commonly, certain vitamin A-related compounds, are recognized contributors to idiopathic intracranial hypertension in susceptible children, and a thorough medication history, applied with the same systematic rigor this book emphasizes for other etiologic evaluations, is a necessary component of the evaluation; identifying a contributing medication carries direct management significance, since discontinuation of the offending agent, where clinically feasible, is itself a component of treatment alongside the other management strategies addressed in the broader idiopathic intracranial hypertension literature.

Vision Monitoring and the Urgency of Ophthalmologic Coordination

The primary long-term morbidity risk in idiopathic intracranial hypertension is permanent visual loss from sustained papilledema and optic nerve compromise, making coordinated, serial ophthalmologic monitoring, including formal visual field testing, a central, ongoing component of management rather than a one-time consultation at diagnosis; the imaging findings discussed in this section, while informative, do not substitute for this direct, functional visual assessment, and a normal-appearing optic nerve sheath on imaging should never be used to defer or delay recommended ophthalmologic follow-up.

Distinguishing Idiopathic Intracranial Hypertension From Secondary Causes

The diagnostic label idiopathic applies only once the specific secondary causes of elevated intracranial pressure addressed throughout this book, including the structural hydrocephalus discussed earlier in this chapter, cerebral sinovenous thrombosis discussed in Chapter 6, and a mass lesion discussed in Chapters 12 and 13, have been actively excluded through the comprehensive imaging evaluation this section describes; a child ultimately found to have one of these secondary causes does not carry the idiopathic intracranial hypertension diagnosis, regardless of how closely the initial clinical presentation resembled it, underscoring why the exclusionary imaging evaluation is not an optional formality but a genuine, diagnosis-determining step.

Medical and Surgical Management Overview

First-line medical management of idiopathic intracranial hypertension typically centers on acetazolamide, which reduces cerebrospinal fluid production, alongside the weight management and medication-discontinuation strategies discussed elsewhere in this section, while surgical intervention, including cerebrospinal fluid diversion procedures or, in selected cases, the venous sinus stenting discussed above, is reserved for medically refractory cases or those with rapidly progressive visual loss; this management landscape, while belonging substantially to the neuro-ophthalmology and neurosurgery literature beyond this chapter's primary imaging focus, is worth outlining briefly so the reader understands how the imaging and diagnostic framework this section develops connects to the subsequent treatment pathway a confirmed diagnosis initiates.

Distinguishing Papilledema From Pseudopapilledema

Not every optic disc appearance suggestive of papilledema on funduscopic examination reflects true, pressure-related disc swelling, since a range of benign anatomic variants, most notably optic disc drusen, can produce a similar elevated, blurred disc appearance without any underlying elevated intracranial pressure; distinguishing true papilledema from this pseudopapilledema mimic, using ancillary ophthalmologic techniques including optical coherence tomography and, where genuinely ambiguous, orbital ultrasound or CT to identify calcified drusen, is an essential step before a full, resource-intensive idiopathic intracranial hypertension evaluation is pursued, applying the same diagnostic-precision-before-extensive-workup principle this book emphasizes throughout.

Recurrence and Long-Term Monitoring

Idiopathic intracranial hypertension can recur or relapse even after apparently successful initial treatment, particularly if weight regain occurs in a child whose initial presentation was weight-associated, or if a contributing medication is inadvertently reintroduced, and structured, longitudinal monitoring, incorporating periodic ophthalmologic reassessment even after symptom resolution, is a component of comprehensive long-term management rather than a concern limited to the acute presentation alone; a family should understand this recurrence possibility explicitly at the time of initial treatment, so a return of symptoms is recognized promptly rather than dismissed as unrelated to the prior, apparently resolved diagnosis.

Idiopathic intracranial hypertension, elevated intracranial pressure without a demonstrable structural cause on imaging, presents a distinct diagnostic and imaging challenge from the structural hydrocephalus discussed in the preceding sections, since the diagnosis depends substantially on excluding a structural cause rather than confirming a specific positive imaging finding. The exclusionary imaging framework, the characteristic secondary findings, and the vision-focused management priority developed across this section together define a diagnostic and counseling approach that differs meaningfully from the more structurally anchored hydrocephalus discussion earlier in this chapter.

Figure 10.2: Secondary Imaging Findings of Idiopathic Intracranial Hypertension

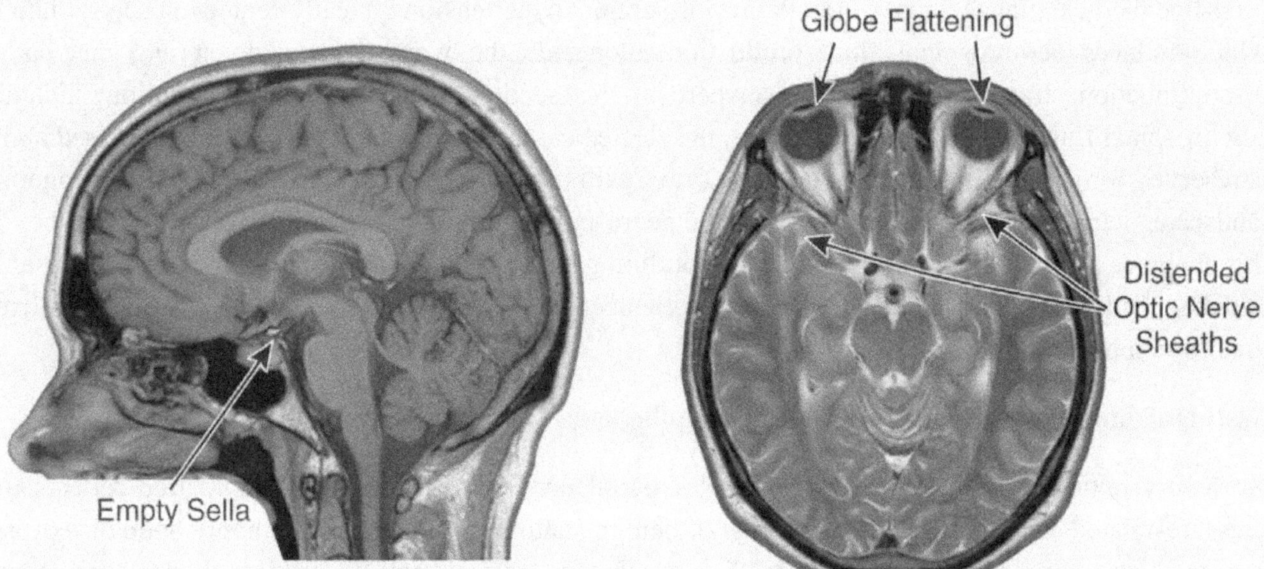

Arachnoid Cysts and Incidental CSF Space Findings

This closing section addresses the specific evaluation and management framework for arachnoid cysts and related incidental cerebrospinal fluid space findings, building directly on the introduction to arachnoid cysts in Chapter 2 and translating that foundational discussion into the more detailed, decision-oriented framework this chapter's clinical focus warrants.

Typical Locations and Imaging Appearance

Arachnoid cysts most commonly occur in the middle cranial fossa, followed in frequency by the posterior fossa and suprasellar region, and characteristically follow cerebrospinal fluid signal precisely on every imaging sequence, including complete suppression on FLAIR, without diffusion restriction, distinguishing them from an epidermoid cyst, a mimicking entity that shows restricted diffusion and does not fully suppress on FLAIR despite a superficially similar simple-cyst appearance on conventional sequences; correctly applying this diffusion and FLAIR-based distinction prevents mistaking a diffusion-restricting epidermoid, an entity with distinct surgical and pathologic significance, for a benign, incidental arachnoid cyst. Middle fossa arachnoid cysts are further subclassified by their degree of temporal lobe involvement and communication with the surrounding subarachnoid space, a classification that carries some prognostic weight regarding growth likelihood and is worth noting explicitly in the structured report for a newly identified cyst in this location.

Natural History and Stability Over Time

The great majority of incidentally discovered arachnoid cysts remain stable in size over long-term follow-up, and this expected stability itself functions as a component of appropriate management, since a documented, stable size on interval imaging, when follow-up imaging is pursued, provides reassurance beyond a single-timepoint assessment alone; a minority of cysts do enlarge over time, particularly in younger children, underscoring why an initial follow-up study, though not necessarily indefinite serial imaging, is a reasonable component of management for a newly identified, incidental arachnoid cyst rather than a single study followed by no further imaging at all. A single confirmatory follow-up study, typically obtained six to twelve months after the initial identification, is generally sufficient for a small, asymptomatic cyst without concerning features; a cyst demonstrating stability at this follow-up interval rarely requires the more extended, indefinite serial imaging surveillance this book reserves for higher-risk or actively evolving findings elsewhere.

Indications for Neurosurgical Evaluation

An arachnoid cyst warrants neurosurgical evaluation, rather than continued observation alone, when it produces mass effect on adjacent brain parenchyma with associated midline shift, when it is large enough to produce macrocephaly or a visible cranial asymmetry, when it demonstrates interval growth on follow-up imaging, or when it is directly implicated in a specific clinical symptom such as new headache with a clear temporal and anatomic correlation, or seizures arising from the immediately adjacent cortex; the great majority of small, incidental, asymptomatic cysts without these specific features do not meet this threshold and are appropriately managed with observation alone, applying the low-yield-intervention reasoning developed in Chapter 3 to this specific surgical, rather than purely imaging, decision. Applying each of these criteria explicitly and individually to a given cyst, rather than relying on cyst size alone as a proxy for all of them, prevents both unnecessary referral of a large but genuinely asymptomatic, stable cyst and, conversely, under-referral of a smaller cyst that nonetheless produces a clear, directly attributable symptom.

Arachnoid Cyst Rupture and Hemorrhage

A recognized, though uncommon, complication of arachnoid cysts is spontaneous or minor-trauma-associated rupture with resulting subdural hemorrhage or hygroma, related to the abnormal, stretched bridging veins that traverse the interface between the cyst and adjacent brain; this specific complication risk is a component of family counseling for a child with a known arachnoid cyst, particularly regarding activity modification in cysts felt to carry elevated risk, such as a large middle fossa cyst in a child engaged in contact sports, a decision made collaboratively between the family and the treating neurosurgeon rather than dictated by a fixed, universal restriction applied to every arachnoid cyst regardless of size or location.

Suprasellar Arachnoid Cysts and Associated Endocrine Findings

Suprasellar arachnoid cysts, though less common than the middle fossa location discussed above, carry a distinct associated risk of hydrocephalus from third ventricular obstruction and of endocrine dysfunction from direct hypothalamic-pituitary compression, and a child with a suprasellar arachnoid cyst therefore warrants the same proactive endocrine evaluation discussed in Chapter 8 for other midline structural findings, applying the coordinated, anticipatory multidisciplinary evaluation principle this book emphasizes across multiple chapters rather than treating this specific cyst location as equivalent in risk profile to the more common, generally lower-risk middle fossa location. Bobble-head doll syndrome, a distinctive, rhythmic head-bobbing movement occasionally associated with a large suprasellar cyst obstructing the anterior third ventricle, is a further, specific clinical clue worth recognizing given its strong anatomic association with this particular cyst location.

Choroid Fissure and Other Uncommon Cyst Locations

Beyond the classic locations discussed above, arachnoid cysts occurring along the choroid fissure or in other less common intracranial locations require the same fundamental evaluation principles applied throughout this section, correct differentiation from a mimicking entity, assessment for mass effect and growth, and correlation with any directly attributable clinical symptom, even though published normative and outcome data specific to these less common locations is comparatively limited; applying the same underlying evaluative framework to an unfamiliar cyst location, rather than requiring a location-specific published series before proceeding with a reasoned evaluation, reflects the transferable, principle-based diagnostic approach this book has developed throughout its full range of chapters.

Communicating Incidental Findings to Families

An incidentally discovered arachnoid cyst, identified on imaging obtained for an unrelated indication, presents a specific communication challenge distinct from the diagnostic reasoning emphasized elsewhere in this chapter: applying the honest, proportionate communication framework developed throughout this book, a family should be told clearly that the finding is common, generally benign, and does not explain the symptom that prompted the original imaging, while avoiding language that either dismisses the finding entirely, which can feel invalidating if the family later researches the term independently, or overstates its significance in a way that generates disproportionate ongoing anxiety about a finding that, in the great majority of cases, will never require intervention.

Surgical Options When Intervention Is Indicated

When an arachnoid cyst meets one of the intervention criteria discussed earlier in this section, surgical options include cyst fenestration, either open microsurgical or endoscopic, allowing the cyst to communicate with and drain into the surrounding subarachnoid space, and, less commonly favored given the associated hardware complication risks discussed earlier in this chapter, cystoperitoneal shunting; the specific surgical approach selected depends on cyst location, size, and the surgeon's assessment of which technique offers the most durable decompression with the lowest complication risk for that specific anatomic circumstance, a decision made collaboratively between the neurosurgical team and the family once intervention has been determined to be warranted.

Distinguishing an Arachnoid Cyst From Other Cystic Lesions

Beyond the epidermoid cyst discussed earlier in this section, the arachnoid cyst differential includes a neuroglial cyst, generally located within the brain parenchyma rather than the extra-axial space an arachnoid cyst occupies, and a porencephalic cyst, discussed in Chapter 7 as an acquired lesion lined by gliotic white matter rather than the thin, translucent arachnoid membrane characteristic of a true arachnoid cyst; applying the systematic location-and-lining-based differential reasoning developed throughout this book, rather than labeling every simple-appearing cystic intracranial finding an arachnoid cyst by default, ensures the correct entity, with its correct associated management pathway, is identified.

Sports and Activity Counseling for a Known Arachnoid Cyst

Beyond the rupture and hemorrhage risk discussed earlier in this section, families of a child with a known arachnoid cyst frequently ask directly about sports participation, and providing a clear, individualized recommendation, rather than a generic, one-size-fits-all restriction, requires weighing the specific cyst size, location, and any associated risk factors against the child's specific sport and its collision risk; documenting this counseling conversation explicitly, including the specific reasoning behind the recommendation given, protects both the family's ability to make an informed decision and the clinical record should the recommendation later be revisited as the child grows or the cyst's characteristics change on interval imaging.

This closing section addresses the specific evaluation and management framework for arachnoid cysts and related incidental cerebrospinal fluid space findings, building directly on the introduction to arachnoid cysts in Chapter 2 and translating that foundational discussion into the more detailed, decision-oriented framework this chapter's clinical focus warrants. The FLAIR-and-diffusion discrimination from mimicking entities, the stability-over-time natural history, and the specific intervention criteria developed across this section together equip the reader to manage the full spectrum of arachnoid cyst presentations, from purely incidental to genuinely symptomatic, with the same calibrated, evidence-based confidence this book has emphasized throughout, closing this chapter's progression from acute, surgically urgent hydrocephalus through to the calmest, most reassuring incidental finding a pediatric neuroimaging study can produce.

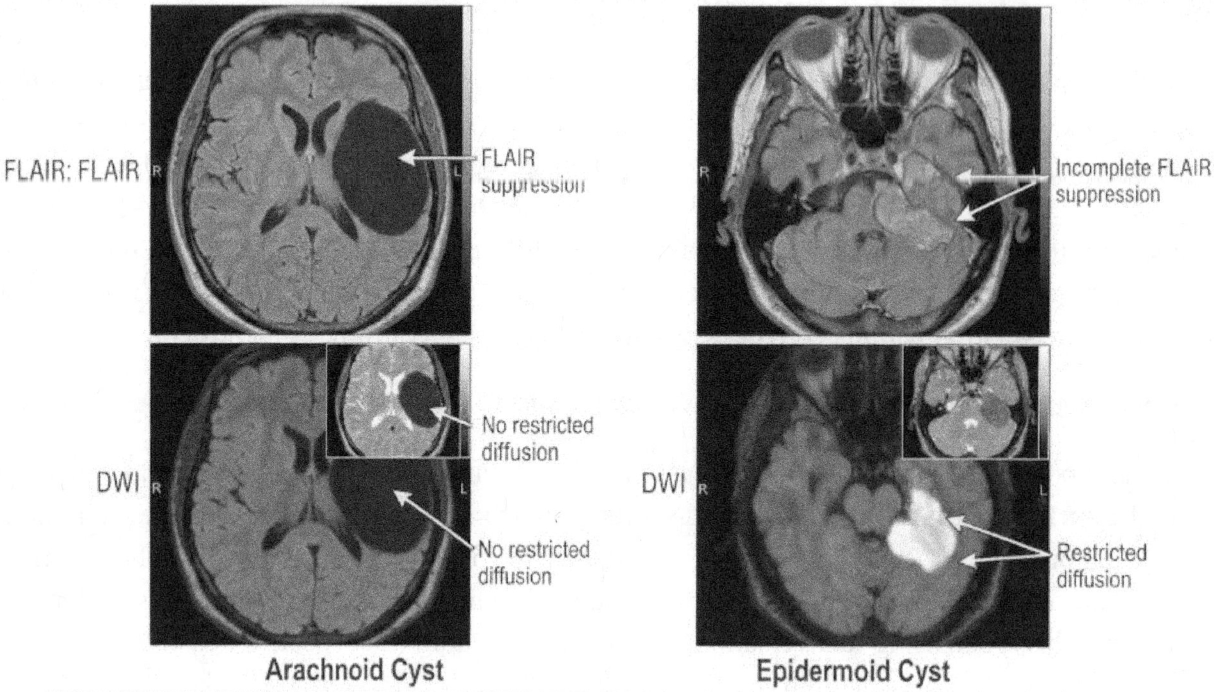

Figure 10.3: Arachnoid Cyst Versus Epidermoid Cyst

Case Presentation: Postinfectious Loculated Hydrocephalus

A four-month-old with a history of bacterial meningitis, discussed in Chapter 15, and an existing ventriculoperitoneal shunt presents with recurrent, asymmetric ventricular enlargement not fully responsive to shunt revision. Applying the reasoning developed in this chapter, dedicated imaging demonstrates compartmentalized, loculated hydrocephalus with septations dividing the ventricular system into separately pressurized components, only one of which is effectively decompressed by the existing single-catheter shunt. Neurosurgery proceeds with endoscopic fenestration of the septations combined with shunt revision, applying the complex-pattern management approach discussed in this chapter, and postoperative imaging confirms improved, more uniform decompression across the previously isolated compartments, illustrating why recognizing loculation specifically, rather than treating this as a routine single-catheter malfunction, directly changed the surgical approach pursued. This case reinforces why the ventricular-pattern-based mechanistic reasoning developed at the start of this chapter remains essential even in a child already carrying an established hydrocephalus diagnosis and existing shunt hardware.

Case Presentation: Idiopathic Intracranial Hypertension in an Adolescent

A fifteen-year-old girl with obesity presents with headache and transient visual obscurations, and funduscopic examination reveals bilateral papilledema. Brain MRI with dedicated venous imaging, applying the exclusionary evaluation framework developed in this chapter, demonstrates no mass lesion, normal ventricular size, and no evidence of venous sinus thrombosis, though bilateral transverse sinus stenosis and a partially empty sella are noted as supportive secondary findings. Lumbar puncture confirms elevated opening pressure with normal cerebrospinal fluid composition, establishing the diagnosis of idiopathic intracranial hypertension. Applying the reasoning developed in this chapter, urgent ophthalmology referral for formal visual field assessment is arranged alongside medical management, and the family is counseled regarding weight management as a component of treatment while being reassured that the imaging findings, though notable, reflect the elevated pressure itself rather than an alternative structural diagnosis requiring separate evaluation.

Case Presentation: An Incidental Arachnoid Cyst Requiring Only Reassurance

A nine-year-old undergoes brain MRI following a minor concussion, applying the imaging criteria discussed in Chapter 19, and the study incidentally identifies a two-centimeter left middle fossa arachnoid cyst without midline shift, mass effect, or any associated parenchymal abnormality. Applying the reasoning developed in this chapter, the interpreting radiologist confirms complete FLAIR suppression and absence of diffusion restriction, excluding an epidermoid cyst, and the finding is reported explicitly as an incidental, benign arachnoid cyst not related to the presenting concussion. The family is counseled using the communication framework developed in this section, explaining clearly that this common, generally stable finding does not explain the child's presenting symptoms and does not require neurosurgical referral or activity restriction beyond the standard concussion return-to-play guidance already in place, illustrating the calibrated reassurance this chapter's incidental-finding framework is designed to provide.

Case Presentation: Congenital Aqueductal Stenosis Managed With Endoscopic Third Ventriculostomy

A six-month-old presents with progressive macrocephaly and a bulging fontanelle, and MRI demonstrates dilated lateral and third ventricles with a normal-sized fourth ventricle, localizing an obstruction to the level of the cerebral aqueduct. Applying the obstructive-pattern reasoning developed in this chapter, further imaging confirms a focal aqueductal web without an associated posterior fossa malformation, and genetics evaluation for L1CAM-related hydrocephalus, applying the reasoning discussed earlier in this chapter, returns negative. Given the discrete, focal nature of the obstruction and the infant's age, the neurosurgical team proceeds with endoscopic third ventriculostomy rather than shunt placement, and postoperative flow-sensitive imaging confirms adequate cerebrospinal fluid flow through the newly created stoma, with subsequent clinical and imaging follow-up demonstrating stable, non-progressive ventricular size without the need for lifelong shunt hardware, illustrating the shunt-independent management pathway this chapter discusses for appropriately selected obstructive cases.

Crossing 1 Recap: In a child with known chronically small, slit-like ventricles, unchanged ventricular size does not exclude shunt malfunction; clinical presentation and shunt series findings are weighted more heavily in this specific population.

Chapter Anchor: Hydrocephalus mechanism, communicating versus obstructive, versus overproduction, is localized directly from the ventricular pattern on imaging, while idiopathic intracranial hypertension and incidental arachnoid cysts each require their own specific, structured evaluation framework distinguishing them from true structural hydrocephalus requiring surgical intervention.

Summary and Key Concepts

Hydrocephalus is classified as communicating (uniform ventricular enlargement, impaired resorption) or obstructive (proximal enlargement only, mechanical blockage); the specific ventricular pattern localizes the mechanism and, in obstructive cases, the level of obstruction, and choroid plexus overproduction is a distinct, less common mechanism worth recognizing when an intraventricular mass is present.

Shunt malfunction is primarily identified by ventricular size increase compared to the child's own baseline; slit ventricle syndrome and loculated hydrocephalus are important exceptions requiring modified interpretation, and distal catheter complications, programmable valve MRI considerations, and shunt infection each warrant their own dedicated evaluation.

Idiopathic intracranial hypertension is a clinical and cerebrospinal-fluid-pressure diagnosis for which imaging serves primarily an exclusionary function; characteristic secondary findings support but do not establish the diagnosis, pseudopapilledema is an important mimic to exclude, and urgent ophthalmologic vision monitoring is the central, ongoing management priority.

Arachnoid cysts are distinguished from epidermoid, neuroglial, and porencephalic cyst mimics by complete FLAIR suppression and absent diffusion restriction plus lining characteristics; most are stable, incidental findings managed with observation, while mass effect, growth, suprasellar location, or a directly attributable symptom warrant neurosurgical evaluation.

Across this chapter, precise mechanistic and anatomic classification, not a generic label of hydrocephalus or cyst, directly determines the surgical approach, the imaging surveillance plan, and the family counseling that follows, and endoscopic third ventriculostomy offers a shunt-independent alternative for appropriately selected obstructive cases.

CHAPTER 11: NEUROIMAGING IN PEDIATRIC EPILEPSY

Learning Objectives

1. Construct a dedicated epilepsy MRI protocol and explain why a routine brain protocol is inadequate for this indication, including the specific role of coronal oblique hippocampal sequencing.
2. Recognize the imaging features of focal cortical dysplasia and describe its subtype-specific detection challenges, including the transmantle sign and bottom-of-sulcus variants.
3. Describe the components of presurgical epilepsy evaluation, including functional imaging and localization techniques, and the role of the multidisciplinary epilepsy surgery conference.
4. Recognize the acute imaging findings of status epilepticus and distinguish peri-ictal change from a primary structural process.

MRI Epilepsy Protocols and Hippocampal Imaging

Neuroimaging in pediatric epilepsy serves a fundamentally different purpose than the acute, diagnostic imaging emphasized in earlier chapters of this book: for the child with newly diagnosed or established epilepsy, the imaging question is not simply whether a structural abnormality is present, but whether a specific, surgically addressable epileptogenic lesion can be identified and precisely localized, a distinction that shapes every aspect of protocol design discussed in this opening section. This distinction, imaging to detect versus imaging to precisely localize and characterize, recurs as the organizing theme across every section of this chapter, from protocol design through presurgical multimodal integration.

Why a Routine Brain Protocol Is Inadequate

Building directly on the protocol-customization principle established in Chapter 1, a routine, non-dedicated brain MRI protocol, even when technically unremarkable, frequently fails to detect the subtle structural abnormalities responsible for medically refractory focal epilepsy, particularly focal cortical dysplasia and hippocampal sclerosis, both discussed at length in this chapter; a normal routine brain MRI in a child with focal epilepsy should therefore prompt a dedicated epilepsy-protocol study before the child is labeled as having non-lesional epilepsy, since a genuine, surgically relevant lesion may simply have been missed by the lower-resolution, non-targeted sequences a routine protocol employs.

Core Sequence Requirements for the Epilepsy Protocol

A dedicated epilepsy protocol requires thin-section, high-resolution three-dimensional T1-weighted imaging permitting multiplanar reformatting, coronal oblique T2 and FLAIR sequences oriented perpendicular to the long axis of the hippocampus specifically to optimize hippocampal evaluation, and, where available, specialized sequences sensitive to the subtle gray-white matter blurring characteristic of focal cortical dysplasia; this combination of sequences, acquired with attention to the specific technical parameters this section develops, distinguishes a genuine epilepsy protocol from a routine brain protocol relabeled without the corresponding technical adjustments this indication actually requires. Susceptibility-weighted imaging is frequently added to this core sequence set specifically to identify a cavernous malformation, discussed in Chapter 18, as a further recognized cause of focal epilepsy that the standard T1 and T2/FLAIR sequences alone can under-detect given its characteristic blooming artifact, which is most conspicuous on susceptibility-sensitive sequences.

Hippocampal Anatomy and the Basis of Sclerosis Detection

Detecting hippocampal sclerosis, discussed in detail in the next subhead, depends on precise assessment of hippocampal volume, internal architecture, and signal characteristics, each of which requires imaging obtained in a plane specifically aligned to the hippocampal long axis rather than the standard axial and coronal planes used for general brain imaging; a hippocampus imaged in a non-optimized plane can appear falsely normal or falsely abnormal due to partial volume averaging across its curved anatomic course, underscoring why the coronal oblique orientation discussed above is not a minor technical preference but a genuine prerequisite for reliable hippocampal assessment. The technologist performing the study should be provided explicit, written prescription instructions for this specific oblique angulation rather than relying on an unwritten institutional convention, since a plane that varies even modestly from true perpendicular alignment can meaningfully degrade the reliability of the resulting hippocampal assessment.

Mesial Temporal (Hippocampal) Sclerosis

Hippocampal sclerosis, characterized by volume loss, loss of the normal internal architecture, and T2/FLAIR hyperintensity within the hippocampus, is among the most common identifiable causes of temporal lobe epilepsy and one of the most favorable lesions for surgical outcome when correctly identified and correlated with electroencephalographic seizure onset; recognizing this specific triad of findings, rather than any single feature in isolation, since volume loss alone can reflect a normal anatomic variant and signal change alone can be subtle or technically confounded, provides the most reliable basis for this diagnosis. A history of a prolonged febrile seizure or febrile status epilepticus in early childhood, discussed further in this chapter's closing section, is a recognized risk factor frequently elicited in a child later diagnosed with hippocampal sclerosis, and actively asking about this specific early history, rather than waiting for it to be volunteered, can support the diagnosis when the imaging findings themselves are borderline or equivocal.

Quantitative and Volumetric Hippocampal Assessment

Beyond qualitative visual assessment, quantitative hippocampal volumetry, comparing the affected hippocampus both to its contralateral counterpart and to age-matched normative volumes, adds objective, reproducible support to a qualitative impression of asymmetry or volume loss, particularly valuable in bilateral or subtle cases where visual asymmetry assessment alone leaves genuine interpretive uncertainty; several centers now incorporate automated or semi-automated volumetric analysis software into routine epilepsy protocol interpretation specifically to standardize this assessment across readers and over serial studies. T2 relaxometry, a further quantitative technique measuring the specific T2 relaxation time within the hippocampus rather than relying on visual signal impression alone, offers additional objective support in cases where qualitative signal assessment remains genuinely ambiguous, though its availability, like several of the advanced techniques discussed in this chapter, remains concentrated at specialized epilepsy imaging centers.

Dual Pathology and Its Detection Implications

A meaningful proportion of children with hippocampal sclerosis harbor a second, coexisting epileptogenic lesion elsewhere in the brain, a phenomenon termed dual pathology, most often a subtle focal cortical dysplasia in the temporal or adjacent extratemporal cortex; failing to actively search for this second lesion once hippocampal sclerosis has been identified, rather than concluding the evaluation upon finding the first, more obvious abnormality, risks an incomplete presurgical picture and can meaningfully affect the surgical outcome if the second, unrecognized lesion is not addressed at the time of resection. A deliberate, systematic search of the entire temporal lobe and immediately adjacent extratemporal cortex, applied as a standing habit whenever hippocampal sclerosis is identified rather than only when a specific additional finding is suspected, is the most reliable way to detect this second, easily overlooked pathology.

Timing of Imaging Relative to Seizure Onset

Optimal epilepsy-protocol imaging is generally obtained in the interictal state, well removed from the immediate peri-ictal period, since acute, seizure-related signal change, discussed further in this chapter's closing section on status epilepticus, can transiently mimic or obscure a genuine structural lesion; when imaging must be obtained acutely for another clinical reason during or shortly after a seizure, the interpreting clinician should explicitly consider whether an observed finding reflects transient peri-ictal change or a true structural abnormality, and interval follow-up imaging once the child has returned to a stable interictal baseline resolves this ambiguity when it is not otherwise clear from the acute study alone.

Sedation Considerations Specific to the Epilepsy Protocol

The epilepsy protocol's longer acquisition time relative to a routine brain MRI, driven by the multiple dedicated sequences discussed throughout this section, carries direct sedation implications in the younger child, extending the anesthetic exposure duration discussed in Chapter 1; balancing the need for a technically complete, diagnostically adequate epilepsy protocol against the goal of minimizing sedation duration requires careful sequence prioritization, and coordinating with the anesthesia team in advance regarding the specific, full sequence list planned, applying the coordination principle from Chapter 1, helps ensure the study is not prematurely truncated before the highest-yield sequences have been acquired.

Repeat Epilepsy Protocol Imaging Over Time

A child with an initially non-lesional epilepsy protocol study may benefit from repeat, updated epilepsy-protocol imaging later in their clinical course, particularly as MRI technology, field strength, and sequence sophistication continue to advance, or as the child's seizures evolve in a way that refines the suspected localization and therefore the specific region requiring closest scrutiny; a repeat study is not merely a redundant repetition of the original but an opportunity to apply updated technical capability and a more refined clinical hypothesis to the same diagnostic question, consistent with the evolving-evidence and reanalysis principle developed in Chapter 7 for genetic testing, applied here to imaging technology instead.

Structured Reporting for Epilepsy Protocol Studies

Applying the structured reporting discipline established in Chapter 1, an epilepsy protocol report should explicitly address hippocampal volume and signal bilaterally, the presence or absence of gray-white blurring or a transmantle sign in each lobe, and any other malformation or lesion identified, using standardized descriptive language rather than a brief, unstructured impression; this structured approach ensures the epilepsy surgery conference discussed later in this chapter receives complete, systematically organized information rather than depending on the referring team to infer completeness from a report that may have addressed some but not all of the relevant structures this section has emphasized.

Comparing Epilepsy Protocols Across Vendors and Field Strengths

Because the specific sequence parameters and acquisition times for an epilepsy protocol vary meaningfully across MRI vendors and field strengths, a child transferring care between institutions or seeking a second opinion at a specialized epilepsy center may require a repeat, site-specific epilepsy protocol rather than relying on an outside study performed to a different institution's technical specifications; communicating this potential need for repeat imaging early in the referral process, rather than only once the outside images prove technically inadequate for the receiving center's specific review standards, sets appropriate expectations for the family regarding both the timeline and the additional sedation exposure a repeat study may involve.

Figure 11.1: Coronal Oblique Hippocampal Imaging Technique

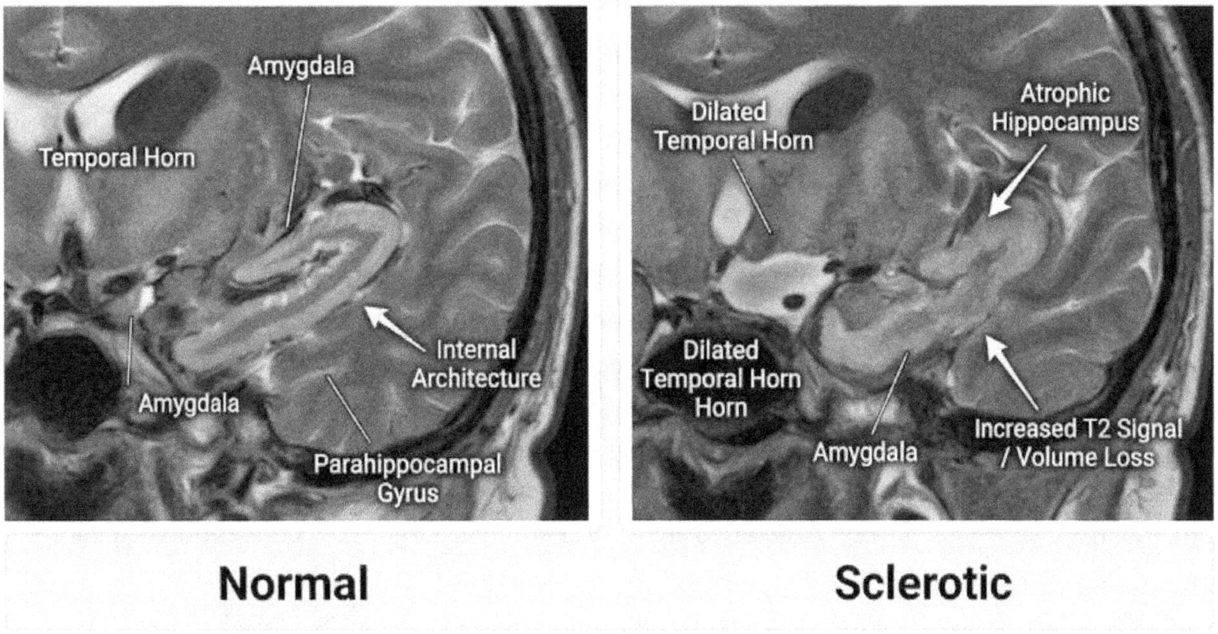

Sequence	Purpose	Key Technical Requirement
3D T1	Volumetric anatomy, multiplanar reformatting	Thin-section, isotropic voxels
Coronal oblique T2/FLAIR	Hippocampal architecture and signal	Perpendicular to hippocampal long axis
High-resolution FLAIR	Gray-white blurring of focal cortical dysplasia	Thin-section, high in-plane resolution

Focal Cortical Dysplasia and Epileptogenic Lesions

Building directly on the focal cortical dysplasia discussion in Chapter 7, this section develops the specific detection challenges and subtype-based imaging reasoning most relevant to the presurgical epilepsy evaluation this chapter addresses, extending that chapter's embryologic framework into this chapter's surgically focused, localization-driven context.

The ILAE Classification and Its Imaging Correlates

The International League Against Epilepsy classification divides focal cortical dysplasia into type I, isolated architectural or cytological abnormality without balloon cells, type II, architectural dysplasia with dysmorphic neurons and, in the more severe type IIb, balloon cells, and type III, cortical dysplasia adjacent to another principal lesion such as hippocampal sclerosis or a tumor; type II lesions, particularly type IIb with its characteristic transmantle sign, an extension of abnormal signal from the cortex toward the ventricle, are generally the most conspicuous and reliably detected on imaging, while type I lesions are frequently subtle or entirely occult even on a well-performed dedicated epilepsy protocol. This classification system, while primarily histopathologic in origin, correlates meaningfully enough with imaging conspicuity that referring to a lesion by its likely ILAE subtype, based on its imaging characteristics, is a useful shorthand for communicating expected detection difficulty and surgical planning complexity among the multidisciplinary team discussed later in this chapter, even before histopathologic confirmation is available.

MRI-Negative Focal Epilepsy

A substantial proportion of children with focal, medically refractory epilepsy have no visible structural lesion even on a properly performed dedicated epilepsy protocol, a circumstance termed MRI-negative or non-lesional epilepsy; this does not necessarily indicate the absence of a true focal cortical dysplasia, since, as discussed above, type I lesions in particular can remain occult on even high-quality conventional imaging, and this population frequently requires the advanced imaging and invasive localization techniques discussed later in this chapter to identify a surgical target that conventional imaging alone cannot resolve. Surgical outcomes in genuinely MRI-negative epilepsy, once a target has been identified through the multimodal techniques this chapter describes, are generally less favorable on average than in clearly lesional cases, information that is appropriately incorporated into the family counseling conversation from the earliest stages of the presurgical evaluation rather than only once surgery is imminent.

The Transmantle Sign in Detail

The transmantle sign, a funnel-shaped band of abnormal T2/FLAIR hyperintensity extending from the cortical surface toward the ventricular margin, reflects the histopathologic radial extension of dysplastic tissue characteristic of type IIb focal cortical dysplasia and is considered among the most specific individual imaging findings in this chapter for localizing a surgically resectable epileptogenic zone; recognizing this sign requires deliberately tracing the white matter signal from the cortical surface inward on the high-resolution sequences discussed in the previous section, rather than examining the cortex and white matter as separate, unrelated regions of interest. Because the transmantle sign can be subtle even when present, deliberately searching for it as a distinct, named finding, rather than only noting it if it happens to be conspicuous on an otherwise unremarkable-appearing study, meaningfully improves detection sensitivity, a discipline worth incorporating explicitly into any systematic epilepsy protocol review checklist.

Postprocessing and Voxel-Based Morphometry

Beyond visual inspection alone, computational postprocessing techniques, including voxel-based morphometry, which statistically compares an individual child's cortical thickness and gray-white junction characteristics against a normative population database to flag subtle regions of abnormality, offer an increasingly available adjunct for detecting focal cortical dysplasia that visual review alone may miss; these tools function as a second, complementary reader rather than a replacement for expert visual interpretation, and a flagged region identified only on postprocessing, without any corroborating visual or electroencephalographic finding, warrants cautious, correlative interpretation rather than automatic acceptance as the surgical target.

Other Epileptogenic Lesions Beyond Focal Cortical Dysplasia

Beyond focal cortical dysplasia and hippocampal sclerosis, a range of other lesions identified elsewhere in this book carry recognized epileptogenic potential, including low-grade tumors such as dysembryoplastic neuroepithelial tumor and ganglioglioma discussed in Chapter 12, cavernous malformations discussed in Chapter 18, and periventricular nodular heterotopia discussed in Chapter 7; recognizing that the epilepsy evaluation this chapter describes applies to any of these lesion types, not exclusively to focal cortical dysplasia, and that the specific lesion identified shapes the expected seizure semiology and surgical approach, reinforces this book's broader principle that precise lesion identification, not a generic label of epileptogenic lesion, drives clinical decision-making. A long-term epilepsy-associated tumor, such as ganglioglioma or dysembryoplastic neuroepithelial tumor, is frequently indolent and slow-growing, and its imaging characterization emphasizes precise localization for resection planning over the aggressive-versus-indolent grading considerations that dominate the broader pediatric brain tumor discussion in Chapter 12.

Correlating Lesion Location With Seizure Semiology

The clinical semiology of a child's seizures, the specific pattern of motor, sensory, autonomic, or behavioral change observed during an ictal event, frequently provides a strong clue to the likely seizure onset zone even before imaging is reviewed, and correlating this clinical localization against the imaging findings, applying the same clinical-imaging correlation principle this book's Crosswalk System embodies throughout, either reinforces confidence in an identified lesion as the true epileptogenic focus or, when the two sources of information conflict, prompts reconsideration of whether the imaging finding is genuinely responsible for the child's seizures or represents an incidental, non-epileptogenic finding.

Genetic Testing in Focal Cortical Dysplasia

A substantial proportion of focal cortical dysplasia, particularly type II, arises from somatic, brain-limited mosaic mutations in the mTOR pathway, mutations present only within the dysplastic tissue itself and not detectable on standard peripheral blood genetic testing, a mechanism distinct from the germline mutations discussed in Chapter 7 for the migration and organization disorders; when genetic confirmation is pursued, testing of the resected surgical tissue itself, rather than blood alone, is frequently necessary to identify the causative somatic variant, and this distinction is worth explaining clearly to a family who might otherwise expect a standard blood-based genetic test to provide a definitive answer before surgery has even occurred.

Tuberous Sclerosis Complex and Multifocal Cortical Tubers

Tuberous sclerosis complex, discussed further in Chapter 14, produces multiple cortical tubers, lesions histologically and, to a substantial degree, radiologically related to focal cortical dysplasia given their shared underlying mTOR pathway dysregulation, and a child with tuberous sclerosis and medically refractory epilepsy presents a specific localization challenge given the presence of multiple potentially epileptogenic tubers rather than a single, isolated lesion; identifying which specific tuber, among several, is the true epileptogenic focus responsible for the child's clinical seizures depends heavily on the electroencephalographic and functional imaging correlation techniques developed later in this chapter, since structural imaging alone cannot reliably distinguish an epileptogenic tuber from an incidental, non-epileptogenic one in this specific multifocal population. A tuber demonstrating interval calcification, cystic change, or a distinctly different signal characteristic from the child's other, presumably stable tubers on serial imaging may itself be a clue worth correlating against the electrographic data, since such a change can, in some cases, correspond to the specific tuber driving the clinical seizures.

mTOR Inhibitor Therapy as a Medical Alternative

Given the shared mTOR pathway dysregulation underlying both tuberous sclerosis complex and a substantial proportion of focal cortical dysplasia, targeted mTOR inhibitor therapy has emerged as a disease-modifying medical treatment option in selected cases, distinct from the symptomatic antiseizure medications used more broadly across epilepsy management, and imaging characterization of tuber or dysplasia burden and location remains relevant even for a child pursuing this medical rather than surgical pathway, since treatment response monitoring benefits from the same structured, baseline-and-follow-up imaging comparison this book emphasizes throughout for other longitudinally managed conditions.

Bottom-of-Sulcus Dysplasia as a Detection-Challenging Subtype

Bottom-of-sulcus dysplasia, a specific, small-volume variant of focal cortical dysplasia located at the depth of a cortical sulcus rather than at the more readily visualized cortical surface, presents a particular detection challenge given both its small size and its location, which can be obscured by normal sulcal folding on standard imaging planes; deliberately reviewing sulcal depths on thin-section imaging using multiplanar reformatting, rather than relying on standard axial and coronal planes alone, and maintaining specific awareness of this subtype's characteristic bottom-of-sulcus location, improves detection of this otherwise easily overlooked lesion category. This lesion is frequently a leading candidate explanation when a child's electroencephalographic and semiology data localize confidently to a specific lobe but the initial structural review of that lobe appears unremarkable, prompting the specific, sulcus-focused re-review this subhead describes.

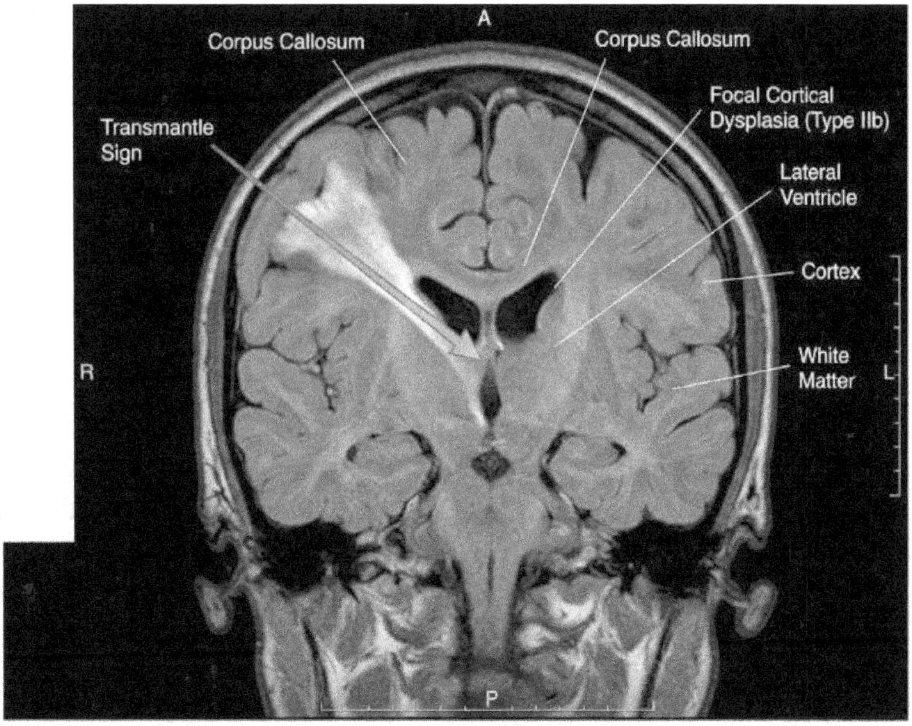

Figure 11.2: Transmantle Sign of Type IIb Focal Cortical Dysplasia

THE CLINICAL-IMAGING CROSSWALK SYSTEM — A Flagged Postprocessing Region Without Visual or Electrographic Correlation

The Crossing: Voxel-based morphometry postprocessing flags a small region of the right frontal lobe as statistically abnormal in a child with left-hemisphere-predominant seizure semiology and electroencephalographic findings.

Presentation Signature: A child undergoing presurgical epilepsy evaluation whose postprocessing analysis identifies a region discordant with the clinical and electrographic lateralization already established.

Imaging Correlate: The flagged region is reviewed carefully on the original high-resolution sequences and does not show a convincing transmantle sign, gray-white blurring, or any other visually corroborating feature of focal cortical dysplasia.

Trap Logic: Accepting a discordant postprocessing flag as the surgical target without visual or electrographic corroboration risks directing surgical planning toward an incorrect, non-epileptogenic region while the true left-hemisphere focus responsible for the child's seizures remains unaddressed.

Crossing Anchor: A postprocessing-flagged region without visual imaging correlation or electroencephalographic concordance should not be accepted as the surgical target; postprocessing serves as an adjunct to, not a replacement for, correlated clinical, electrographic, and visual imaging assessment.

Presurgical Evaluation and Functional Imaging

For the child with medically refractory focal epilepsy being considered for surgical resection, presurgical evaluation integrates structural imaging with electroencephalographic and functional localization techniques into a single, coherent surgical plan, the multimodal integration process this section develops in detail.

Scalp Video-EEG Monitoring as the Foundation

Inpatient video-electroencephalography monitoring, capturing multiple typical seizure events with simultaneous video and electrographic recording, remains the foundational component of presurgical evaluation, establishing both the clinical semiology and the scalp-based electrographic seizure onset zone against which every other component of the evaluation, structural imaging, functional imaging, and, where pursued, invasive monitoring, is correlated; a presurgical evaluation proceeding without this foundational video-EEG characterization lacks the clinical and electrographic anchor the remaining components of the evaluation depend upon for meaningful interpretation. Reducing antiseizure medication during this monitoring admission, under close inpatient supervision, is frequently necessary to capture a sufficient number of typical seizure events within a reasonable admission length, a practice that requires careful safety planning and continuous monitoring given the recognized risks of medication reduction in a hospitalized child with epilepsy.

Ictal and Interictal SPECT

Ictal and interictal single-photon emission computed tomography, introduced in Chapter 1, localizes the seizure onset zone through the regional cerebral blood flow changes accompanying seizure activity, with the ictal study, requiring precisely timed radiotracer injection at seizure onset, showing focal hyperperfusion at the true onset zone while the interictal baseline study shows the resting-state perfusion pattern against which the ictal study is subtracted; this subtraction technique, termed SISCOM when co-registered with structural MRI, provides a powerful localizing tool particularly valuable in the MRI-negative epilepsy population discussed earlier in this chapter. The precision of injection timing relative to true electrographic seizure onset, rather than relative to the clinically apparent onset, which frequently lags the true electrographic start, directly determines the reliability of the resulting ictal study, making close coordination between the epilepsy monitoring unit nursing staff and the nuclear medicine team a genuine technical prerequisite for a diagnostically useful result.

FDG-PET in Presurgical Localization

Interictal fluorodeoxyglucose positron emission tomography, exploiting the characteristic interictal hypometabolism frequently observed at a chronic epileptogenic focus, offers a complementary localizing technique to the perfusion-based SPECT discussed above, and co-registration of PET findings with the structural MRI, applying the same multimodal integration principle developed in Chapter 7 for structural-functional correlation, can reveal a subtle hypometabolic region corresponding to an otherwise MRI-occult lesion, particularly valuable in the type I focal cortical dysplasia population in whom conventional structural imaging most frequently fails to identify a visible lesion. PET-MRI co-registration software, increasingly standard at dedicated pediatric epilepsy centers, allows overlay of the functional hypometabolism map directly onto the high-resolution structural sequences discussed earlier in this chapter, a visual integration that substantially improves a reader's ability to correlate the two modalities compared to independent, side-by-side review of separately acquired studies.

Magnetoencephalography for Source Localization

Magnetoencephalography, measuring the magnetic fields generated by neuronal electrical activity with excellent temporal and, when co-registered with structural MRI, good spatial resolution, offers a noninvasive source-localization technique particularly valuable for characterizing interictal epileptiform discharges and their relationship to eloquent cortex, complementing rather than replacing the electroencephalographic and perfusion-based techniques discussed elsewhere in this section; availability of this specialized technique remains limited to a smaller number of tertiary epilepsy centers, and referral for magnetoencephalography, when not locally available, is a reasonable component of a comprehensive presurgical evaluation for an appropriately complex case. Because magnetoencephalography requires the child to remain still for an extended recording session, the same motion-reduction and, where age-appropriate, preparation strategies developed in Chapter 1 for MRI apply with equal relevance to this distinct imaging and electrophysiologic modality.

Functional MRI for Eloquent Cortex Mapping

Functional MRI, applying the blood-oxygen-level-dependent technique to map language, motor, and, less commonly in routine clinical practice, memory function relative to a planned resection site, is a standard component of presurgical planning whenever the epileptogenic zone lies near or within classically eloquent cortex, providing noninvasive functional localization that complements the more invasive techniques discussed below; functional MRI in children requires task cooperation that can be genuinely challenging to obtain reliably in a younger or cognitively impaired child, and age-appropriate task design, coordinated with a child life specialist or neuropsychologist experienced in pediatric functional imaging, meaningfully improves the reliability of the resulting functional maps. Language lateralization by functional MRI has, in many centers, substantially reduced but not entirely eliminated the need for the more invasive Wada test, an intracarotid amobarbital procedure historically used for this specific purpose, and understanding which children still require Wada testing despite functional MRI, generally those with ambiguous or discordant functional MRI lateralization results, is a further, specific component of comprehensive presurgical planning.

Invasive Monitoring: Stereo-EEG and Subdural Grids

When noninvasive evaluation leaves genuine localization uncertainty, invasive intracranial monitoring, using either stereotactically placed depth electrodes (stereo-EEG) or, less commonly favored in contemporary practice given its greater surgical morbidity, subdural grid and strip electrodes, provides direct, high-resolution electrographic recording from the brain surface or deep structures to definitively localize the seizure onset zone and map its relationship to eloquent cortex through direct cortical stimulation; the specific electrode placement plan is derived directly from the noninvasive evaluation's hypothesized onset zone, making the imaging and electroencephalographic reasoning developed throughout this chapter a direct determinant of where invasive electrodes are ultimately placed, rather than an independent, disconnected prior step.

Neuropsychological Evaluation as a Complementary Component

Comprehensive neuropsychological evaluation, assessing baseline cognitive, language, and memory function before any surgical intervention, is a standard, complementary component of presurgical evaluation that both informs the risk-benefit discussion regarding a planned resection near eloquent or memory-related structures and establishes a genuine preoperative baseline against which postoperative outcome can be meaningfully compared; a resection proceeding without this baseline assessment loses the ability to reliably attribute a postoperative cognitive change specifically to the surgery itself, since without a documented baseline, a family and care team cannot distinguish a surgery-related change from a pre-existing deficit that was simply not previously formally characterized. This baseline evaluation also frequently reveals functional impairment the family had attributed to the child's general temperament or academic effort rather than to the underlying seizure disorder itself, information that can meaningfully reshape both educational planning and the family's overall understanding of the epilepsy's functional impact.

The Multidisciplinary Epilepsy Surgery Conference

The multiple, independently generated data sources discussed throughout this section, structural and functional imaging, electroencephalography, neuropsychological assessment, and, where obtained, invasive monitoring results, are most effectively integrated through a formal, multidisciplinary epilepsy surgery conference bringing together epileptology, neurosurgery, neuroradiology, and neuropsychology to review the complete case together before a final surgical recommendation is made; this collaborative review format, rather than a single specialist synthesizing the full dataset independently, reduces the risk that a single perspective's interpretation goes unchallenged and improves the overall reliability of the final surgical target identified.

Surgical Outcome Counseling and Seizure Freedom Rates

Seizure freedom rates following resective epilepsy surgery vary substantially by the specific lesion identified and the completeness of its resection, with lesional epilepsy, particularly hippocampal sclerosis and well-localized focal cortical dysplasia with complete resection, generally showing the most favorable outcomes, while non-lesional epilepsy and cases requiring resection near eloquent cortex, where a more limited, function-preserving resection may be necessary, show correspondingly more variable outcomes; presenting this lesion-specific, rather than generic, outcome data to a family during the counseling process, applying the honest, proportionate communication principle developed throughout this book, allows the family to make a genuinely informed decision regarding whether to proceed with the invasive evaluation and surgery this chapter has described.

Laser Interstitial Thermal Therapy as a Minimally Invasive Alternative

For selected, well-localized lesions, particularly deep or difficult-to-access targets such as certain hypothalamic hamartomas or a discrete mesial temporal focus, laser interstitial thermal therapy, a minimally invasive stereotactic technique that ablates the target lesion through precisely delivered thermal energy under real-time MRI thermography guidance, offers an alternative to open resective surgery with a shorter recovery period, though generally more limited long-term outcome data relative to the more extensively studied open resection techniques discussed elsewhere in this chapter; precise preoperative imaging characterization of the target lesion's size, shape, and relationship to adjacent critical structures is equally, if not more, essential for this technique given the smaller margin for error inherent to a precisely targeted ablation compared to a wider open resection. Real-time thermography monitoring during the ablation itself represents a further, distinct imaging application beyond the diagnostic and presurgical planning imaging emphasized throughout the remainder of this chapter, extending imaging's role directly into the intraoperative period.

Figure 11.3: Multimodal Presurgical Localization Integration

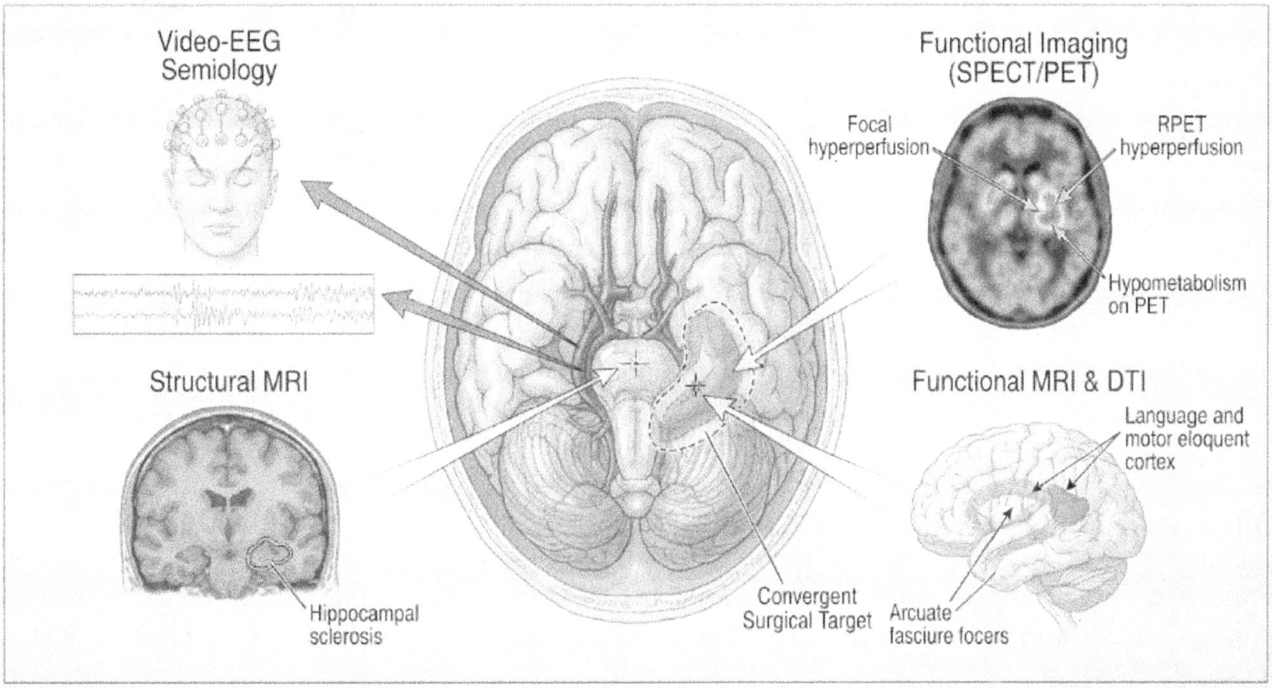

Status Epilepticus: Acute Imaging Findings

This closing section addresses the acute imaging findings that can accompany prolonged or repetitive seizure activity, findings that must be correctly distinguished from a primary structural process precipitating the seizures, applying the same acute-versus-chronic and cause-versus-consequence reasoning this book emphasizes throughout.

Peri-Ictal Signal Change: Mechanism and Appearance

Prolonged or repetitive seizure activity can itself produce transient, reversible signal change on MRI, most characteristically cortical and, at times, subcortical T2/FLAIR hyperintensity with variable diffusion restriction in the region of maximal seizure activity, reflecting a combination of cytotoxic edema from the intense metabolic demand of sustained seizure activity and, in some cases, vasogenic edema from disrupted autoregulation in the same region; recognizing this pattern as a physiologic consequence of the seizure itself, rather than a primary structural lesion that caused the seizure, depends on correlating the imaging finding's location and timing against the clinical seizure semiology and electroencephalographic focus. Contralateral cerebellar diaschisis, a pattern of reduced perfusion and, at times, signal change in the cerebellar hemisphere contralateral to a supratentorial seizure focus, is a further, less commonly recognized peri-ictal phenomenon worth naming explicitly so it is not mistaken for a separate, primary cerebellar process when identified alongside a more classic supratentorial peri-ictal pattern.

Distinguishing Peri-Ictal Change From a Primary Causative Lesion

The key distinguishing features supporting a peri-ictal, rather than primary causative, mechanism include a distribution that corresponds anatomically to the known or suspected seizure onset zone rather than an unrelated vascular territory, resolution or substantial improvement on follow-up imaging obtained once the acute seizure activity has resolved, and the absence of the specific findings, restricted diffusion in a vascular distribution, hemorrhage, or an enhancing mass, that would instead suggest a primary structural process such as the acute stroke discussed in Chapter 18 or the infectious or inflammatory processes discussed in Chapters 15 and 16; when this distinction remains genuinely ambiguous on the acute study, follow-up imaging once the child has stabilized is the most reliable way to resolve it. Documenting the specific reasoning supporting a peri-ictal interpretation explicitly in the acute report, rather than a bare descriptive statement of the finding without accompanying interpretive context, helps the treating team avoid an unnecessary escalation of workup for what is, in fact, an expected physiologic consequence of the seizure itself.

Hippocampal Injury From Prolonged Status Epilepticus

Prolonged, particularly convulsive, status epilepticus carries a recognized risk of acute hippocampal injury, visible as diffusion restriction and T2 signal change within the hippocampus on imaging obtained during or shortly after a prolonged seizure episode, a finding with direct relevance to this chapter's earlier discussion of hippocampal sclerosis, since this specific acute injury pattern is hypothesized, though not definitively proven in every case, to represent a potential precursor to the chronic hippocampal sclerosis discussed earlier in this chapter in at least a subset of affected children; recognizing acute hippocampal injury at the time of a prolonged seizure episode therefore carries both immediate and potential long-term prognostic significance worth communicating to the family and incorporating into subsequent long-term epilepsy surveillance planning. Applying the same coronal oblique hippocampal imaging technique developed earlier in this chapter to this acute setting, rather than relying on a routine, non-hippocampus-optimized acute protocol, improves the reliability of this specific finding's detection even in the urgent, acute-care context this section addresses.

Imaging Indications During Acute Status Epilepticus Management

Acute imaging during active status epilepticus is generally reserved for a child without a known epilepsy diagnosis presenting with new-onset prolonged seizures, in whom an acute structural cause, including the stroke, infection, or trauma discussed elsewhere in this book, must be actively excluded, or for a child with established epilepsy whose status epilepticus presentation is atypical for their known seizure pattern, raising concern for a new, superimposed process; a child with a well-established epilepsy diagnosis experiencing a seizure pattern fully consistent with their known baseline does not automatically require acute imaging for every breakthrough seizure or brief status episode, applying the same evidence-based, low-yield-presentation reasoning developed in Chapter 3 to this specific epilepsy-management context. Applying this threshold consistently, rather than defaulting to imaging for every status epilepticus presentation regardless of clinical context, both protects the child from unnecessary sedation and radiation exposure and preserves imaging resources for the presentations in which a genuine, actionable finding is more likely to be identified.

Follow-Up Imaging After Status Epilepticus

When acute peri-ictal or hippocampal injury signal change is identified during a status epilepticus episode, scheduled follow-up imaging once the child has clinically stabilized, typically several weeks to a few months later, is warranted both to confirm the expected resolution of a purely peri-ictal, reversible pattern and, where the initial injury was more substantial, to assess for the development of chronic changes including hippocampal or cortical volume loss that might inform long-term seizure and cognitive outcome counseling; this follow-up imaging is a direct application of the longitudinal, serial-comparison surveillance principle this book has applied throughout to numerous other acute injury patterns.

Febrile Status Epilepticus and the FEBSTAT Findings

Prolonged febrile status epilepticus, distinct from the simple febrile seizure discussed in Chapter 3, has been specifically studied for its association with acute hippocampal injury and subsequent hippocampal sclerosis, with published prospective cohort data demonstrating that a meaningful proportion of children with prolonged febrile status epilepticus show acute hippocampal signal abnormality on imaging obtained shortly after the event, and that a subset of this group subsequently develops hippocampal sclerosis on longer-term follow-up; this specific body of evidence has meaningfully shaped current understanding of the relationship between prolonged early-childhood seizures and subsequent temporal lobe epilepsy, and imaging following a genuinely prolonged febrile status epilepticus episode, unlike the simple febrile seizure discussed in Chapter 3, is an appropriate component of the evaluation given this specific, evidence-based association. Families of a child who has experienced this specific, prolonged presentation benefit from proactive counseling regarding this documented association and the plan for longer-term epilepsy surveillance it warrants, rather than learning of this connection only if and when a subsequent seizure disorder eventually develops.

Nonconvulsive Status Epilepticus and Its Imaging Correlates

Nonconvulsive status epilepticus, in which prolonged electrographic seizure activity occurs without the overt motor convulsion characteristic of convulsive status epilepticus, can be substantially more difficult to recognize clinically and is frequently identified only through continuous electroencephalographic monitoring in a child with unexplained, persistent altered mental status; imaging findings in this circumstance can be subtler or entirely absent compared to convulsive status epilepticus, reinforcing that a normal or near-normal imaging study does not exclude ongoing nonconvulsive seizure activity as an explanation for persistent altered mental status, and continuous electroencephalographic monitoring, not imaging, is the definitive diagnostic tool for this specific presentation.

New-Onset Refractory Status Epilepticus

New-onset refractory status epilepticus, a severe presentation in a previously healthy child without a prior epilepsy history who develops prolonged, treatment-resistant status epilepticus without an immediately identifiable cause, warrants an especially thorough evaluation extending beyond the acute imaging discussed throughout this section, including comprehensive infectious, autoimmune, and metabolic workup, since a substantial proportion of cases ultimately prove to have an autoimmune encephalitis, discussed further in Chapter 16, or another specific, treatable underlying cause; imaging in this specific, severe presentation, while following the same peri-ictal-versus-primary-lesion reasoning developed throughout this section, is understood as one component of a broader, urgent, multidisciplinary diagnostic effort rather than a study expected to provide a standalone, complete explanation on its own.

Communicating Acute Imaging Findings During an Active Emergency

Because status epilepticus is a genuine medical emergency, imaging findings identified during active management require immediate, direct verbal communication to the treating team rather than a written report reviewed asynchronously, applying the urgent-communication principle established in Chapter 1 with particular force given the acuity of this specific clinical scenario; a finding suggesting an acute structural cause requiring immediate intervention, such as a mass with impending herniation or an acute stroke potentially eligible for time-sensitive treatment, must reach the treating team within minutes, not hours, and institutional protocols ensuring this rapid communication pathway is reliably available around the clock are an essential component of comprehensive status epilepticus management infrastructure. Even a reassuring, peri-ictal-consistent finding benefits from timely direct communication in this acute context, since confirming the absence of an alternative structural explanation allows the treating team to proceed confidently with standard status epilepticus management protocols without an unresolved diagnostic question complicating the acute treatment course.

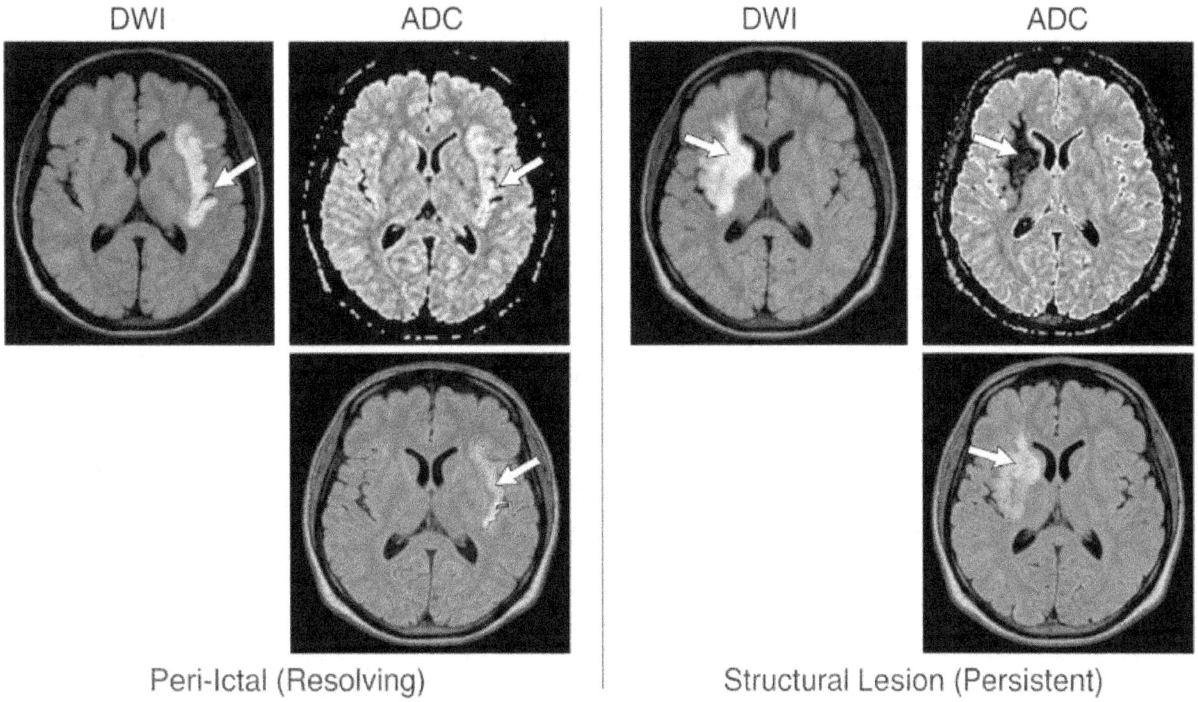

Figure 11.4: Peri-Ictal Signal Change Versus Acute Structural Lesion

Case Presentation: MRI-Negative Epilepsy Localized by SISCOM and PET

A nine-year-old with medically refractory focal epilepsy and a normal dedicated epilepsy-protocol MRI undergoes comprehensive presurgical evaluation. Video-EEG monitoring establishes a right frontal electrographic onset zone concordant with the child's clinical seizure semiology. Applying the reasoning developed in this chapter, ictal SPECT with SISCOM co-registration and interictal FDG-PET are obtained given the MRI-negative status, and both studies concordantly localize a small right frontal hypometabolic, hyperperfusing focus not visible on the original structural MRI. Targeted re-review of the structural MRI at the specific location flagged by SISCOM and PET reveals a subtle area of gray-white blurring not initially appreciated, illustrating how functional imaging can direct a more focused re-review that ultimately identifies a subtle structural correlate. Stereo-EEG is placed targeting this concordant region, confirms it as the true seizure onset zone, and the child proceeds to successful resection, illustrating the complete multimodal integration process this chapter has developed. Neuropsychological evaluation obtained before surgery establishes a documented baseline, and postoperative follow-up assessment at one year demonstrates seizure freedom without a new cognitive deficit relative to that baseline, completing the full arc of presurgical planning through postoperative outcome confirmation this chapter has emphasized throughout.

Case Presentation: Peri-Ictal Change Mistaken for Acute Stroke

A seven-year-old with known focal epilepsy presents to the emergency department following a prolonged focal seizure with associated transient hemiparesis, and acute MRI demonstrates cortical diffusion restriction and T2 signal change in the left parietal region corresponding to her known seizure focus. The covering emergency physician initially raises concern for acute stroke given the diffusion restriction and associated hemiparesis. Applying the reasoning developed in this chapter, child neurology is consulted and notes that the affected region corresponds precisely to the child's previously established seizure onset zone rather than a vascular territory, and that the transient hemiparesis is consistent with a postictal Todd paralysis rather than a new, acute focal deficit. Follow-up MRI obtained two weeks later demonstrates complete resolution of the diffusion and signal abnormality, confirming the peri-ictal mechanism and avoiding what would otherwise have been an unnecessary acute stroke evaluation, including the thrombolysis consideration discussed in Chapter 18, in a child whose presentation was in fact fully explained by her known epilepsy.

Case Presentation: Dual Pathology Identified on Careful Review

A fourteen-year-old with medically refractory temporal lobe epilepsy undergoes epilepsy-protocol MRI demonstrating clear right hippocampal sclerosis with the classic triad of volume loss, architectural disruption, and T2 hyperintensity discussed earlier in this chapter. Applying the dual-pathology reasoning developed in this chapter, the interpreting radiologist does not conclude the search upon identifying this clear, expected finding, and systematic review of the remaining temporal and adjacent extratemporal cortex identifies a subtle area of gray-white blurring in the adjacent temporal neocortex, distinct from the hippocampus itself, consistent with a coexisting focal cortical dysplasia. This second finding is incorporated explicitly into the surgical planning discussion, and the resection is extended beyond a standard mesial temporal resection to address both the hippocampal sclerosis and the adjacent dysplastic cortex, illustrating why concluding the imaging search after identifying the first, more obvious lesion would have left a second, surgically relevant abnormality unaddressed. Postoperative histopathology confirms both entities, validating the imaging-based dual-pathology identification and reinforcing this chapter's central discipline of systematic, complete review rather than stopping at the first satisfying answer.

THE CLINICAL-IMAGING CROSSWALK SYSTEM — Epileptogenic Lesion Recognition and Presurgical Localization

---

Crossing 1 Recap: A postprocessing-flagged region without visual imaging correlation or electroencephalographic concordance should not be accepted as the surgical target; postprocessing is an adjunct to, not a replacement for, correlated assessment.

Chapter Anchor: Epilepsy neuroimaging requires a dedicated protocol distinct from routine brain imaging, and localizing the true epileptogenic zone depends on converging multiple independent data sources, structural imaging, semiology, electroencephalography, and functional imaging, rather than any single modality in isolation; acute peri-ictal signal change must be distinguished from a primary causative lesion by its anatomic concordance with the known seizure focus and its resolution on follow-up.

Summary and Key Concepts

A dedicated epilepsy MRI protocol, with thin-section 3D T1 and coronal oblique hippocampal-optimized T2/FLAIR sequences, is required to reliably detect hippocampal sclerosis and focal cortical dysplasia; a normal routine protocol does not exclude a surgically relevant lesion.

Focal cortical dysplasia type IIb, with its characteristic transmantle sign, is the most reliably detected subtype; type I lesions are frequently MRI-occult, and dual pathology should be actively excluded once one lesion is identified.

Presurgical evaluation integrates video-EEG semiology and electrographic localization with structural MRI, SPECT/PET functional imaging, functional MRI eloquent cortex mapping, and, when needed, invasive stereo-EEG monitoring into a single, converging surgical target.

Peri-ictal signal change from prolonged seizure activity mimics but is distinguished from a primary structural lesion by its anatomic concordance with the known seizure focus and its expected resolution on follow-up imaging; hippocampal injury from prolonged status epilepticus carries long-term surveillance significance.

Acute imaging during status epilepticus is reserved for new-onset seizures or an atypical presentation in known epilepsy, applying the same evidence-based imaging-ordering threshold developed in Chapter 3 rather than reflexive imaging for every breakthrough seizure.

CHAPTER 12: PEDIATRIC BRAIN TUMORS — SUPRATENTORIAL AND SELLAR REGION

Learning Objectives

1. Distinguish low-grade from high-grade supratentorial glioma based on imaging characteristics and correlate imaging grade with expected clinical behavior, including the specific role of molecular classification.
2. Generate an age-appropriate differential diagnosis for a sellar or suprasellar mass and describe the associated endocrine and visual evaluation.
3. Distinguish the major pineal region tumor categories and describe their distinct tumor marker and imaging correlates.
4. Distinguish expected postoperative and treatment-related imaging change from tumor recurrence or progression, including pseudoprogression and radiation necrosis.

Low-Grade and High-Grade Supratentorial Gliomas

Gliomas, tumors arising from the supporting glial cells of the central nervous system, represent the most common category of pediatric brain tumor, and distinguishing low-grade from high-grade glioma on imaging, while never a substitute for histopathologic and molecular confirmation, provides essential early information shaping both the urgency of further evaluation and the family's initial understanding of prognosis. This distinction, and the location-specific reasoning it requires across the supratentorial hemispheres, brainstem, sellar region, and pineal region, forms the organizing structure this chapter applies throughout, extending the anatomically precise, mechanism-based diagnostic approach this book has developed across every preceding chapter into the oncologic domain.

Pilocytic Astrocytoma as the Prototypical Low-Grade Glioma

Pilocytic astrocytoma, the most common pediatric low-grade glioma, classically presents as a well-circumscribed, cystic mass with an enhancing mural nodule, most frequently arising in the cerebellum, discussed further in Chapter 13, but also occurring supratentorially, particularly along the optic pathway and hypothalamic region discussed later in this chapter; this specific cystic-with-mural-nodule morphology, combined with the tumor's characteristically indolent behavior and generally favorable prognosis following surgical resection, distinguishes it sharply from the high-grade gliomas discussed later in this section, and recognizing this pattern confidently on initial imaging appropriately calibrates the urgency and tenor of the family's initial counseling conversation. A minority of pilocytic astrocytomas present instead as a solid, non-cystic mass without the classic mural nodule pattern, and maintaining awareness of this less common but recognized presentation prevents dismissing a solid, otherwise well-circumscribed supratentorial mass from consideration as a pilocytic astrocytoma simply because it lacks the more textbook-typical cystic architecture.

Diffuse Low-Grade Gliomas

Beyond the well-circumscribed pilocytic astrocytoma, a further category of diffuse, infiltrative low-grade gliomas, including diffuse astrocytoma, presents a less discrete imaging appearance, characterized by non-enhancing or minimally enhancing T2/FLAIR hyperintense signal abnormality without a well-defined tumor margin, distinguishing them both from the discrete pilocytic astrocytoma discussed above and from the more aggressive high-grade gliomas discussed below; this diffuse, infiltrative growth pattern carries direct surgical implications, since a tumor without a clear margin cannot be as completely resected as a well-circumscribed lesion, and molecular and genetic characterization of the resected or biopsied tissue increasingly refines the specific prognosis and treatment pathway within this broader diffuse low-grade category. A subset of diffuse low-grade gliomas nonetheless follows an indolent, slowly progressive or even radiographically stable course over years, and serial surveillance imaging, rather than a presumption of inevitable progression at the time of initial diagnosis, is often the most appropriate initial management approach for an asymptomatic or minimally symptomatic child with this specific tumor category.

High-Grade Glioma Imaging Characteristics

High-grade gliomas, including diffuse midline glioma discussed further below and other high-grade astrocytic tumors, characteristically show more aggressive imaging features than their low-grade counterparts: irregular, infiltrative margins, heterogeneous or irregular ring enhancement reflecting central necrosis, substantial surrounding vasogenic edema, and, on advanced imaging, elevated perfusion and a spectroscopic profile reflecting the tumor's increased cellularity and metabolic activity; recognizing this constellation of aggressive features, even before histopathologic grading is available, appropriately triggers urgent, rather than routine, referral and family communication given the substantially different management timeline high-grade glioma requires relative to the low-grade tumors discussed above. Restricted diffusion within the solid, enhancing component of a high-grade glioma, reflecting its high cellular density, is a further supportive feature worth actively assessing, since a low-grade tumor characteristically does not show this same degree of diffusion restriction within its solid components.

Diffuse Midline Glioma and the Pontine Predilection

Diffuse midline glioma, most classically arising in the pons, where it was historically termed diffuse intrinsic pontine glioma, but also occurring in the thalamus and spinal cord, represents among the most devastating diagnoses in pediatric neuro-oncology, characteristically presenting with a classic clinical triad of cranial neuropathy, long tract signs, and ataxia reflecting its brainstem location, and an imaging appearance of diffuse, expansile T2/FLAIR signal abnormality effacing the normal pontine architecture, often with only minimal or patchy enhancement despite its high-grade molecular biology; the characteristic imaging appearance combined with the classic clinical presentation is sufficiently distinctive that biopsy, while increasingly pursued at specialized centers specifically for molecular characterization and clinical trial eligibility, is not always required to establish this diagnosis with high confidence.

Communicating this specific diagnosis and its generally poor prognosis to a family is among the most difficult conversations in pediatric neuro-oncology, and the honest, proportionate, uncertainty-acknowledging communication framework developed throughout this book applies with particular weight to this specific circumstance, balancing clear, honest prognostic information against continued hope for the evolving clinical trial and treatment landscape this diagnosis is actively subject to.

Molecular Classification and Its Growing Imaging Correlation

Contemporary tumor classification increasingly incorporates molecular and genetic markers, including IDH mutation status, H3K27M alteration characteristic of diffuse midline glioma, and BRAF alterations common in pilocytic astrocytoma and other low-grade gliomas, alongside traditional histopathologic grading, and specific imaging features are increasingly recognized to correlate, though imperfectly, with these molecular subgroups; while a full discussion of molecular neuro-oncology extends beyond this chapter's imaging focus, the reader should understand that a final, complete diagnosis in contemporary practice integrates imaging, histopathology, and molecular testing together, rather than imaging or histopathology serving as a standalone, sufficient diagnostic endpoint. BRAF-altered low-grade gliomas, in particular, are increasingly eligible for targeted molecular therapy rather than conventional chemotherapy alone, making molecular characterization of a resected or biopsied low-grade glioma directly relevant to treatment selection, not merely an academic or prognostic exercise.

Advanced Imaging Techniques in Glioma Characterization

Beyond conventional structural sequences, advanced techniques introduced in Chapter 1, including perfusion imaging, which assesses tumor vascularity and tends to be elevated in higher-grade lesions, and magnetic resonance spectroscopy, which characterizes the tumor's metabolic profile through elevated choline and reduced N-acetylaspartate relative to normal brain, add complementary information that can refine the imaging-based grade estimate discussed above, particularly valuable when a tumor's conventional imaging appearance falls in an ambiguous, intermediate zone between clearly low-grade and clearly high-grade features. These advanced sequences are added selectively, applying the same adjunct-sequence discipline established in Chapter 1, when the conventional imaging grade assessment is genuinely ambiguous or when the specific perfusion or spectroscopic data will directly change the urgency of referral or the biopsy target selected, rather than obtained reflexively for every newly identified supratentorial mass regardless of how confidently its grade can already be estimated from conventional sequences alone.

Optic Pathway Glioma and Its NF1 Association

Optic pathway glioma, a low-grade glioma variant arising along the optic nerves, chiasm, or tracts, occurs both sporadically and, with substantially increased frequency, in children with neurofibromatosis type 1, discussed further in Chapter 14, and this specific location carries direct visual risk regardless of the tumor's favorable histologic grade, making visual outcome, rather than survival alone, a central consideration in both imaging surveillance and treatment decision-making; a child with neurofibromatosis type 1 undergoes proactive screening for this specific tumor given its markedly increased incidence in this population, applying the same anticipatory, syndrome-directed surveillance principle this book has emphasized throughout for other genetically defined risk populations.

Ganglioglioma and Dysembryoplastic Neuroepithelial Tumor

Ganglioglioma and dysembryoplastic neuroepithelial tumor, both low-grade, well-differentiated tumors with a strong association with medically refractory epilepsy, discussed in Chapter 11, present with a distinctive imaging appearance frequently including a cortically based location, cystic components, and, particularly for dysembryoplastic neuroepithelial tumor, a characteristic bubbly, multicystic appearance without significant surrounding edema or mass effect disproportionate to their size; recognizing these tumors' characteristically indolent behavior and their strong epilepsy association, rather than the more aggressive behavior typical of other glioma categories in this chapter, appropriately calibrates the urgency of the family's initial counseling and directs surgical planning toward the epilepsy-focused resection approach discussed in Chapter 11. Both entities may show a faint, T2-hyperintense cortical rim or a small, curvilinear enhancing component, further distinguishing them from a simple, avascular cortical cyst, and the reader is encouraged to apply the same systematic surface-and-signal characterization habit developed in Chapter 7 when evaluating a cortically based lesion of uncertain nature.

Surgical Resection Extent and Its Prognostic Significance

The extent of surgical resection achieved, whether gross total, near-total, or subtotal, carries direct prognostic significance across essentially every glioma category discussed in this section, and precise, quantitative assessment of residual tumor volume on the early postoperative imaging discussed later in this chapter, rather than a qualitative surgeon's impression alone, provides the most reliable basis for this assessment; a family counseled regarding expected prognosis benefits from understanding this direct relationship between resection completeness and outcome, since it directly explains why the specific early postoperative imaging timing this chapter emphasizes carries genuine clinical, not merely administrative, significance. Standardized, structured residual-volume reporting, using the same reproducible measurement approach across a treating institution's neuro-oncology practice, allows meaningful comparison of outcomes across patients and over time, supporting both individual patient counseling and the institution's own ongoing quality assessment of its surgical outcomes.

Hemispheric Glioma and Extent of Resection Considerations

Supratentorial hemispheric high-grade gliomas, arising within the cerebral hemispheres away from the deep midline structures discussed elsewhere in this chapter, generally offer a more favorable surgical resection opportunity than the midline and brainstem tumors discussed above, since a hemispheric location more often permits an aggressive resection without the same degree of eloquent-structure risk; precise preoperative imaging characterization of the tumor's relationship to eloquent cortex, applying the same functional mapping techniques developed in Chapter 11 for epilepsy surgery, similarly informs the achievable resection extent and expected functional outcome for this specific tumor category. Diffusion tensor tractography, mapping the major white matter tracts adjacent to a planned resection, further complements this functional characterization by identifying critical subcortical pathways, such as the corticospinal tract, that conventional structural and functional MRI localization alone may not fully capture, extending the multimodal presurgical integration principle from Chapter 11 into this chapter's oncologic surgical planning context.

Figure 12.1: Pilocytic Astrocytoma Versus High-Grade Glioma

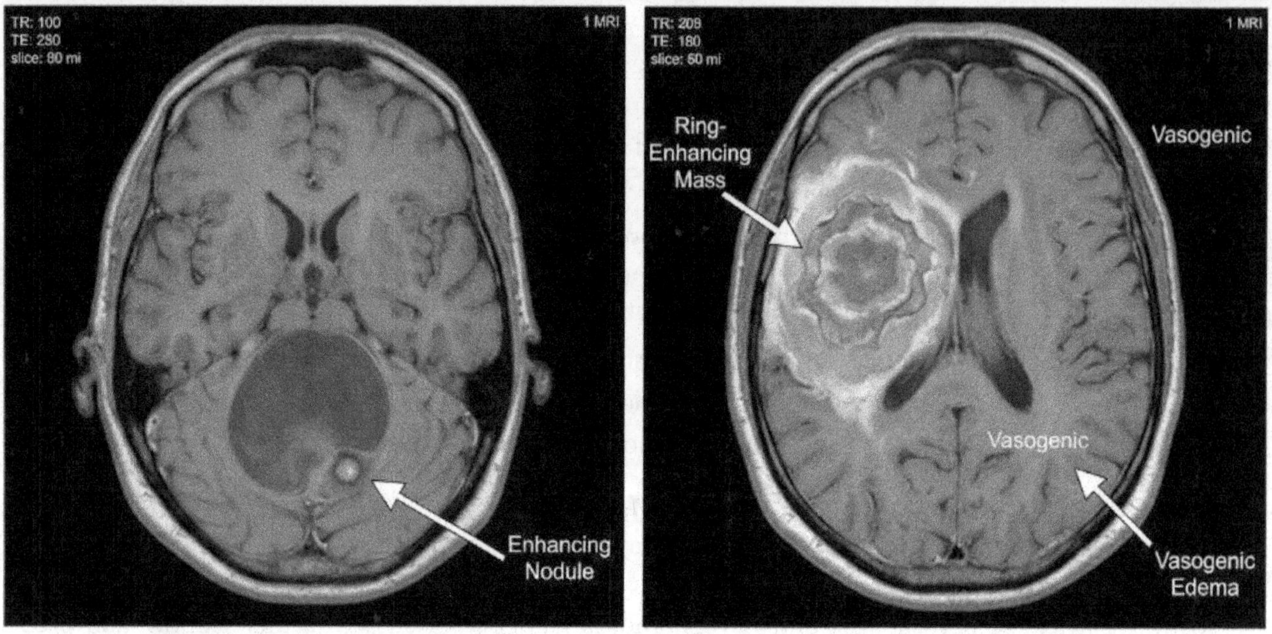

Pilocytic Astrocytoma | High-Grade Glioma

Feature	Low-Grade Glioma	High-Grade Glioma
Margin	Well-circumscribed (pilocytic) or diffuse but non-aggressive	Irregular, infiltrative
Enhancement	Solid nodule (pilocytic) or minimal (diffuse)	Heterogeneous, often ring-enhancing
Edema	Minimal	Substantial vasogenic edema
Perfusion	Low	Elevated

Sellar and Suprasellar Masses

The sellar and suprasellar region hosts a distinctive differential diagnosis shaped by the specific anatomic structures present in this location, the pituitary gland, optic chiasm, hypothalamus, and infundibulum, and correctly narrowing this differential requires the same age-specific and anatomically precise reasoning this book applies throughout. Every entity addressed in this section, whether neoplastic or the non-neoplastic entities discussed alongside them, is distinguished not by a single defining feature but by the specific combination of solid, cystic, calcified, and enhancement characteristics this section develops systematically for each.

Craniopharyngioma

Craniopharyngioma, the most common pediatric sellar and suprasellar tumor, characteristically presents as a mixed solid-cystic mass with calcification, particularly in its more common adamantinomatous histologic subtype, and frequently produces the combination of visual disturbance from optic chiasm compression, endocrine dysfunction from hypothalamic-pituitary involvement, and, when large enough to obstruct the third ventricle, hydrocephalus discussed in Chapter 10; recognizing this specific combination of solid, cystic, and calcified components on imaging, rather than any single feature in isolation, provides the most reliable basis for suspecting this diagnosis before histopathologic confirmation. The less common papillary histologic subtype, occurring predominantly in adults but occasionally in adolescents, typically presents as a more solid, less calcified mass than the classic adamantinomatous pattern, a distinction worth holding in mind when an otherwise suspected craniopharyngioma lacks the calcification this section has emphasized as characteristic.

Germ Cell Tumors of the Suprasellar Region

Germ cell tumors, including germinoma and the less common, more heterogeneous nongerminomatous germ cell tumors, occur in the suprasellar region with a distinct predilection related to the embryologic origin of germ cell tumors along the midline, and this location shares a bimodal distribution with the pineal region germ cell tumors discussed later in this chapter, at times occurring synchronously in both locations (bifocal germinoma); serum and cerebrospinal fluid tumor marker assessment, including alpha-fetoprotein and beta-human chorionic gonadotropin, is a standard, essential component of the evaluation for a suspected suprasellar germ cell tumor, since marker elevation both supports the diagnosis and, particularly for nongerminomatous germ cell tumors, can obviate the need for biopsy in an appropriately characteristic clinical and imaging context. Suprasellar germinoma classically presents with diabetes insipidus, at times preceding any visible mass on imaging by months to years, a specific, well-documented diagnostic pitfall in which a child with unexplained diabetes insipidus and an initially normal-appearing pituitary stalk warrants close interval imaging surveillance rather than a single, reassuring negative study.

Rathke Cleft Cyst

Rathke cleft cyst, a benign, non-neoplastic cystic remnant of the embryologic Rathke pouch, is a common incidental finding within or adjacent to the sella, generally small, simple in signal characteristics, and asymptomatic, though a larger cyst can produce mass effect on the pituitary gland or optic chiasm with resulting endocrine or visual symptoms; distinguishing a Rathke cleft cyst from the cystic component of a craniopharyngioma depends on the absence of solid enhancing components and calcification characteristic of the latter, a distinction with direct management implications given the benign, generally observation-appropriate natural history of an asymptomatic Rathke cleft cyst relative to the more aggressive management craniopharyngioma warrants. A Rathke cleft cyst occasionally contains a small, non-enhancing intracystic nodule, distinct from the solid, enhancing nodule of a true neoplasm, and recognizing this specific, benign nodular variant prevents an unnecessary escalation of concern when this characteristic, non-enhancing internal nodule is identified within an otherwise typical Rathke cleft cyst.

Hypothalamic Hamartoma

Hypothalamic hamartoma, a non-neoplastic, congenital heterotopic mass of normal-appearing gray matter arising from the tuber cinereum or mammillary bodies, presents with a distinctive clinical syndrome of gelastic (laughing) seizures, often the earliest presenting symptom, and, in a subset of affected children, precocious puberty from direct hypothalamic hormonal disruption; recognizing the characteristic imaging appearance, an isointense-to-gray-matter mass without enhancement or growth over time, distinguishes this benign, congenital lesion from the neoplastic sellar and suprasellar masses discussed elsewhere in this section, and the specific surgical or laser ablation approaches discussed in Chapter 11 for this lesion reflect its distinct, non-neoplastic nature. Beyond gelastic seizures, hypothalamic hamartoma is frequently associated with a broader epilepsy syndrome that can evolve to include additional seizure types and progressive cognitive and behavioral decline if left untreated, providing further rationale, beyond seizure control alone, for definitive treatment once this diagnosis is confirmed.

Pituitary Adenoma in Childhood

Pituitary adenoma, while considerably less common in childhood than in adulthood, does occur in the pediatric population, most frequently as a prolactin-secreting or growth-hormone-secreting functional adenoma presenting with the corresponding endocrine syndrome rather than as an incidental finding; a child with a suspected pituitary adenoma requires the same dedicated, thin-section pituitary imaging protocol discussed in Chapter 8, and correlating the imaging findings with the specific endocrine laboratory abnormality identified, rather than relying on imaging characterization alone, most reliably confirms this diagnosis and distinguishes a genuine functional adenoma from the normal pubertal pituitary enlargement discussed in Chapter 2. Given the increased incidence of pituitary adenoma in specific genetic syndromes, including multiple endocrine neoplasia type 1 and certain familial isolated pituitary adenoma syndromes, a confirmed pediatric pituitary adenoma, an uncommon finding at this age relative to adulthood, warrants genetics referral to evaluate for one of these underlying syndromes, applying the same phenotype-directed genetic testing principle developed in Chapter 7.

Endocrine and Visual Evaluation as an Integral Component

Given the shared anatomic location this section's tumor categories occupy, coordinated endocrine and ophthalmologic evaluation is a necessary, integral component of the evaluation for any sellar or suprasellar mass, not an optional adjunct pursued only once a specific symptom has emerged; baseline pituitary hormone panel testing and formal visual field assessment, obtained proactively at the time of initial diagnosis regardless of whether the child has yet reported a specific endocrine or visual symptom, establishes the baseline against which both tumor-related progression and treatment-related change can be reliably tracked over the child's subsequent longitudinal care.

Craniopharyngioma Surgical Approach and Hypothalamic Preservation

Surgical management of craniopharyngioma has evolved to weigh the goal of complete resection against the substantial morbidity risk of aggressive hypothalamic manipulation, since the tumor's frequent close adherence to the hypothalamus can make gross total resection achievable only at the cost of severe, permanent hypothalamic dysfunction including intractable obesity and disrupted temperature and sleep regulation; precise preoperative imaging characterization of the tumor's specific relationship to the hypothalamus, distinguishing a tumor that displaces the hypothalamus from one that has infiltrated it, directly informs this critical surgical risk-benefit calculation and the resulting decision between an aggressive resection strategy and a more conservative, function-preserving approach combined with adjuvant radiation. This specific imaging distinction, displacement versus infiltration, is among the most consequential single interpretive judgments addressed anywhere in this chapter, given its direct bearing on a child's lifelong metabolic and endocrine function, and warrants the same deliberate, unhurried, multidisciplinary review this book has emphasized for other high-stakes structural determinations.

Long-Term Endocrine Surveillance After Sellar Tumor Treatment

Given the near-universal endocrine involvement accompanying sellar and suprasellar tumors and their treatment, whether from the tumor itself, the surgical resection, or radiation therapy, lifelong endocrine surveillance extending well beyond the completion of oncologic treatment is a standard, essential component of long-term care for this population, addressing growth, pubertal development, thyroid function, adrenal function, and, particularly following hypothalamic involvement or injury, the metabolic and weight-regulation dysfunction discussed above; coordinating this surveillance explicitly with endocrinology from the point of diagnosis, rather than allowing it to lapse once active oncologic treatment concludes, protects against these often-delayed but highly consequential long-term effects. A structured, written endocrine surveillance schedule, established jointly by the neuro-oncology and endocrinology teams at the time of diagnosis and shared explicitly with the family, prevents this critical, ongoing surveillance component from being deprioritized once the more visible oncologic treatment phase has concluded.

Vascular Considerations Near the Sellar Region

The sellar and suprasellar region's close anatomic relationship to the circle of Willis and internal carotid arteries means a large sellar or suprasellar mass can produce vascular displacement or, less commonly, direct vascular encasement, findings with direct surgical planning significance given the catastrophic potential of an intraoperative vascular injury in this densely packed anatomic region; dedicated vascular imaging, whether through conventional MR angiography or the vascular-phase information present on a well-performed structural study, is incorporated into the preoperative evaluation whenever a large or unusually located sellar mass raises this specific vascular relationship as a surgical planning concern. Documenting the specific degree of vascular encasement, using a standardized grading scale where the specific surgical team's practice employs one, gives the surgical team a precise, reproducible basis for the approach-selection discussion this finding necessarily prompts, rather than a purely qualitative, potentially variably interpreted descriptive impression.

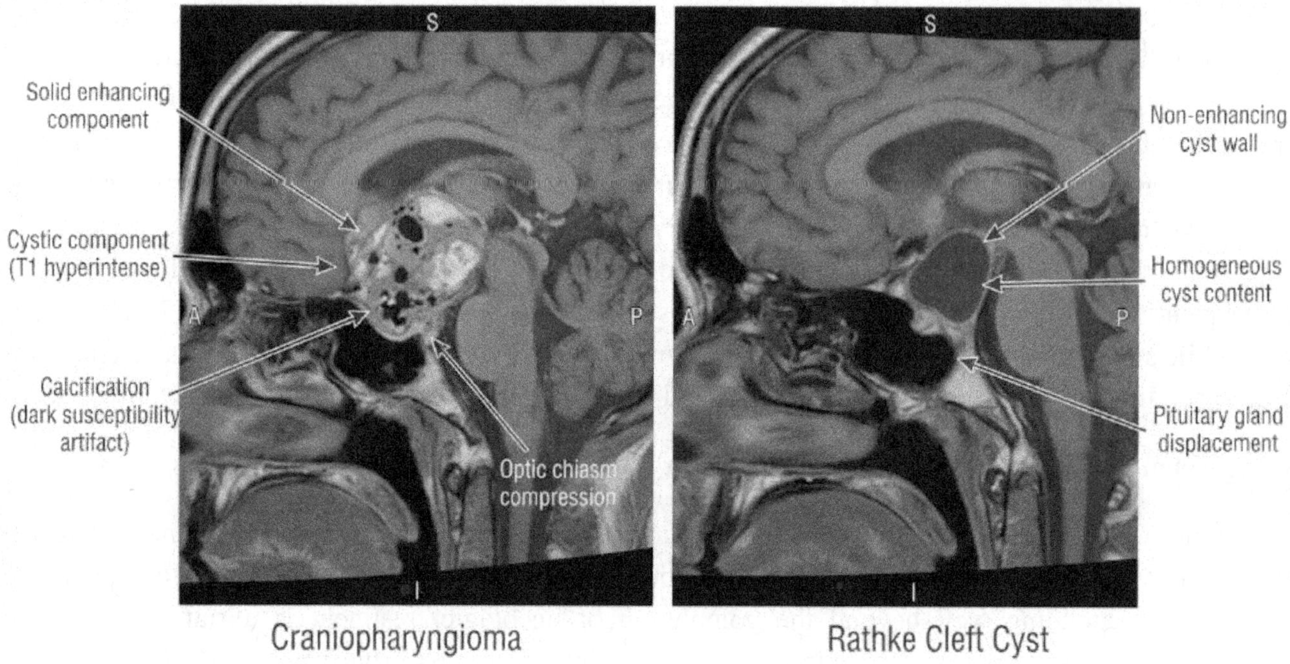

Figure 12.2: Craniopharyngioma Versus Rathke Cleft Cyst

THE CLINICAL-IMAGING CROSSWALK SYSTEM — A Suprasellar Mass With Elevated Tumor Markers

The Crossing: A twelve-year-old boy presents with new diabetes insipidus and a suprasellar mass on MRI, and serum beta-human chorionic gonadotropin is mildly elevated.

Presentation Signature: A school-age or adolescent child with diabetes insipidus, a suprasellar mass, and an elevated serum tumor marker.

Imaging Correlate: The suprasellar mass shows homogeneous enhancement without the calcification and mixed cystic architecture characteristic of craniopharyngioma; cerebrospinal fluid tumor marker assessment and dedicated pineal region imaging are obtained given the recognized bifocal germinoma pattern discussed in this chapter, and pineal region imaging identifies a second, synchronous lesion.

Trap Logic: Attributing a suprasellar mass with diabetes insipidus reflexively to craniopharyngioma without first assessing tumor markers risks missing a germ cell tumor, a diagnosis with a distinct treatment pathway, including radiation-sensitive chemoradiotherapy protocols, and a search for synchronous pineal involvement that would otherwise be omitted.

Crossing Anchor: A suprasellar mass with diabetes insipidus warrants serum and cerebrospinal fluid tumor marker assessment before presuming craniopharyngioma; elevated markers should prompt dedicated pineal region imaging to evaluate for bifocal germinoma.

Pineal Region Tumors

The pineal region hosts a distinct tumor differential shaped by the region's unique embryology, encompassing both germ cell tumors sharing the midline origin discussed in the preceding section and tumors arising from the pineal parenchyma itself, and this section develops the specific imaging and tumor marker reasoning that distinguishes these categories.

Germinoma of the Pineal Region

Germinoma, the most common pineal region tumor, characteristically presents as a well-defined, homogeneously enhancing mass, often engulfing rather than displacing the normal pineal gland calcification, a distinctive pattern sometimes termed the exploded pineal gland sign; germinoma is exquisitely radiosensitive, and this favorable radiosensitivity, combined with typically normal or only mildly elevated tumor markers, distinguishes it prognostically from the nongerminomatous germ cell tumors discussed below, though tissue or cerebrospinal fluid confirmation remains standard practice before committing to a specific treatment pathway given the significant treatment differences between these categories. Germinoma shows a marked male predominance in the pineal region, the reverse of the sex distribution more typically seen in suprasellar germinoma, a demographic detail worth holding alongside the imaging and marker findings discussed throughout this section when constructing the overall differential for a newly identified pineal or suprasellar mass in a specific child.

Nongerminomatous Germ Cell Tumors

Nongerminomatous germ cell tumors, a heterogeneous category including yolk sac tumor, choriocarcinoma, embryonal carcinoma, and mixed germ cell tumors, typically present with more substantially elevated tumor markers than germinoma, alpha-fetoprotein for yolk sac tumor and beta-human chorionic gonadotropin for choriocarcinoma, and carry a less favorable prognosis than pure germinoma, generally requiring more intensive multimodal treatment; the specific pattern and magnitude of marker elevation, correlated against the imaging appearance, substantially narrows this heterogeneous category even before histopathologic confirmation and directly informs the treatment intensity a family should be counseled to expect. Mixed germ cell tumors, containing more than one histologic component within a single lesion, present a particular marker-interpretation challenge, since the resulting marker profile reflects the combined contribution of each component present, and a marker pattern that does not neatly fit a single, pure histologic category should prompt consideration of this specific, combined possibility rather than being forced into one of the purer diagnostic categories this section has named individually.

Pineoblastoma and Pineocytoma

Pineoblastoma, a highly aggressive embryonal tumor arising from pineal parenchymal cells, and pineocytoma, its far more indolent, well-differentiated counterpart, represent opposite ends of the pineal parenchymal tumor spectrum, and their imaging appearances correspondingly diverge: pineoblastoma typically shows an aggressive, invasive, heterogeneously enhancing mass with a propensity for early leptomeningeal dissemination requiring full craniospinal staging imaging, while pineocytoma typically shows a smaller, well-circumscribed, homogeneously enhancing mass without the invasive features or dissemination risk characteristic of its aggressive counterpart; correctly distinguishing these two entities on initial imaging, while ultimately requiring histopathologic confirmation, substantially shapes the initial urgency of the evaluation and staging pursued. An intermediate-grade category, pineal parenchymal tumor of intermediate differentiation, occupies a histologic and, correspondingly, an imaging middle ground between these two extremes, underscoring that the pineocytoma-to-pineoblastoma spectrum, like several other categories addressed throughout this book, is better understood as a continuum than as two sharply separated, mutually exclusive diagnostic categories.

Pineal Cyst Versus Pineal Tumor

Building directly on the benign pineal cyst discussion in Chapter 2, distinguishing a simple, benign pineal cyst from a true pineal region tumor depends on the specific imaging features developed throughout that earlier chapter and reinforced here: a simple cyst shows a thin wall, no solid enhancing component, and stability on any follow-up imaging obtained, while a true tumor shows a more substantial solid, enhancing component and, frequently, associated mass effect on adjacent structures including the tectum, with resulting obstructive hydrocephalus from aqueductal compression; applying this same discrimination framework consistently, whether the pineal region finding is identified incidentally, as in Chapter 2, or as the primary focus of a dedicated tumor evaluation, as in this chapter, ensures a benign cyst is not mistaken for a tumor requiring aggressive intervention, and the reverse. A pineal cyst with a mildly thickened wall or faint peripheral enhancement, an intermediate appearance falling short of the more substantial solid component that would clearly indicate a tumor, is reasonably managed with a single, confirmatory follow-up study rather than either immediate biopsy or indefinite dismissal, applying the same proportionate, graduated response this book has emphasized for other genuinely borderline imaging findings.

Obstructive Hydrocephalus as a Common Presenting Feature

Given the pineal region's direct anatomic relationship to the cerebral aqueduct, a pineal region tumor of any category discussed in this section frequently presents with obstructive hydrocephalus from direct aqueductal compression, applying the obstructive hydrocephalus reasoning developed in Chapter 10, and Parinaud syndrome, a specific pattern of upward gaze palsy and convergence-retraction nystagmus reflecting direct compression of the dorsal midbrain tectum; recognizing this specific combined presentation, hydrocephalus plus Parinaud syndrome, should prompt immediate consideration of a pineal region mass as the underlying cause, directing dedicated pineal region imaging as the appropriate next diagnostic step.

Cerebrospinal Fluid Cytology and Staging Imaging

Given the recognized leptomeningeal dissemination risk carried by several pineal region tumor categories discussed in this section, particularly pineoblastoma and, to a lesser degree, germ cell tumors, cerebrospinal fluid cytology and full craniospinal staging imaging, extending the imaging field of view to the entire spinal axis applying the field-of-view extension principle established in Chapter 1, are standard components of the initial evaluation once a pineal region tumor is suspected, performed before, or in careful coordination with, any surgical intervention that might otherwise transiently elevate intracranial pressure and complicate safe lumbar cerebrospinal fluid sampling. Drop metastases identified on this staging spine imaging, discrete, enhancing nodules along the spinal cord surface or cauda equina reflecting cerebrospinal-fluid-borne tumor spread, carry direct implications for both overall staging and the radiation field ultimately selected, since a child with confirmed spinal dissemination requires craniospinal, rather than focal, radiation coverage.

Biopsy Versus Empiric Treatment for Suspected Germinoma

Because germinoma is exquisitely radiosensitive and carries an excellent prognosis with appropriate treatment, a clinical debate exists regarding whether a highly characteristic imaging and tumor marker presentation, in the appropriate demographic context, justifies proceeding directly to empiric radiation therapy rather than pursuing surgical biopsy first, weighing the surgical risk of biopsy in this deep, midline location against the diagnostic certainty biopsy provides before committing to a specific treatment pathway; practice varies across specialized centers regarding this specific question, and a family should understand that this represents a genuine area of clinical judgment rather than a single, universally agreed-upon standard, consistent with the honest acknowledgment of areas of clinical controversy this book's broader framework requires.

Pineal Region Surgical Approach Considerations

The pineal region's deep, midline location surrounded by critical venous structures, including the internal cerebral veins and vein of Galen, makes surgical approach to this region among the more technically demanding in pediatric neurosurgery, and precise preoperative imaging characterization of the tumor's relationship to these venous structures, along with the deep cerebral veins and the tectum itself, directly shapes the specific surgical corridor selected, whether an infratentorial supracerebellar or occipital transtentorial approach, each offering different advantages depending on the tumor's precise anatomic relationships as characterized on the preoperative imaging this chapter has emphasized throughout. Preoperative venous-phase imaging, applying the venous imaging principles introduced in Chapter 6, is therefore a standard, essential component of pineal region tumor characterization, not an optional adjunct, given the catastrophic potential of unplanned venous injury during surgery in this specific anatomic corridor.

Figure 12.3: Germinoma With the Exploded Pineal Gland Sign

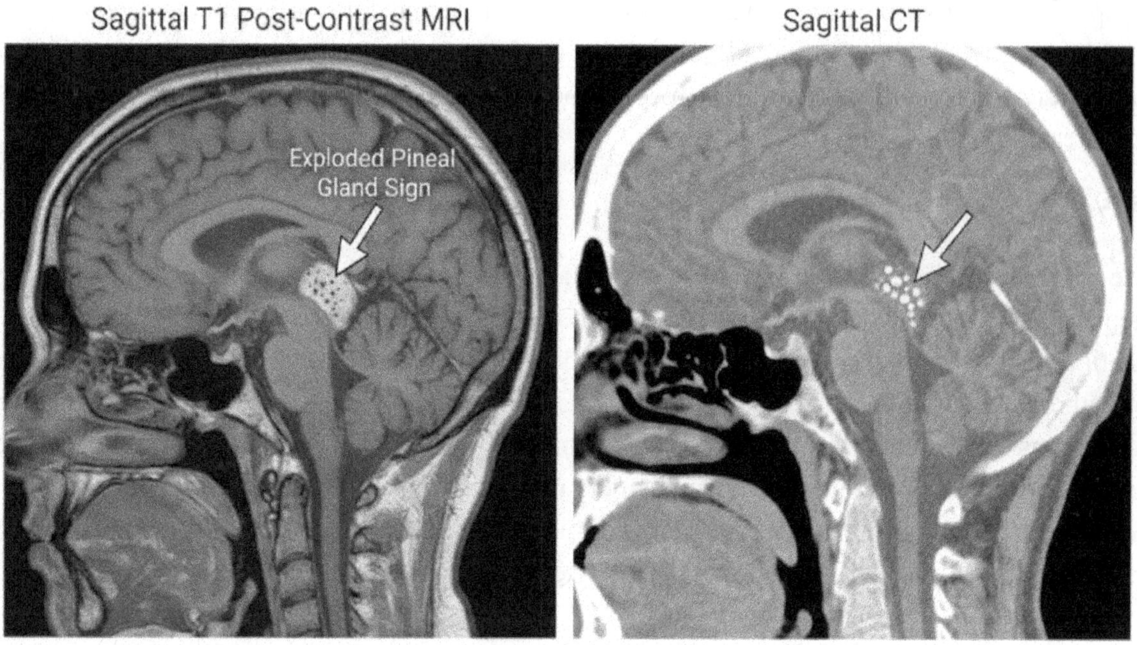

Postoperative and Treatment-Related Imaging Change

This closing section addresses the distinct, essential skill of distinguishing expected postoperative and treatment-related imaging change from genuine tumor recurrence or progression, a discrimination task with direct, ongoing significance across the entire longitudinal course of pediatric brain tumor management.

Early Postoperative Imaging and Its Specific Purpose

Early postoperative MRI, typically obtained within forty-eight to seventy-two hours of resection, serves a specific, time-limited purpose distinct from later surveillance imaging: establishing the extent of resection achieved and identifying any acute surgical complication, before the expected postsurgical enhancement discussed below has had time to develop and potentially confound the assessment of residual tumor; obtaining this study within the specific early window this section identifies, rather than at an arbitrary later postoperative time point, is essential to its diagnostic reliability for extent-of-resection assessment specifically. A study obtained even a few days beyond this window can already show early, confounding postsurgical enhancement that makes distinguishing residual tumor from expected surgical change meaningfully more difficult, underscoring why scheduling this specific study within the correct window is a genuine clinical priority rather than a flexible administrative convenience.

Expected Postsurgical Enhancement and Its Timeline

Benign, expected postsurgical enhancement along the resection margin develops over the days to weeks following surgery, reflecting a combination of disrupted blood-brain barrier and reactive granulation tissue at the surgical site, and can persist for weeks to several months before gradually resolving; this expected enhancement pattern, thin, smooth, and linear along the resection cavity margin, is distinguished from nodular, thick, or progressively enlarging enhancement, which instead raises concern for residual or recurrent tumor, a distinction requiring the same careful, structured comparison against prior imaging this book emphasizes throughout for other longitudinal surveillance contexts. Blood products and hemosiderin staining along the resection margin, expected findings on susceptibility-weighted or gradient-echo sequences following any craniotomy, should similarly not be mistaken for a separate, concerning finding, and distinguishing this expected postsurgical blood-product pattern from a new, unexpected hemorrhage elsewhere in the brain is a further discrimination this section's early postoperative imaging is specifically positioned to make.

Radiation-Related Imaging Change

Radiation therapy produces its own distinct spectrum of imaging change over a timeline extending well beyond the immediate postoperative period discussed above, including pseudoprogression, a transient increase in enhancement and edema occurring typically within the first few months after radiation completion that can closely mimic true tumor progression, and, over a longer timeline measured in years, radiation necrosis, a delayed, progressive change that similarly can be difficult to distinguish from recurrent tumor on conventional imaging alone; advanced imaging techniques, including perfusion imaging and spectroscopy discussed earlier in this chapter, assist in this discrimination, since radiation-related change typically shows lower perfusion and a different metabolic profile than viable, recurrent tumor, though genuine diagnostic ambiguity in an individual case sometimes ultimately requires biopsy for definitive resolution. Amino acid PET tracers, an emerging complementary technique at specialized centers, offer a further tool for this specific discrimination, since tumor tissue characteristically shows increased amino acid uptake relative to radiation-related change, though availability of this specific technique remains limited outside dedicated neuro-oncology imaging programs.

Structured Surveillance Imaging Schedules

Following the immediate postoperative and treatment period, structured surveillance imaging at defined intervals, typically more frequent in the first one to two years following treatment when recurrence risk is highest and progressively less frequent thereafter, is standard practice for essentially every pediatric brain tumor category discussed in this chapter, with the specific interval and total surveillance duration tailored to the tumor's histologic and molecular risk profile; applying a consistent, protocol-driven surveillance schedule, rather than an ad hoc, individually improvised imaging interval, ensures recurrence is identified at the earliest possible point across a family's entire treatment journey. Coordinating this surveillance schedule explicitly with the family, including providing a written, forward-looking schedule of anticipated future studies rather than scheduling each study reactively only shortly before it is due, helps the family plan around this recurring commitment and reduces the anxiety an unpredictable, ad hoc scheduling pattern can otherwise compound.

Chemotherapy-Related Imaging Findings

Beyond the surgical and radiation-related changes discussed above, chemotherapy carries its own recognized imaging associations, including posterior reversible encephalopathy syndrome related to certain chemotherapeutic agents and the hypertension they can induce, and, less commonly, treatment-related leukoencephalopathy from certain agents' direct white matter toxicity; recognizing these specific, agent-associated patterns, and correlating a new imaging finding against the specific treatment regimen a child is actively receiving, prevents misattributing a treatment-related complication to tumor progression, a distinction with direct implications for whether treatment is continued, modified, or discontinued. Maintaining a current, accessible treatment timeline alongside each child's imaging record, listing every agent received and its administration dates, is a practical documentation habit that directly supports this correlation exercise at the moment a new, unexpected finding is identified, rather than requiring the interpreting clinician to reconstruct this history retrospectively from a fragmented chart.

Communicating Surveillance Imaging Results to Families

Given the substantial anxiety a family of a child with a treated brain tumor experiences around each scheduled surveillance study, sometimes termed scanxiety in the broader oncology literature, clear, prompt communication of results, whether reassuring or concerning, applying the honest, timely communication principles developed throughout this book, meaningfully supports the family through this recurring, high-stress component of long-term survivorship care; establishing a consistent, predictable communication timeline for surveillance results at the outset of a child's treatment course, rather than leaving the family uncertain how or when they will learn each result, is itself a component of comprehensive, family-centered long-term care.

Second Malignancy Risk From Radiation Exposure

Children treated with radiation therapy for a primary brain tumor carry a small but well-documented, long-term risk of a second, radiation-induced malignancy arising within the treatment field many years after treatment completion, a risk that extends the surveillance imaging discussed throughout this section well beyond the primary tumor's own recurrence risk window; a new, unexpected finding arising many years after successful treatment of the original tumor, particularly one occurring within or at the margin of the original radiation field, should prompt consideration of this specific, delayed second-malignancy possibility rather than being presumed to represent either a benign, unrelated finding or a highly unlikely, decades-delayed recurrence of the original tumor. This risk is a further, important component of the informed treatment discussion at the time radiation therapy is initially considered, weighed honestly alongside radiation's substantial therapeutic benefit for the primary tumor, consistent with the balanced, proportionate risk communication this book has emphasized throughout for every major treatment decision it addresses.

Neurocognitive Late Effects and Their Imaging Correlates

Beyond the structural imaging surveillance emphasized throughout this section, children treated for a brain tumor, particularly with radiation therapy at a young age, carry a recognized risk of long-term neurocognitive late effects, and volumetric and diffusion-based imaging techniques have identified correlates of this cognitive impact, including white matter volume reduction and altered diffusion tensor imaging metrics in radiation-exposed regions; while these advanced techniques remain primarily research tools rather than standard clinical surveillance practice, awareness of this documented structural-cognitive correlation supports proactive neuropsychological surveillance, applying the same baseline-and-longitudinal-tracking principle developed in Chapter 11, as a standard, anticipated component of comprehensive long-term survivorship care. Younger age at treatment is consistently associated with greater neurocognitive vulnerability in the published literature, a dose-and-age relationship that has directly motivated efforts to defer or reduce radiation exposure in the youngest affected children whenever an equally effective alternative treatment approach exists.

Transitioning Surveillance Imaging Into Adult Survivorship Care

As a child treated for a brain tumor approaches adulthood, coordinated transition of the surveillance imaging schedule and long-term survivorship monitoring into adult-focused care, ideally through a dedicated survivorship program experienced in the specific late effects this population carries, ensures continuity of the structured, protocol-driven surveillance this chapter has emphasized throughout rather than a gap in monitoring at this vulnerable transition point; providing the young adult and their receiving adult care team with a complete, organized summary of prior treatment, imaging findings, and the specific surveillance schedule still required is a practical, concrete component of this transition that directly protects the continuity of care this book's longitudinal surveillance principle depends upon. This transition summary, prepared well in advance of the actual transfer of care rather than assembled hastily at the final pediatric visit, gives both the young adult and the receiving team adequate time to review the full treatment history and ask clarifying questions before responsibility for ongoing surveillance formally shifts.

Figure 12.4: Expected Postsurgical Change Versus Recurrent Tumor

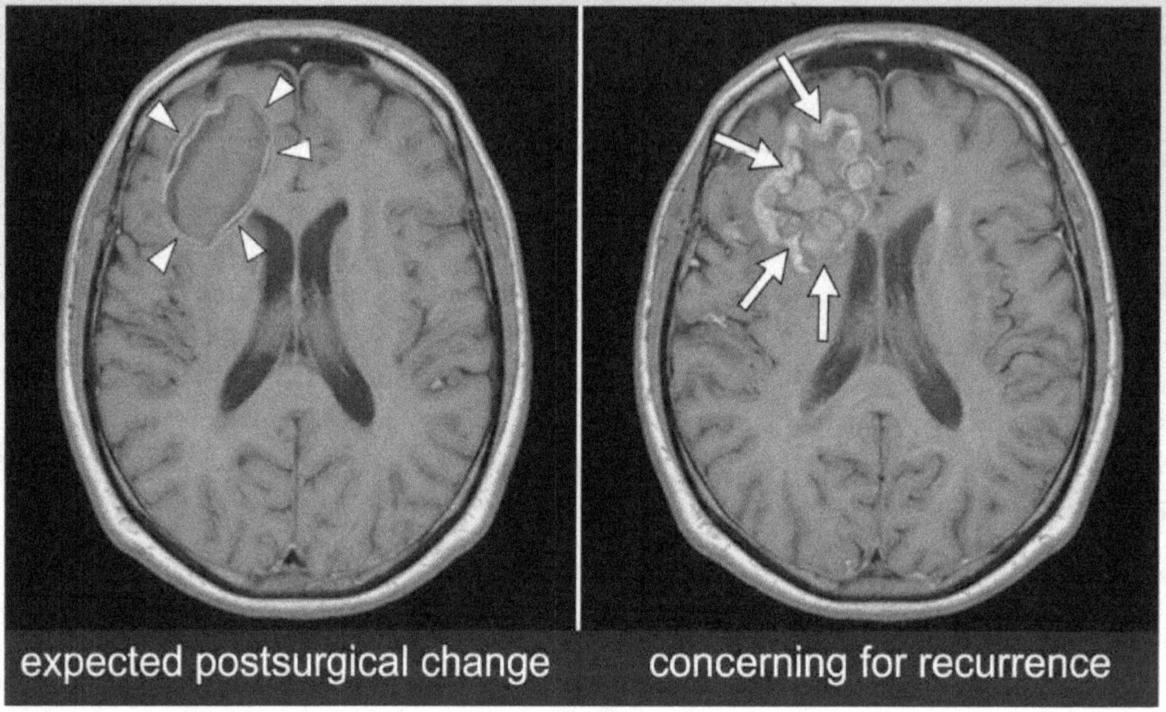

Case Presentation: Optic Pathway Glioma in Neurofibromatosis Type 1

A four-year-old with a known diagnosis of neurofibromatosis type 1 undergoes surveillance brain MRI as part of the proactive screening protocol discussed in this chapter, identifying a new, mildly enlarged, minimally enhancing mass along the left optic nerve. Applying the reasoning developed in this chapter, formal visual acuity and visual field assessment is obtained given the tumor's direct anatomic relationship to the visual pathway, and, given the tumor's small size, absence of chiasmal involvement, and preserved visual function on formal testing, the family and care team elect close observation with serial imaging and visual monitoring rather than immediate treatment, applying the shared decision-making and surveillance-over-immediate-intervention approach appropriate to this specific, favorable low-grade tumor presentation. This case illustrates how the syndrome-specific screening context, rather than a purely incidental discovery, shaped both the early detection and the measured, function-focused management approach applied. Serial imaging over the following two years demonstrates stability without further growth or chiasmal extension, and the family is counseled that this stable trajectory, now confirmed over a meaningful observation period, further supports the continued observation approach rather than a reflexive transition to treatment based on the tumor's mere presence.

Case Presentation: Pseudoprogression After Radiation for High-Grade Glioma

A ten-year-old completes radiation therapy for a supratentorial high-grade glioma, and surveillance MRI obtained six weeks after treatment completion demonstrates increased enhancement and surrounding edema at the treatment site compared to the immediate post-radiation baseline. Applying the reasoning developed in this chapter, the timing of this change, occurring within the classic pseudoprogression window, combined with perfusion imaging showing relatively low perfusion within the enhancing region, favors pseudoprogression over true tumor progression, and the family is counseled honestly regarding this genuine diagnostic uncertainty while a short-interval follow-up study, rather than an immediate change in treatment course, is scheduled to clarify the trajectory. Follow-up imaging eight weeks later demonstrates spontaneous improvement in both enhancement and edema, confirming the pseudoprogression diagnosis retrospectively and illustrating why a single, isolated increase in enhancement in this specific post-radiation timeframe should not automatically be equated with treatment failure.

Case Presentation: Craniopharyngioma With Hypothalamic Involvement

An eight-year-old presents with several months of declining vision, polyuria and polydipsia, and a recent, unexplained rapid weight gain, and brain MRI demonstrates a mixed solid-cystic, calcified suprasellar mass compressing the optic chiasm and third ventricle, with associated mild hydrocephalus. Applying the reasoning developed in this chapter, endocrinology confirms diabetes insipidus and growth hormone deficiency, and formal visual field testing confirms bitemporal hemianopia consistent with chiasmal compression. Preoperative imaging characterization demonstrates the tumor closely adherent to, and likely infiltrating, the hypothalamus rather than simply displacing it, prompting the multidisciplinary team to recommend a planned subtotal resection preserving hypothalamic structures, followed by adjuvant radiation, rather than an aggressive gross total resection carrying substantial hypothalamic injury risk, illustrating the surgical risk-benefit reasoning this chapter has developed specifically for hypothalamic-adherent craniopharyngioma.

THE CLINICAL-IMAGING CROSSWALK SYSTEM — Supratentorial and Sellar Tumor Recognition

---

Crossing 1 Recap: A suprasellar mass with diabetes insipidus warrants tumor marker assessment before presuming craniopharyngioma; elevated markers should prompt dedicated pineal region imaging to evaluate for bifocal germinoma.

Chapter Anchor: Supratentorial, sellar, and pineal region tumors are distinguished by location-specific imaging patterns, calcification, cystic architecture, tumor markers, and enhancement characteristics, each directly shaping the urgency, endocrine and visual evaluation, and treatment pathway; postoperative and treatment-related imaging change must be actively distinguished from recurrence using timing, enhancement pattern, and advanced imaging correlation.

Summary and Key Concepts

Pilocytic astrocytoma presents as a well-circumscribed cystic mass with an enhancing mural nodule and favorable prognosis; diffuse midline glioma, most classically pontine, presents with a classic brainstem clinical triad and diffuse, minimally enhancing signal abnormality despite high-grade molecular biology.

Craniopharyngioma, germ cell tumors, Rathke cleft cyst, hypothalamic hamartoma, and pituitary adenoma each carry a distinct sellar and suprasellar imaging signature; tumor marker assessment and coordinated endocrine and visual evaluation are integral, not adjunct, components of this evaluation.

Pineal germinoma classically engulfs pineal calcification (exploded pineal gland sign) and is exquisitely radiosensitive; nongerminomatous germ cell tumors show higher marker elevation and less favorable prognosis, and pineoblastoma requires full craniospinal staging given its dissemination risk.

A simple pineal or Rathke cleft cyst is distinguished from a true tumor by absence of a solid enhancing component and imaging stability over time; obstructive hydrocephalus and Parinaud syndrome are classic presenting features of a pineal region mass.

Expected postsurgical enhancement is thin, smooth, and resolves over weeks to months; pseudoprogression after radiation mimics recurrence within a characteristic early post-treatment window and is distinguished using timing and perfusion imaging, with short-interval follow-up resolving genuine ambiguity.

CHAPTER 13: PEDIATRIC BRAIN TUMORS — POSTERIOR FOSSA AND SPINAL CORD

Learning Objectives

1. Distinguish medulloblastoma from other embryonal tumors and describe its molecular subgroups and their imaging correlates.
2. Distinguish pilocytic astrocytoma from ependymoma based on posterior fossa location and imaging characteristics.
3. Describe the distinct imaging appearance and clinical implications of focal versus diffuse brainstem glioma.
4. Generate an age-appropriate differential diagnosis for a spinal cord mass and recognize the imaging appearance of drop metastases.

Medulloblastoma and Embryonal Tumors

Medulloblastoma, the most common malignant pediatric brain tumor, arises within the cerebellum and exemplifies this chapter's central theme: posterior fossa and spinal cord tumors are distinguished not by a single feature but by the convergence of location, age, imaging morphology, and, increasingly, molecular subgroup, each of which this section develops in turn.

Classic Imaging Appearance of Medulloblastoma

Medulloblastoma classically arises from the cerebellar vermis, filling and expanding the fourth ventricle, and presents as a solid, hypercellular mass that appears characteristically hyperdense on CT and shows restricted diffusion on MRI reflecting its densely packed small round blue cells, a diffusion pattern that immediately distinguishes it from the more cystic, less cellular pilocytic astrocytoma discussed later in this chapter; heterogeneous enhancement following contrast administration is typical, though the degree of enhancement varies across the molecular subgroups discussed below, and obstructive hydrocephalus from fourth ventricular effacement, applying the reasoning developed in Chapter 10, is a near-universal accompanying finding at presentation given the tumor's characteristic filling of this critical cerebrospinal fluid pathway. This diffusion-restricting, hyperdense, hydrocephalus-producing constellation is sufficiently characteristic that an experienced reader can often suggest medulloblastoma as the leading diagnosis from the initial imaging alone, well before surgical pathology confirms the specific diagnosis and molecular subgroup.

The Four Molecular Subgroups

Contemporary medulloblastoma classification recognizes four molecularly distinct subgroups, WNT-activated, SHH-activated, and the less well-characterized Group 3 and Group 4, each carrying a distinct age distribution, tumor location tendency, and prognosis; WNT-activated medulloblastoma, the rarest but most favorable subgroup, tends to arise more laterally near the cerebellopontine angle and carries an excellent prognosis with appropriately de-escalated therapy, while Group 3 medulloblastoma carries the least favorable prognosis and is disproportionately associated with metastatic disease at diagnosis, making molecular subgrouping, obtained from the resected tissue, as clinically consequential to treatment planning as the histologic diagnosis of medulloblastoma itself. Clinical trials increasingly stratify treatment intensity directly by this molecular subgroup rather than by histology alone, meaning two children with histologically identical medulloblastoma may receive substantially different treatment intensity, and a different radiation field and chemotherapy regimen, once their respective molecular subgroups are known, a point worth explaining clearly to families who may otherwise expect a uniform treatment approach for what they understand as the same diagnosis.

SHH-Activated Medulloblastoma and Its Bimodal Age Distribution

SHH-activated medulloblastoma shows a distinctive bimodal age distribution, occurring both in infants younger than three years and in adolescents and young adults, a pattern reflecting distinct underlying genetic drivers within this single molecular category; SHH-activated tumors tend to arise more laterally within the cerebellar hemispheres than the midline vermian location classically associated with medulloblastoma generally, and recognizing this specific lateral tendency, particularly in an infant, should prompt active consideration of this specific molecular subgroup and its associated germline cancer predisposition syndromes, including Gorlin syndrome, discussed further in the genetic correlates this chapter addresses. The infant and adolescent presentations of SHH-activated medulloblastoma, despite sharing the same underlying molecular driver pathway, differ meaningfully in their specific genetic alterations and, correspondingly, their prognosis, with the infant presentation generally carrying a more favorable outcome than the adolescent and young adult presentation, a further layer of prognostic nuance beyond the subgroup label alone that ongoing molecular research continues to refine.

Atypical Teratoid/Rhabdoid Tumor as a Critical Mimic

Atypical teratoid/rhabdoid tumor, a highly aggressive embryonal tumor that can closely mimic medulloblastoma on conventional imaging, occurs disproportionately in infants and very young children and carries a substantially worse prognosis than medulloblastoma, making its correct distinction a genuine diagnostic priority rather than an academic nicety; a heterogeneous posterior fossa mass in an infant younger than three years, particularly one showing atypical features such as marked heterogeneity, hemorrhage, or an eccentric rather than midline location, should prompt active consideration of this diagnosis, and molecular testing for the characteristic SMARCB1 or, less commonly, SMARCA4 alteration definitively distinguishes it from medulloblastoma when imaging alone leaves genuine ambiguity. Because atypical teratoid/rhabdoid tumor can also arise supratentorially and, less commonly, in the spinal cord, unlike medulloblastoma's strong posterior fossa predilection, an unusually aggressive-appearing embryonal tumor at any of these locations in a very young child should prompt the same molecular testing consideration this section describes for the classic posterior fossa presentation.

Staging and Metastatic Evaluation

Given medulloblastoma's recognized propensity for leptomeningeal dissemination through the cerebrospinal fluid, complete staging at diagnosis requires both full craniospinal MRI, applying the field-of-view extension principle established in Chapter 1, and cerebrospinal fluid cytology, ideally obtained postoperatively once the risk of false-positive cytology from surgical seeding has passed but before adjuvant therapy is initiated; the presence or absence of metastatic disease at diagnosis, together with the extent of surgical resection and the molecular subgroup discussed above, together determine the specific risk stratification, standard-risk versus high-risk, that governs treatment intensity. This risk stratification, integrating imaging staging, surgical outcome, and molecular subgroup into a single composite assessment, exemplifies the multimodal, converging-evidence approach this book has applied throughout, extended here into the specific context of pediatric neuro-oncologic risk classification and treatment planning.

Genetic Predisposition Syndromes

A meaningful proportion of medulloblastoma, particularly the SHH-activated subgroup discussed above, arises in the context of an underlying germline cancer predisposition syndrome, most notably Gorlin syndrome related to germline PTCH1 mutation and Li-Fraumeni syndrome related to germline TP53 mutation, and genetics referral is appropriately pursued for essentially any child with newly diagnosed medulloblastoma, particularly a very young child or one with additional syndromic features on examination, since a confirmed predisposition syndrome carries direct implications for both the specific treatment approach selected, given increased radiation sensitivity in some of these syndromes, and family counseling regarding surveillance for other syndrome-associated tumors and future reproductive planning. Identifying a germline TP53 mutation carries particularly weighty implications, given Li-Fraumeni syndrome's broad, lifelong elevated risk across numerous additional cancer types, and confirming or excluding this specific diagnosis directly shapes both the immediate treatment planning, since standard radiation carries disproportionate secondary malignancy risk in this specific genetic context, and the lifelong, whole-body cancer surveillance program the family and child require going forward.

Other Embryonal Tumors of the Posterior Fossa

Beyond medulloblastoma and atypical teratoid/rhabdoid tumor, a further category of embryonal tumors, collectively grouped under evolving nomenclature as embryonal tumors with multilayered rosettes and related entities, occurs less commonly in the posterior fossa and shares substantial imaging overlap with the more common medulloblastoma; definitive distinction among this heterogeneous, less common embryonal tumor category ultimately depends on histopathologic and molecular characterization rather than imaging alone, and a family should understand that an initial imaging-based working diagnosis of probable medulloblastoma may be refined or revised once complete pathologic characterization of the resected tissue is available.

Group 3 and Group 4 Medulloblastoma

Group 3 and Group 4 medulloblastoma, the two less molecularly well-characterized subgroups relative to the more clearly defined WNT-activated and SHH-activated categories, together account for the majority of medulloblastoma cases and both characteristically arise from the midline cerebellar vermis, producing the classic fourth-ventricle-filling appearance described earlier in this section; Group 3 medulloblastoma carries a disproportionate association with MYC amplification and metastatic disease at diagnosis, findings that together drive its comparatively less favorable prognosis relative to Group 4, and ongoing research continues to refine the specific imaging and clinical features that might eventually allow more confident subgroup prediction before molecular testing results become available.

Clinical Presentation and the Role of Early Recognition

Medulloblastoma classically presents with the signs and symptoms of obstructive hydrocephalus discussed in Chapter 10, morning headache, vomiting, and, in the young child, progressive macrocephaly or a bulging fontanelle, together with cerebellar signs including truncal ataxia and gait disturbance reflecting direct vermian involvement; the relatively nonspecific nature of these presenting symptoms, particularly in a young child who cannot reliably report headache, means a meaningful proportion of children experience a diagnostic delay of weeks to months before imaging is obtained, underscoring the value of the evidence-based imaging threshold developed in Chapter 3 applied specifically to a young child with new, persistent vomiting and morning-predominant symptoms, a presentation pattern that should prompt more urgent consideration of intracranial pathology than an isolated, non-progressive symptom would warrant. A careful, targeted history specifically asking about symptom timing relative to waking and sleep, rather than a general inquiry about headache alone, can help elicit this specific morning-predominant pattern that a family may not otherwise think to volunteer, applying the same active, structured questioning discipline this book has emphasized throughout for other presentations in which a specific detail meaningfully shifts the clinical threshold.

Figure 13.1: Medulloblastoma Filling the Fourth Ventricle

SAGITTAL T1 POSTCONTRAST AXIAL DWI

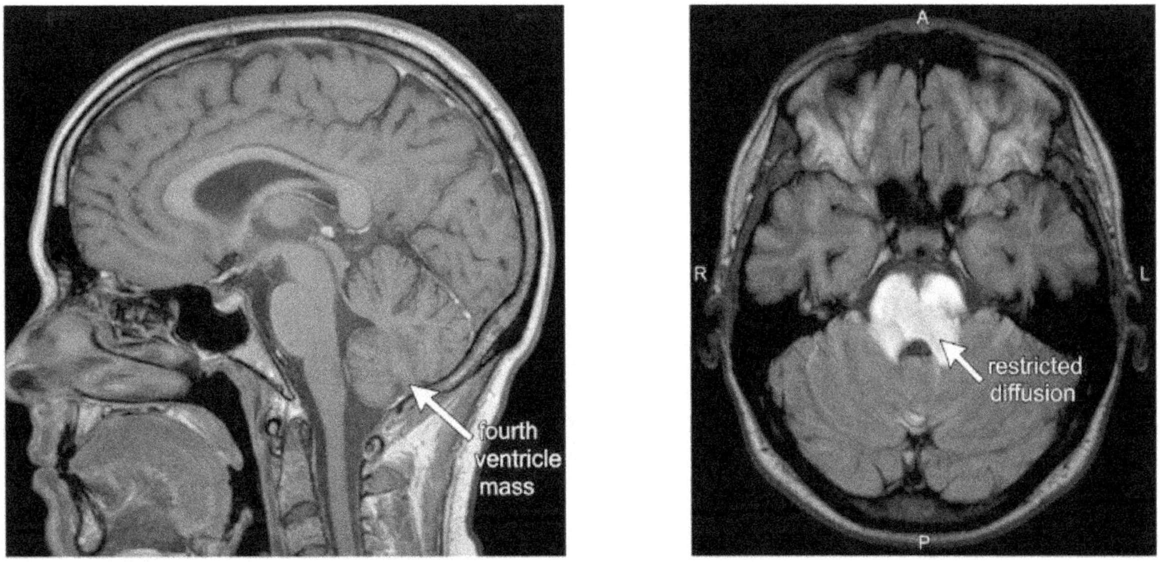

SAGITTAL T1 POSTCONTRAST AXIAL DWI

Molecular Subgroup	Typical Age	Typical Location	Prognosis
WNT-activated	Older children	Midline, cerebellopontine angle	Excellent
SHH-activated	Infants and adolescents (bimodal)	Lateral cerebellar hemisphere	Intermediate, varies by subtype
Group 3	Infants and young children	Midline	Least favorable
Group 4	Children and adolescents	Midline	Intermediate

Pilocytic Astrocytoma and Ependymoma

Pilocytic astrocytoma and ependymoma represent the two other most common posterior fossa tumor categories in childhood, and distinguishing them from each other and from the medulloblastoma discussed above depends on a specific combination of location within the posterior fossa, imaging morphology, and growth pattern this section develops systematically.

Cerebellar Pilocytic Astrocytoma

Cerebellar pilocytic astrocytoma, building on the general pilocytic astrocytoma discussion in Chapter 12, is the most common posterior fossa tumor overall and classically presents as a well-circumscribed cystic mass with an enhancing mural nodule arising within the cerebellar hemisphere, distinguishing it both by its lateral hemispheric location, in contrast to the midline vermian predilection of medulloblastoma, and by its well-circumscribed, cystic-with-nodule morphology, in contrast to medulloblastoma's solid, hypercellular, diffusion-restricting appearance; this combination of favorable location and favorable histology makes cerebellar pilocytic astrocytoma the posterior fossa tumor category most amenable to complete surgical cure, and a family can be counseled with genuine, well-supported optimism once this specific diagnosis is confidently suspected on imaging. A subset of pilocytic astrocytomas show a solid, rather than mural-nodule, enhancement pattern with only minimal cyst formation, and while this presentation is somewhat less classic, the tumor's still well-circumscribed margin and lack of the diffusion restriction and hydrocephalus-producing midline filling characteristic of medulloblastoma continue to support the favorable pilocytic astrocytoma diagnosis over the more concerning alternative.

Ependymoma: Location and Growth Pattern

Ependymoma arises from the ependymal lining of the ventricular system and, in the posterior fossa, characteristically originates from the floor of the fourth ventricle, producing a distinctive plastic, mold-like growth pattern that extends through the fourth ventricular outlet foramina, the foramen of Luschka laterally and the foramen of Magendie inferiorly, into the adjacent cerebellopontine angle cisterns and cervical spinal canal; recognizing this specific extrusive growth pattern, tumor extending through and beyond the normal ventricular boundaries rather than remaining confined within an expanded ventricle as medulloblastoma characteristically does, is among the most reliable imaging features distinguishing ependymoma from the other posterior fossa tumors discussed in this chapter. This characteristic plastic growth pattern, sometimes described as toothpaste-like as the tumor extrudes through the available foraminal openings, directly explains why complete surgical resection of ependymoma is technically more demanding than resection of a confined mass, since achieving a gross total resection requires following the tumor into these narrow, cranial-nerve-rich extensions rather than removing a single, contained mass.

Calcification and Heterogeneity in Ependymoma

Ependymoma frequently shows heterogeneous signal characteristics reflecting a combination of calcification, cystic change, and, at times, hemorrhage, a heterogeneous, mixed-signal appearance that further distinguishes it from the more homogeneous, hypercellular appearance of medulloblastoma; susceptibility-weighted or gradient-echo sequences, applying the technique introduced in Chapter 1, are particularly useful for characterizing this specific heterogeneity, since calcification and hemorrhage each produce a characteristic susceptibility artifact that a standard T1 and T2 sequence combination alone may not fully capture. The presence of calcification specifically, while not absolutely specific to ependymoma among posterior fossa tumors, is distinctly more common in ependymoma than in medulloblastoma, and its identification on a susceptibility-sensitive sequence or CT, where available, adds further supportive weight to an ependymoma diagnosis when considered alongside the extrusive growth pattern discussed above.

Cerebellopontine Angle Extension and Cranial Nerve Involvement

Ependymoma's characteristic extension through the foramen of Luschka into the cerebellopontine angle, discussed above, places the tumor in direct anatomic proximity to the facial and vestibulocochlear cranial nerves traversing this same region, and a child with ependymoma presenting with facial weakness or hearing change reflects this specific, mechanistically explicable anatomic relationship rather than an unrelated, coincidental cranial neuropathy; precise preoperative imaging characterization of this specific cerebellopontine angle extension and its relationship to the adjacent cranial nerves directly informs the surgical team's approach to this technically demanding region and the family's counseling regarding the specific cranial nerve preservation risk this particular extension pattern carries.

Molecular Classification of Ependymoma

Similar to the molecular subgrouping discussed for medulloblastoma above, contemporary ependymoma classification incorporates molecular markers, most notably the presence or absence of a posterior fossa group A versus group B molecular signature, which carry distinct prognostic and age-distribution implications, with posterior fossa group A ependymoma, more common in younger children, generally carrying a less favorable prognosis than group B; this molecular refinement, obtained from the resected tissue, increasingly supplements the traditional histologic grading in guiding both prognosis and the specific intensity of adjuvant treatment recommended following surgical resection.

Extent of Resection as the Dominant Prognostic Factor

Across both pilocytic astrocytoma and ependymoma, the extent of surgical resection achieved is among the strongest single prognostic factors, and this holds with particular force for ependymoma given its characteristic extension into the cerebellopontine angle and cervical spinal canal discussed above, regions where achieving a complete resection carries meaningfully greater technical difficulty and risk to adjacent cranial nerves and brainstem structures than the more surgically accessible cerebellar hemispheric location typical of pilocytic astrocytoma; precise preoperative imaging characterization of the tumor's specific extent and its relationship to these critical adjacent structures is therefore a direct determinant of both the achievable resection extent and the family's expected surgical risk-benefit counseling. A staged surgical approach, in which an initial, safer resection is followed by a planned second-look procedure once postoperative swelling has resolved and residual disease can be more clearly characterized, is sometimes pursued specifically for ependymoma given this technical complexity, illustrating that achieving a complete resection is, for this specific tumor, sometimes better understood as a staged process than a single definitive operation.

Postoperative Complications Specific to Posterior Fossa Surgery

Posterior fossa tumor resection carries a specific complication risk profile beyond the general postoperative considerations discussed in Chapter 12, most notably posterior fossa syndrome, also termed cerebellar mutism syndrome, a delayed-onset constellation of mutism, emotional lability, and ataxia emerging days after an initially uneventful surgery, believed to relate to disruption of the cerebello-cerebral pathways discussed in Chapter 5; recognizing this specific, well-characterized postoperative syndrome, rather than mistaking its delayed onset for a new surgical complication or tumor-related deterioration, allows appropriate counseling and supportive management, since the syndrome, while often prolonged, is generally though not universally followed by meaningful, if sometimes incomplete, recovery over subsequent months.

Cystic Versus Solid Ependymoma Presentations

While ependymoma is more frequently solid or predominantly solid with the heterogeneous calcified and hemorrhagic features discussed above, a minority of ependymomas show a substantial cystic component that can superficially resemble the cystic-with-mural-nodule appearance of pilocytic astrocytoma discussed earlier in this section; careful attention to the specific growth pattern, whether the mass remains confined to the cerebellar hemisphere as pilocytic astrocytoma characteristically does, or instead arises from and extends through the fourth ventricle as ependymoma characteristically does, remains the more reliable distinguishing feature in this specific, potentially confusing cystic-appearing subset than cyst presence or absence alone. This diagnostic overlap between cystic ependymoma and pilocytic astrocytoma is a specific, recurring interpretive pitfall worth naming explicitly, since the two entities carry meaningfully different prognosis and treatment intensity, making the growth-pattern-based distinction developed in this section a genuinely consequential interpretive skill rather than an academic refinement.

Radiation Therapy Considerations for Ependymoma

Given ependymoma's comparatively lower propensity for cerebrospinal fluid dissemination relative to medulloblastoma, radiation therapy for localized ependymoma is generally directed at the tumor bed and a defined margin rather than the full craniospinal axis reserved for disseminated disease or the higher-dissemination-risk tumors discussed elsewhere in this chapter, an important distinction shaping both treatment planning and family counseling regarding anticipated radiation-related late effects; precise postoperative imaging characterization of the resection cavity and any residual disease, applying the early postoperative imaging principles developed in Chapter 12, directly defines the radiation target volume this focused treatment approach requires. This more targeted radiation field, relative to the craniospinal field medulloblastoma frequently requires, generally translates into a somewhat more favorable late-effects profile for ependymoma survivors, though the cognitive and endocrine surveillance principles developed in Chapter 12 remain equally applicable and essential for this population.

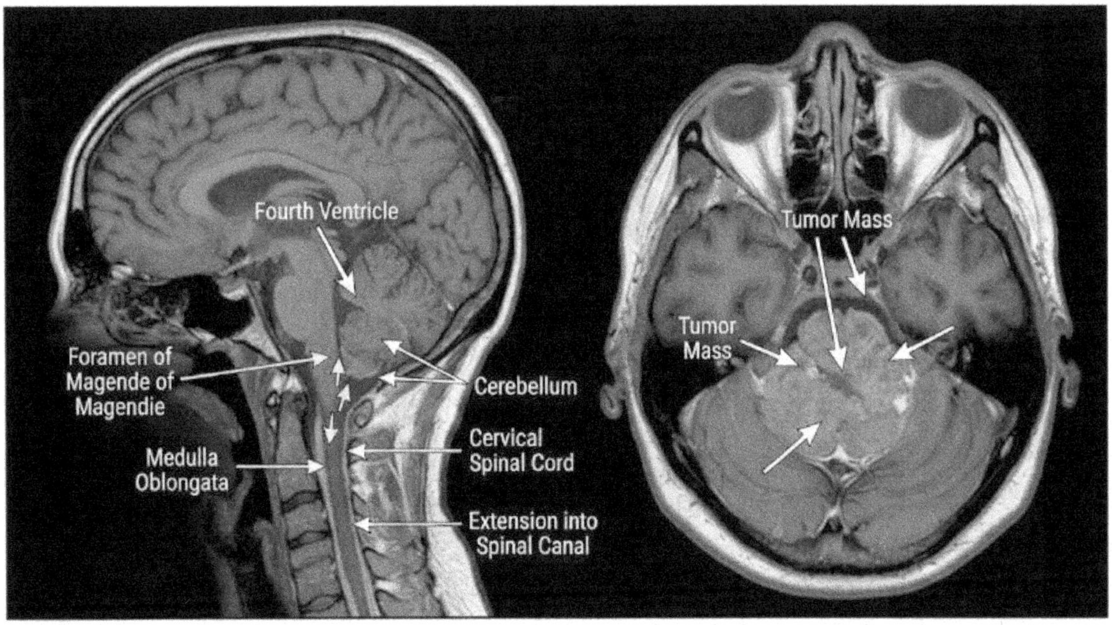

Figure 13.2: Ependymoma Extending Through the Fourth Ventricular Outlet

THE CLINICAL-IMAGING CROSSWALK SYSTEM — Delayed Mutism After Uneventful Posterior Fossa Surgery

The Crossing: A seven-year-old undergoes apparently uncomplicated resection of a cerebellar pilocytic astrocytoma, and on postoperative day two develops new mutism, emotional lability, and worsened ataxia.

Presentation Signature: A child with a delayed, rather than immediate, onset of mutism and behavioral change following posterior fossa tumor resection, occurring after an initially reassuring early postoperative course.

Imaging Correlate: Postoperative imaging is reviewed and confirms an appropriate resection cavity without evidence of a new structural complication, hemorrhage, or hydrocephalus, supporting a diagnosis of posterior fossa (cerebellar mutism) syndrome rather than a new surgical complication.

Trap Logic: The delayed onset of this syndrome, emerging days after an uneventful early postoperative course, can be mistaken for a new, acute complication requiring urgent additional intervention if the clinician is unfamiliar with this specific, well-characterized syndrome's typical timeline.

Crossing Anchor: Delayed-onset mutism and emotional lability following posterior fossa tumor resection, in the absence of a new structural finding on imaging, is characteristic of posterior fossa syndrome; supportive management and family counseling regarding the generally favorable, though sometimes prolonged, recovery trajectory is the appropriate response.

Brainstem Gliomas

Brainstem gliomas span a spectrum from the devastating diffuse midline glioma introduced in Chapter 12 to a group of far more favorable, focal brainstem tumors, and this section develops the specific imaging distinctions that separate these dramatically different prognostic categories within a single anatomic region.

Diffuse Intrinsic Pontine Glioma Revisited

Diffuse midline glioma of the pons, introduced in Chapter 12 given its shared molecular biology with thalamic and spinal cord diffuse midline glioma, is revisited here with specific attention to its brainstem imaging characteristics: diffuse, expansile T2/FLAIR signal abnormality involving greater than fifty percent of the pons, often encasing rather than displacing the basilar artery, a specific finding that helps distinguish this diffuse, infiltrative pattern from the focal, exophytic tumors discussed below; the diffuse, infiltrative margin and the absence of a discrete, resectable tumor mass are the defining imaging features that place this specific presentation into the poor-prognosis diffuse midline glioma category rather than the far more favorable focal categories this section addresses next. The basilar artery encasement sign specifically, in which the normally free-floating basilar artery becomes embedded within the expanded, infiltrated pons, is a particularly reliable discriminating feature, since a focal, exophytic brainstem tumor characteristically displaces or drapes over the basilar artery rather than encasing it directly within its own substance.

Focal Tectal Glioma

Focal tectal glioma, a distinct, low-grade brainstem tumor arising specifically within the dorsal midbrain tectum, presents an entirely different clinical and imaging picture from diffuse pontine glioma: a small, well-circumscribed, non-enhancing or minimally enhancing lesion typically identified incidentally during evaluation of obstructive hydrocephalus from aqueductal compression, applying the reasoning developed in Chapter 10, with a characteristically indolent, often radiographically stable course over years of observation; correctly identifying this specific, favorable diagnosis, rather than conflating it with the far more ominous diffuse midline glioma simply because both occur within the brainstem, is among the most consequential distinctions this chapter addresses, given the dramatically different prognosis and management approach, often simple cerebrospinal fluid diversion alone without tumor-directed treatment, that focal tectal glioma warrants. A tectal glioma occasionally shows very gradual, slow growth over many years of surveillance without ever meeting the threshold for active tumor-directed intervention, illustrating that even documented growth, when sufficiently slow and the tumor remains otherwise typical in appearance, does not automatically necessitate a change from the observation-based management this favorable diagnosis generally supports.

Exophytic Dorsal Brainstem Glioma

Exophytic dorsal brainstem glioma, a further focal, generally low-grade tumor arising from the dorsal brainstem surface and growing outward into the fourth ventricle rather than infiltrating diffusely within the pons itself, similarly carries a substantially more favorable prognosis than diffuse midline glioma, and its predominantly exophytic, well-demarcated growth pattern, often amenable to at least partial surgical resection given its more accessible dorsal surface location, further distinguishes both its imaging appearance and its management pathway from the diffuse, non-resectable pontine glioma discussed earlier in this section. This exophytic growth pattern, protruding outward into the fourth ventricular cavity rather than infiltrating the surrounding pontine parenchyma, can occasionally be mistaken on a cursory review for a medulloblastoma or ependymoma filling the same ventricular space, and careful attention to the tumor's point of origin, the dorsal brainstem surface itself rather than the ventricular floor or the vermis, resolves this potential confusion.

Diffusion Tensor Imaging in Brainstem Tumor Characterization

Diffusion tensor imaging, applying the technique introduced in Chapter 1 and developed further in Chapter 8, offers a further, complementary characterization tool specifically valuable in the brainstem given its dense concentration of critical white matter tracts, allowing visualization of whether these tracts are displaced, a pattern more consistent with a focal, extrinsic or exophytic process, or infiltrated and disrupted, a pattern more consistent with the diffuse, infiltrative process characteristic of diffuse midline glioma; this tractography-based distinction adds a further, complementary line of evidence to the conventional imaging features this section has emphasized throughout for distinguishing the favorable focal brainstem tumor categories from diffuse midline glioma.

Cervicomedullary Glioma

Cervicomedullary glioma, arising at the junction of the medulla and upper cervical spinal cord, represents a further focal, generally favorable brainstem glioma variant, presenting with a distinct clinical picture often including lower cranial nerve dysfunction and long tract signs referable to this specific junctional location, and an imaging appearance of a focal, often partially exophytic mass at the cervicomedullary junction distinguishable from the diffuse pontine infiltration characteristic of diffuse midline glioma; recognizing this specific junctional location and its generally favorable focal, rather than diffuse infiltrative, growth pattern again places this tumor into the more favorable prognostic category this section has developed as a recurring theme across its focal, non-diffuse brainstem tumor subtypes. Because this tumor spans the anatomic boundary between the brainstem proper and the upper cervical spinal cord, imaging characterization must extend the field of view to fully capture both the intracranial and upper spinal extent of the lesion, applying the field-of-view extension principle from Chapter 1 to this specific junctional anatomy.

Long-Term Functional Outcome Across Brainstem Tumor Categories

Even among the favorable, focal brainstem tumor categories this section has emphasized, long-term functional outcome depends substantially on the specific brainstem structures involved and the degree to which surgical intervention, when pursued, can be achieved without injury to these densely packed critical pathways, meaning a favorable histologic and molecular prognosis does not automatically translate into an entirely uncomplicated functional outcome; coordinated, longitudinal rehabilitation assessment, incorporating speech and swallowing evaluation given the brainstem's role in these functions, is therefore a standard, anticipated component of comprehensive care for this population regardless of which specific focal brainstem tumor category a child carries.

The Critical Distinction Between Focal and Diffuse Patterns

The overarching, unifying principle this section has developed across its several focal brainstem tumor subtypes, tectal glioma, exophytic dorsal glioma, and cervicomedullary glioma, is that a well-circumscribed, focal growth pattern, regardless of the exact brainstem subregion involved, carries a fundamentally more favorable prognosis than the diffuse, infiltrative pattern characteristic of diffuse midline glioma, and this focal-versus-diffuse distinction, rather than brainstem location alone, is the single most important imaging determination this chapter's brainstem tumor discussion requires the reader to make confidently and correctly. A reader who internalizes this single organizing principle, rather than memorizing each named focal subtype independently, is equipped to correctly classify a brainstem tumor presentation this chapter has not specifically named, applying the same durable, transferable reasoning habit this book has cultivated across every preceding chapter.

Biopsy Considerations in Brainstem Tumors

Biopsy of a brainstem lesion, historically approached with substantial caution given the density of critical structures traversing this small anatomic region, has become increasingly feasible at specialized centers using stereotactic technique, and is increasingly pursued for a classic diffuse midline glioma presentation specifically to obtain molecular characterization for clinical trial eligibility, even though the diagnosis itself, as discussed above, is often confidently made on imaging and clinical grounds alone; for the focal, favorable brainstem tumor subtypes discussed in this section, biopsy or resection, where anatomically feasible, additionally provides the histopathologic confirmation that further supports the more optimistic prognostic counseling these focal categories warrant, distinct from the primarily imaging-and-clinical-based diagnostic approach more commonly applied to classic diffuse pontine glioma.

Serial Imaging Surveillance for Focal Brainstem Tumors

The favorable, indolent natural history characteristic of the focal brainstem tumor subtypes discussed throughout this section, tectal glioma in particular, is confirmed and reinforced through scheduled serial imaging surveillance demonstrating stability over time, applying the same longitudinal, baseline-and-follow-up comparison principle this book emphasizes throughout; a documented pattern of genuine radiographic stability across multiple, carefully compared serial studies provides a family with concrete, accumulating reassurance beyond what a single, favorable-appearing initial study alone can offer, and any deviation from this expected stable trajectory, growth, new enhancement, or a change in signal characteristics, prompts reconsideration of the original favorable classification rather than being dismissed as an insignificant imaging variation.

Family Counseling Across the Brainstem Glioma Spectrum

Given the dramatically divergent prognosis this section has developed between diffuse midline glioma and the several favorable focal brainstem tumor variants, precise, confident imaging classification at the time of initial diagnosis directly determines the entire subsequent tenor of family counseling, from the profound, difficult conversation diffuse midline glioma requires to the genuinely reassuring conversation appropriate for a confirmed focal tectal glioma; a clinician communicating an initial brainstem mass finding to a family before this specific focal-versus-diffuse classification has been confidently established should communicate honestly that this classification, not the bare fact of a brainstem mass alone, is what will determine the prognosis, avoiding either premature alarm or premature reassurance before the imaging characterization this section has developed is complete.

Figure 13.3: Diffuse Pontine Glioma Versus Focal Tectal Glioma

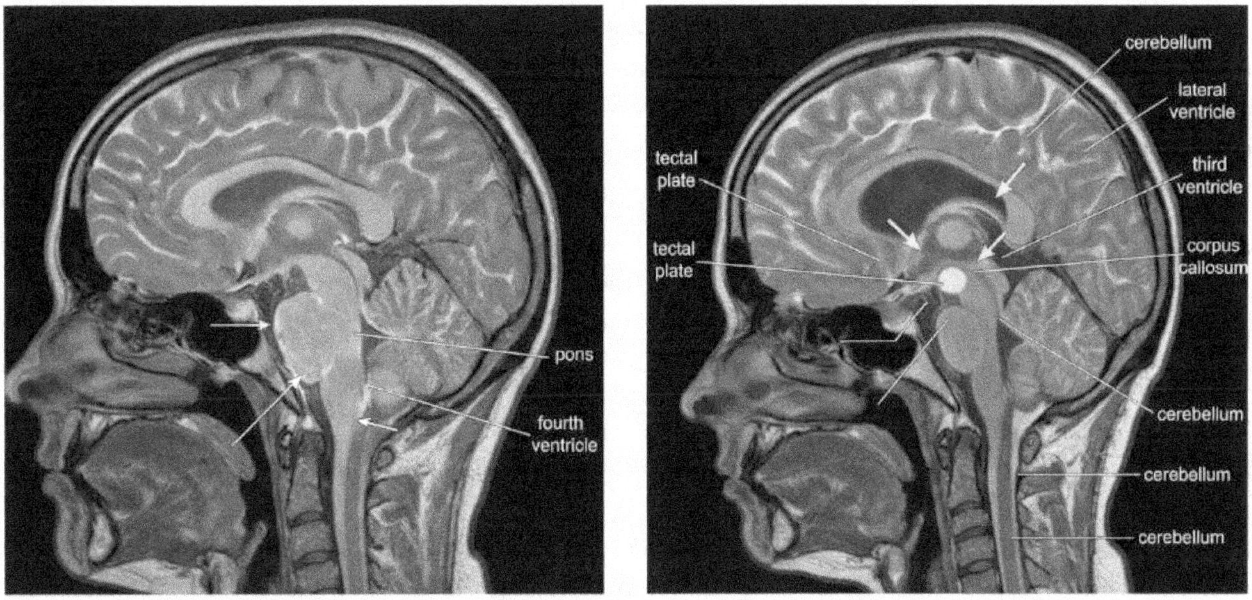

diffuse pontine glioma focal tectal glioma

Spinal Cord Tumors and Drop Metastases

This closing section addresses the distinct differential diagnosis of an intramedullary spinal cord mass and the specific imaging recognition of drop metastases, cerebrospinal-fluid-borne spread from an intracranial primary tumor, extending this chapter's posterior fossa focus into the spinal axis these tumors frequently involve.

Astrocytoma as the Most Common Intramedullary Tumor

Astrocytoma, spanning the same low-grade-to-high-grade spectrum discussed in Chapter 12 for supratentorial gliomas, is the most common primary intramedullary spinal cord tumor in childhood, typically presenting as a fusiform expansion of the spinal cord over multiple vertebral segments with variable enhancement depending on tumor grade; a long-segment, expansile intramedullary signal abnormality with an ill-defined margin is characteristic of this diffuse, infiltrative growth pattern, and, as with its supratentorial counterpart, distinguishing low-grade from high-grade features on imaging, enhancement pattern, associated edema, and margin definition, provides essential early prognostic information. The full extent of cord involvement should be characterized using sagittal imaging spanning the entire suspected tumor length rather than a limited field of view, since underestimating the cranial-caudal extent of a fusiform astrocytoma directly risks an incomplete surgical or radiation planning target that fails to address the tumor's true full extent.

Ependymoma of the Spinal Cord

Spinal cord ependymoma, distinct from the posterior fossa ependymoma discussed earlier in this chapter though sharing the same underlying ependymal cell origin, more commonly presents as a well-circumscribed, centrally located intramedullary mass, frequently accompanied by a rostral or caudal syrinx, discussed in relation to Chiari malformation in Chapter 8, and, at times, a hemosiderin cap reflecting chronic microhemorrhage at the tumor margin; this more discrete, well-circumscribed morphology, in contrast to the fusiform, infiltrative pattern of astrocytoma discussed above, both aids diagnostic distinction and, given its more surgically favorable, well-demarcated margin, generally permits a more complete resection than the infiltrative astrocytoma. The specific molecular subtype myxopapillary ependymoma, occurring characteristically in the conus medullaris and filum terminale region rather than more rostrally within the cord itself, represents a further, distinct spinal ependymoma variant with its own characteristic location and generally favorable behavior, worth recognizing as anatomically and, to some degree, behaviorally distinct from the ependymoma arising more rostrally within the cervical or thoracic cord.

Distinguishing Neoplastic From Non-Neoplastic Intramedullary Signal Change

An intramedullary spinal cord signal abnormality is not always neoplastic, and the differential diagnosis must actively include transverse myelitis and other inflammatory or demyelinating processes discussed in Chapter 16, and, less commonly in the pediatric population, a vascular malformation; distinguishing a true intramedullary tumor from these non-neoplastic mimics depends on the specific pattern of cord expansion, the presence or absence of a discrete mass with associated enhancement, and, critically, the clinical trajectory, since a tumor typically produces a more gradual, progressive clinical course while an inflammatory process more often presents acutely or subacutely, a distinction this chapter's broader clinical-imaging correlation framework applies directly to this specific spinal cord context. When this distinction remains genuinely ambiguous after the initial evaluation, cerebrospinal fluid analysis for inflammatory markers and, where the clinical picture supports it, a trial of corticosteroid therapy with close interval follow-up imaging can help resolve the ambiguity, since a genuine inflammatory process would be expected to show meaningful improvement on this specific management trial in a way a true neoplasm would not.

Extramedullary and Extradural Spinal Masses

Beyond the intramedullary tumors emphasized throughout this section, extramedullary intradural masses, including schwannoma and meningioma, both less common in children than in adults but occurring particularly in the context of neurofibromatosis type 2 discussed in Chapter 14, and extradural masses, including neuroblastoma and other pediatric solid tumors capable of spinal extension, present with a distinct imaging compartment localization, outside rather than within the spinal cord parenchyma itself, that fundamentally reorganizes the differential diagnosis; correctly localizing a spinal mass to its specific anatomic compartment, intramedullary, intradural extramedullary, or extradural, applying the same anatomic precision this book emphasizes throughout, is therefore the essential first step before any further differential diagnostic reasoning is pursued for a newly identified spinal mass. The specific imaging sign most useful for this compartmental localization is the relationship between the mass and the cord itself, widening of the subarachnoid space and displacement of the cord away from an intradural extramedullary mass, versus the smooth, expansile widening of the cord itself characteristic of a true intramedullary process, a distinction requiring careful attention to the specific margin and displacement pattern on high-resolution sagittal and axial imaging.

Drop Metastases: Imaging Recognition

Drop metastases, discrete nodules of tumor spread via the cerebrospinal fluid from an intracranial primary, most classically medulloblastoma but also occurring with the other embryonal and pineal region tumors discussed in this chapter and Chapter 12, appear as discrete, enhancing nodules studding the spinal cord surface, cauda equina, or thecal sac, requiring the dedicated, thin-section, postcontrast spine imaging discussed in this chapter's staging section to reliably detect, since these small, surface-based nodules can be easily overlooked on a non-dedicated or lower-resolution spine study; systematically reviewing the entire spinal axis specifically for this finding, applying a deliberate, structured search pattern rather than a cursory overall impression, is essential given the direct staging and treatment-field implications a positive finding carries. A diffuse, smooth, linear pattern of leptomeningeal enhancement coating the cord surface, rather than the discrete, nodular pattern this section has emphasized, represents a related but distinct pattern of cerebrospinal-fluid-disseminated disease, and both patterns, nodular and diffuse linear, are actively searched for and separately documented whenever staging imaging for a disseminating tumor category is performed.

Timing of Spinal Staging Relative to Surgery

As introduced earlier in this chapter, spinal staging imaging for a suspected medulloblastoma or other cerebrospinal-fluid-disseminating tumor is ideally obtained preoperatively whenever clinically feasible, since postoperative blood products and surgical change within the intracranial and spinal cerebrospinal fluid spaces can produce artifactual enhancement that mimics or obscures true leptomeningeal or drop metastatic disease; when preoperative staging is not feasible given clinical urgency, delaying the definitive postoperative staging study by the interval this section's postoperative discussion recommends, rather than obtaining it in the immediate, blood-product-confounded postoperative window, improves its diagnostic reliability. This preoperative-versus-postoperative timing consideration mirrors, in the spinal staging context specifically, the same early-postoperative-imaging-window discipline developed in Chapter 12 for extent-of-resection assessment, reinforcing that timing relative to surgery is a recurring, cross-cutting theme in pediatric neuro-oncologic imaging that this book has now developed across three consecutive chapters.

Clinical Presentation of Spinal Cord Tumors

Spinal cord tumors classically present with a progressive, rather than static, pattern of back pain, gait disturbance, and, as the tumor enlarges, bladder and bowel dysfunction, a clinical trajectory that shares the progressive quality emphasized in Chapter 9 for tethered cord but reflects a fundamentally different underlying mechanism, mass effect and cord compression rather than mechanical tethering; back pain in a young child, less commonly a benign, self-limited symptom than in an older child or adult, warrants a somewhat lower threshold for spinal imaging, particularly when accompanied by any of the progressive neurologic or urologic features this section has emphasized, applying the age-and-symptom-specific imaging threshold reasoning developed in Chapter 3 to this specific spinal cord tumor context. Scoliosis, particularly when atypical in its curve pattern, rapidly progressive, or accompanied by pain, a presentation distinct from the more common, painless idiopathic scoliosis of adolescence discussed in Chapter 9, is a further, sometimes overlooked presenting feature of an underlying spinal cord tumor, and this atypical scoliosis pattern should prompt spinal cord imaging rather than orthopedic bracing alone.

Surgical and Adjuvant Treatment Considerations

Surgical resection of an intramedullary spinal cord tumor requires intraoperative neurophysiologic monitoring to protect the cord's motor and sensory pathways during tumor removal, applying a functional-preservation principle analogous to the eloquent-cortex mapping discussed in Chapters 11 and 12 but adapted to the spinal cord's specific anatomy, and the achievable extent of resection, similarly to the posterior fossa tumors discussed earlier in this chapter, depends heavily on whether the tumor presents the discrete, well-circumscribed margin characteristic of ependymoma or the infiltrative, poorly demarcated margin characteristic of astrocytoma; adjuvant radiation and chemotherapy decisions for spinal cord tumors similarly follow the same grade-and-resection-extent-driven framework this chapter has applied throughout to its other tumor categories. A myelotomy, the surgical incision through the posterior median sulcus used to access an intramedullary tumor, is planned with precise preoperative imaging guidance regarding the tumor's exact dorsal-ventral position within the cord, since even a small deviation from the optimal entry point can risk unnecessary injury to normal, functioning cord tissue during the surgical approach itself.

Figure 13.4: Drop Metastases Along the Spinal Cord Surface

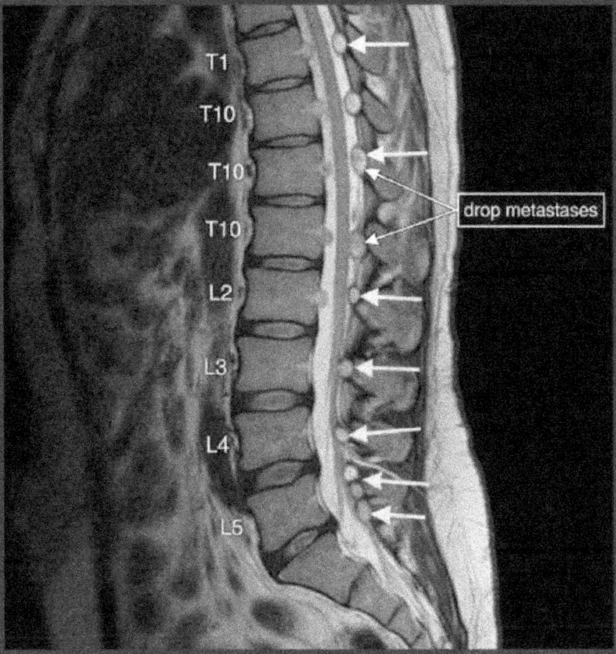

Case Presentation: SHH-Activated Medulloblastoma in an Infant

A fourteen-month-old presents with vomiting and increasing head circumference, and brain MRI demonstrates a laterally located left cerebellar hemispheric mass with restricted diffusion and associated obstructive hydrocephalus. Applying the reasoning developed in this chapter, the lateral, rather than midline vermian, location raises specific consideration of SHH-activated medulloblastoma given this subgroup's characteristic infant age distribution and lateral hemispheric tendency discussed in this chapter. Following resection, molecular testing confirms SHH activation, and genetics evaluation identifies a germline PTCH1 mutation consistent with Gorlin syndrome. The family is counseled regarding both the child's medulloblastoma treatment plan, incorporating awareness of Gorlin syndrome's associated radiation sensitivity into treatment planning, and the broader syndrome-associated surveillance and family counseling implications this genetic diagnosis carries, illustrating the direct connection this chapter has developed between imaging location, molecular subgroup, and genetic predisposition evaluation. The family is further counseled regarding lifelong dermatologic surveillance for the basal cell carcinomas characteristic of Gorlin syndrome, a specific, actionable component of long-term care that the genetic diagnosis, rather than the medulloblastoma diagnosis alone, has directly generated.

Case Presentation: Ependymoma With Cerebellopontine Angle Extension

A three-year-old presents with ataxia and new-onset facial asymmetry, and brain MRI demonstrates a heterogeneous, partially calcified mass arising from the floor of the fourth ventricle with extension through the right foramen of Luschka into the cerebellopontine angle, closely abutting the facial and vestibulocochlear nerve complex. Applying the reasoning developed in this chapter, this specific plastic growth pattern and cerebellopontine angle extension strongly favor ependymoma over medulloblastoma, and the facial asymmetry is recognized as a direct, anatomically explicable consequence of this specific extension pattern rather than an unrelated finding. The surgical team, informed by this precise preoperative anatomic characterization, counsels the family regarding the specific facial nerve preservation risk this extension pattern carries and the possibility that achieving gross total resection may require accepting some risk to facial nerve function, a risk-benefit discussion made possible only by the detailed anatomic imaging characterization this chapter has emphasized throughout. Molecular testing of the resected tissue confirms posterior fossa group B ependymoma, the more favorable of the two molecular subgroups discussed earlier in this chapter, informing a correspondingly measured, rather than maximally intensive, adjuvant treatment recommendation.

Case Presentation: Incidental Focal Tectal Glioma

A six-year-old undergoes brain MRI for evaluation of headache, and the study identifies mild ventriculomegaly with a small, well-circumscribed, non-enhancing lesion within the dorsal midbrain tectum. Applying the reasoning developed in this chapter, the interpreting radiologist recognizes this as a classic focal tectal glioma rather than raising alarm about a diffuse brainstem process, given its small size, sharp margins, and absence of the diffuse, expansile signal abnormality characteristic of diffuse midline glioma. The family is counseled regarding the generally indolent, often radiographically stable natural history this specific diagnosis carries, and management proceeds with cerebrospinal fluid diversion for the mild hydrocephalus alone, without tumor-directed biopsy or treatment, alongside scheduled serial imaging surveillance to confirm the expected stability over time, illustrating the dramatically different management pathway this specific, favorable brainstem tumor subtype warrants relative to the diffuse pontine glioma discussed elsewhere in this chapter. Surveillance imaging at one and three years confirms the expected stability, and the family, now equipped with this accumulated reassurance, transitions to a less frequent, longer-interval surveillance schedule, consistent with the risk-adapted, longitudinal surveillance framework this book has applied throughout to conditions demonstrating a confirmed, stable trajectory over time.

THE CLINICAL-IMAGING CROSSWALK SYSTEM — Posterior Fossa and Spinal Cord Tumor Recognition

---

Crossing 1 Recap: Delayed-onset mutism and emotional lability following posterior fossa tumor resection, without a new structural finding, is characteristic of posterior fossa syndrome, not a new surgical complication.

Chapter Anchor: Posterior fossa and spinal cord tumors are distinguished by the convergence of precise anatomic location, growth pattern (confined versus extrusive, focal versus diffuse), and, increasingly, molecular subgroup; the focal-versus-diffuse distinction in brainstem glioma and the anatomic compartment localization of a spinal mass are the single most consequential imaging determinations this chapter requires.

Summary and Key Concepts

Medulloblastoma fills the fourth ventricle with a solid, diffusion-restricting mass and is classified into four molecular subgroups with distinct age, location, and prognostic implications; atypical teratoid/rhabdoid tumor is a critical, more aggressive mimic in infants requiring molecular distinction.

Cerebellar pilocytic astrocytoma presents as a well-circumscribed cystic mass with a favorable prognosis; ependymoma shows a characteristic plastic growth pattern extending through the fourth ventricular outlet foramina, and extent of resection is the dominant prognostic factor for both.

Diffuse midline (pontine) glioma shows diffuse, infiltrative, basilar-artery-encasing signal change with poor prognosis; focal tectal glioma, exophytic dorsal glioma, and cervicomedullary glioma are well-circumscribed, favorable variants requiring confident distinction from diffuse disease.

Astrocytoma and ependymoma are the most common intramedullary spinal cord tumors, distinguished by fusiform-infiltrative versus well-circumscribed morphology respectively; correct anatomic compartment localization (intramedullary, intradural extramedullary, extradural) is the essential first step for any spinal mass.

Drop metastases appear as discrete, enhancing surface nodules requiring dedicated postcontrast spine imaging, ideally obtained preoperatively to avoid postsurgical blood-product artifact confounding true leptomeningeal disease detection.

CHAPTER 14: THE NEUROCUTANEOUS SYNDROMES

Learning Objectives

1. Describe the diagnostic criteria and imaging surveillance protocol for neurofibromatosis type 1 and distinguish it from neurofibromatosis type 2, including the specific tumor spectrum unique to each.
2. Recognize the characteristic imaging findings of tuberous sclerosis complex and their relationship to the epilepsy reasoning developed in Chapter 11, including the growth-based criterion for subependymal giant cell astrocytoma.
3. Recognize the imaging findings of Sturge-Weber syndrome and describe the associated seizure and stroke-like episode risk, and the predictive value of the facial cutaneous distribution.
4. Describe the central nervous system manifestations of von Hippel-Lindau disease and the imaging features of other phakomatoses, including PHACE and Klippel-Trenaunay syndromes.

Neurofibromatosis Type 1 and Type 2

Neurofibromatosis type 1 and type 2, despite their similar names, are genetically and clinically distinct disorders, and this section develops both entities in parallel specifically to reinforce that this naming similarity should never be allowed to obscure their fundamentally different underlying genetics, tumor spectrum, and surveillance requirements. Each entity is addressed in turn, beginning with the more common neurofibromatosis type 1 and its associated tumor and cutaneous spectrum, before turning to the far less common but distinct neurofibromatosis type 2 and its own hallmark bilateral vestibular schwannoma finding.

Diagnostic Criteria for Neurofibromatosis Type 1

Neurofibromatosis type 1, caused by mutation in the NF1 tumor suppressor gene, is diagnosed clinically using a defined set of criteria requiring at least two of several features, including six or more café-au-lait macules, two or more neurofibromas of any type or one plexiform neurofibroma, axillary or inguinal freckling, optic pathway glioma, two or more Lisch nodules (iris hamartomas), a distinctive osseous lesion, and a first-degree relative with confirmed neurofibromatosis type 1; recognizing that this is a clinical diagnosis built from a constellation of findings, rather than a diagnosis requiring genetic confirmation in every case, matters directly for imaging practice, since a child meeting clinical criteria warrants the imaging surveillance this section develops regardless of whether confirmatory genetic testing has yet been obtained. A young child with only café-au-lait macules and no other criterion met at initial presentation, a common early presentation given that several diagnostic features, including Lisch nodules and neurofibromas, typically emerge later in childhood, is appropriately followed with scheduled reassessment as additional criteria may become apparent with age, rather than either premature diagnostic closure or premature diagnostic exclusion based on an incomplete picture at a single early evaluation.

Optic Pathway Glioma Screening Protocol

Building directly on the optic pathway glioma discussion in Chapter 12, children with neurofibromatosis type 1 undergo proactive screening for this specific tumor, and current practice increasingly favors clinical, particularly ophthalmologic, surveillance as the primary screening tool, reserving MRI for a child with an abnormal visual finding or other clinical concern, rather than universal, reflexive baseline MRI in every asymptomatic child with neurofibromatosis type 1; this evolving, more selective screening approach reflects accumulated evidence that clinically silent optic pathway gliomas identified only on screening imaging frequently do not progress to threaten vision, and that the resource and sedation burden of universal imaging screening may outweigh its benefit relative to a well-executed clinical surveillance program with imaging reserved for a specific, actionable clinical trigger. Annual, structured ophthalmologic examination through early childhood, the peak age window for this tumor's clinical emergence, therefore functions as the primary screening modality this section endorses, with MRI serving a confirmatory and treatment-planning role once a clinical abnormality has been identified rather than as the initial, universal screening tool itself.

T2 Hyperintensities (Unidentified Bright Objects)

A characteristic and extremely common incidental finding in neurofibromatosis type 1, T2 hyperintensities, historically and still colloquially termed unidentified bright objects, appear as focal, non-enhancing, non-mass-like areas of T2/FLAIR signal abnormality most commonly within the basal ganglia, thalami, brainstem, and cerebellum, believed to represent regions of abnormal myelin vacuolization rather than a neoplastic or otherwise pathologic process; recognizing these lesions as a benign, expected finding in this specific population, typically most numerous in early-to-mid childhood and frequently diminishing or resolving by adolescence, prevents an unnecessary and anxiety-provoking evaluation for an alternative, more concerning explanation for this exceptionally common incidental finding. The absence of mass effect, the absence of enhancement, and the characteristic, non-progressive or spontaneously improving trajectory on any interval imaging obtained are the specific features that distinguish these benign T2 hyperintensities from a genuinely concerning finding, and a family encountering this specific term in their child's radiology report benefits from a clear, direct explanation using this section's reasoning, since the term itself, unidentified bright object, can sound alarming despite describing an entirely expected, benign finding.

Plexiform Neurofibroma

Plexiform neurofibroma, a diffuse, infiltrative peripheral nerve sheath tumor that can involve any peripheral nerve and frequently extends along multiple fascicles in a characteristic serpentine, multinodular pattern often described as a bag of worms appearance, carries a lifetime risk of malignant transformation to malignant peripheral nerve sheath tumor, making baseline characterization and, for a lesion causing pain, rapid growth, or a new neurologic deficit, prompt reevaluation for this specific transformation risk an essential component of long-term surveillance; whole-body MRI, increasingly incorporated into comprehensive neurofibromatosis type 1 surveillance protocols at specialized centers, allows more complete characterization of plexiform neurofibroma burden than the more limited, symptom-directed imaging a purely reactive approach would provide. A plexiform neurofibroma is present in a substantial minority of children with neurofibromatosis type 1 from birth or early infancy, often growing disproportionately during periods of rapid childhood growth and puberty, and establishing a documented baseline characterization early, before this expected growth-phase enlargement, provides the most reliable reference point for later distinguishing expected, syndrome-typical growth from the more concerning, disproportionate growth pattern that would instead raise malignant transformation concern.

Malignant Peripheral Nerve Sheath Tumor as a Critical Complication

Malignant transformation of a plexiform neurofibroma to malignant peripheral nerve sheath tumor represents the most serious oncologic complication of neurofibromatosis type 1, and specific imaging features, including new or accelerating growth, heterogeneous signal with areas of necrosis, loss of the target sign characteristic of a benign plexiform lesion, and, on advanced imaging, elevated metabolic activity on PET, should prompt urgent biopsy given the substantially worse prognosis this transformed, malignant tumor carries relative to its benign precursor; a family with a known plexiform neurofibroma should be counseled explicitly regarding the specific warning signs, new pain, rapid growth, or a new neurologic deficit, that should prompt urgent reevaluation rather than waiting for a scheduled surveillance interval. The target sign, a specific imaging pattern in which a benign peripheral nerve sheath tumor shows central low signal on T2-weighted imaging surrounded by a peripheral rim of higher signal, reflecting the tumor's internal architecture, is a reassuring feature whose loss, replaced instead by a more heterogeneous, disorganized internal signal pattern, is itself among the most specific individual imaging findings supporting malignant transformation over benign plexiform disease.

Diagnostic Criteria and Imaging Findings in Neurofibromatosis Type 2

Neurofibromatosis type 2, caused by mutation in the distinct NF2 tumor suppressor gene and clinically and genetically unrelated to neurofibromatosis type 1 despite the shared naming convention, is defined by bilateral vestibular schwannomas as its hallmark finding, together with an increased risk of meningioma, ependymoma, and other schwannomas throughout the central and peripheral nervous system; a child or adolescent presenting with hearing loss, tinnitus, or balance disturbance and a family history of neurofibromatosis type 2 warrants dedicated, thin-section internal auditory canal imaging specifically to evaluate for bilateral vestibular schwannoma, the imaging finding that most reliably establishes this diagnosis and immediately distinguishes it from the entirely different tumor spectrum characteristic of neurofibromatosis type 1. Neurofibromatosis type 2 typically presents somewhat later than neurofibromatosis type 1, often in adolescence or early adulthood rather than early childhood, and a child from a known neurofibromatosis type 2 family undergoes baseline and periodic surveillance imaging beginning in later childhood, timed to this syndrome's characteristic, somewhat later age of clinical onset relative to the earlier-presenting neurofibromatosis type 1.

Distinguishing the Two Syndromes in Practice

Given the frequency with which these two conditions are conflated by families and, at times, non-specialist clinicians simply because of their shared name, explicitly and repeatedly clarifying that neurofibromatosis type 1 and type 2 are different genes, different tumor spectrums, and different surveillance protocols is a recurring, necessary component of family education this chapter emphasizes as a distinct communication task in its own right, separate from the medical imaging reasoning this section has developed; a family who understands this distinction clearly is better equipped to engage meaningfully in the specific, syndrome-appropriate surveillance plan their child actually requires rather than conflating guidance intended for one syndrome with their child's genuinely different diagnosis.

Genetic Testing and Mosaicism in Neurofibromatosis

Genetic confirmation of neurofibromatosis type 1 or type 2, while not required to establish a clinical diagnosis meeting the criteria discussed above, becomes particularly valuable when clinical features are limited or atypical, and segmental or mosaic neurofibromatosis, in which the causative mutation is confined to a subset of the body's cells rather than present in every cell, produces a localized, asymmetric distribution of clinical findings that can otherwise confound the standard diagnostic criteria; recognizing this mosaic presentation pattern, and pursuing genetic testing of affected, rather than unaffected, tissue when mosaicism is suspected, improves diagnostic yield in this specific, atypical presentation and carries distinct, generally lower recurrence risk implications for future offspring relative to non-mosaic, fully germline disease.

Coordinating Multidisciplinary Neurofibromatosis Care

Comprehensive care for a child with either neurofibromatosis type 1 or type 2 is best delivered through a dedicated, multidisciplinary neurofibromatosis clinic bringing together neurology, genetics, ophthalmology, dermatology, and, where relevant, orthopedics and oncology, applying the same coordinated, multidisciplinary team principle this book has developed for other complex, multisystem conditions; this team-based model reduces the fragmentation a family might otherwise experience navigating each specialty independently and ensures the specific, syndrome-appropriate surveillance protocol this section has developed is applied consistently over the child's entire course of care rather than depending on any single clinician remembering each component in isolation. Orthopedic involvement, in particular, addresses the skeletal manifestations neurofibromatosis type 1 can produce, including scoliosis and long-bone dysplasia, further findings belonging to this syndrome's broader manifestation spectrum beyond the central nervous system and cutaneous findings this section has primarily emphasized.

Figure 14.1: Optic Pathway Glioma and T2 Hyperintensities in NF1

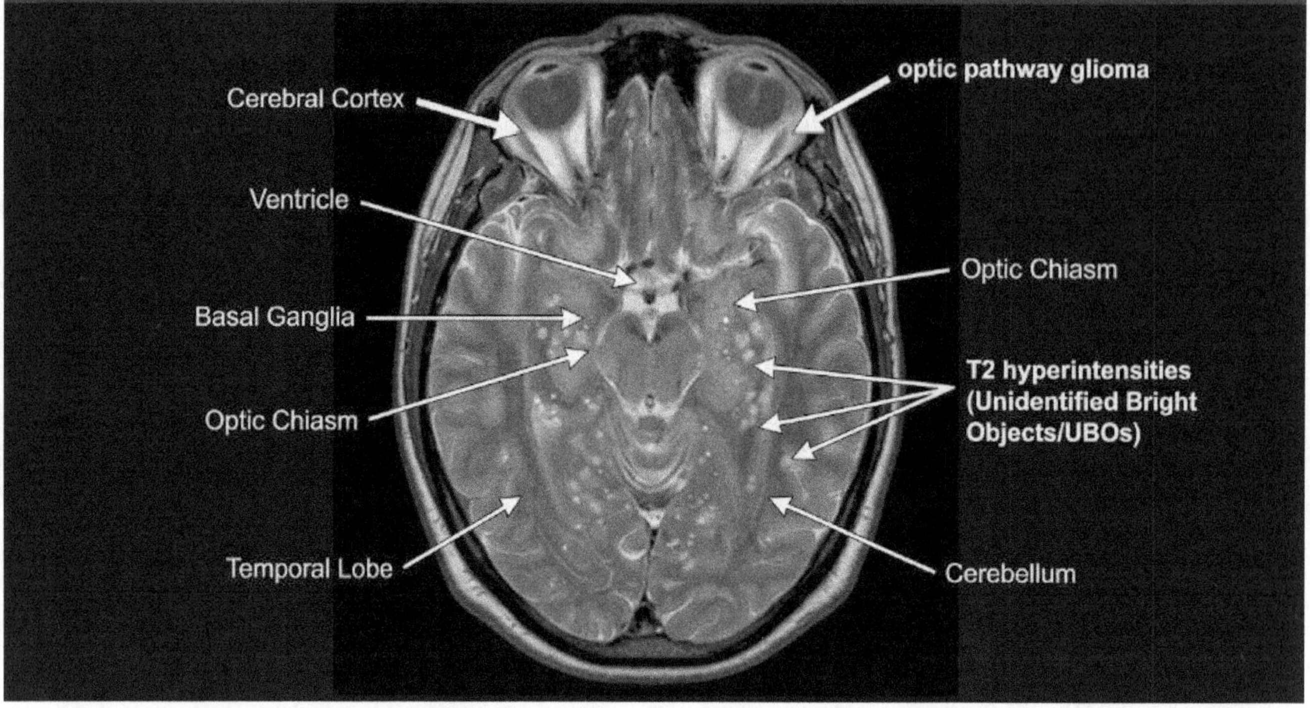

Feature	Neurofibromatosis Type 1	Neurofibromatosis Type 2
Gene	NF1	NF2
Hallmark tumor	Optic pathway glioma, plexiform neurofibroma	Bilateral vestibular schwannoma
Skin findings	Café-au-lait macules, neurofibromas, axillary freckling	Generally absent
Key surveillance imaging	Clinically directed MRI, whole-body MRI for plexiform burden	Internal auditory canal MRI

Tuberous Sclerosis Complex

Tuberous sclerosis complex, introduced in Chapter 11 for its central role in medically refractory epilepsy, is developed comprehensively in this section, extending that earlier, epilepsy-focused discussion into the syndrome's full central nervous system and multisystem imaging spectrum. The cortical tubers, subependymal nodules, and radial migration lines addressed in the following subheads share a common underlying mTOR pathway mechanism, and understanding this shared mechanism, rather than memorizing each finding as an independent, unrelated entity, gives the reader a durable, transferable framework for recognizing this syndrome's full brain imaging spectrum.

Cortical Tubers Revisited

Cortical tubers, the defining brain lesion of tuberous sclerosis complex and discussed in Chapter 11 primarily for their epileptogenic potential, appear on imaging as areas of cortical thickening and abnormal T2/FLAIR signal, frequently with a characteristic wedge-shaped configuration extending from the cortical surface toward the ventricle, a pattern sharing conceptual and, at times, visual similarity to the transmantle sign of focal cortical dysplasia discussed in Chapter 11, reflecting the shared underlying mTOR pathway dysregulation between these two entities; the total tuber burden, quantified and tracked over serial imaging, correlates broadly, though imperfectly, with both epilepsy severity and cognitive outcome, making systematic tuber counting and characterization a standard, structured component of tuberous sclerosis complex imaging reporting. Tuber signal characteristics evolve somewhat with age, becoming relatively more T1-hyperintense and less T2-hyperintense as myelination of the surrounding normal brain progresses through infancy and early childhood, applying the same age-specific interpretive framework established in Chapter 2 to this specific, syndrome-associated lesion type.

Subependymal Nodules

Subependymal nodules, small, calcified or non-calcified nodules lining the ventricular walls, represent a further characteristic and highly common brain finding in tuberous sclerosis complex, generally asymptomatic in themselves but requiring ongoing surveillance specifically because a subset can transform into the subependymal giant cell astrocytoma discussed in the next subhead; distinguishing a stable subependymal nodule from an enlarging one warrants the same structured, quantitative, serial-comparison surveillance approach this book has emphasized throughout for other conditions requiring longitudinal size tracking, since the transition point at which a nodule is reclassified as a giant cell astrocytoma depends substantially on demonstrated growth over time rather than size at a single time point alone. Standard surveillance protocols for children with tuberous sclerosis complex typically recommend brain MRI at defined intervals through childhood and adolescence, with the specific interval and total surveillance duration informed by the number, size, and location of subependymal nodules identified on baseline imaging, giving the reader a further concrete example of risk-stratified, individualized surveillance planning applied to a specific neurocutaneous syndrome.

Subependymal Giant Cell Astrocytoma

Subependymal giant cell astrocytoma, a low-grade tumor arising specifically from a subependymal nodule located near the foramen of Monro, carries direct clinical significance beyond its generally favorable histologic grade because its specific location places it at risk of producing obstructive hydrocephalus through direct foraminal obstruction, applying the obstructive hydrocephalus reasoning developed in Chapter 10; serial imaging surveillance specifically targeting this foramen of Monro region, with attention to both nodule size and any accompanying ventricular size change, is a standard, structured component of tuberous sclerosis complex surveillance, and mTOR inhibitor therapy, discussed in Chapter 11 as a targeted medical treatment option for this molecular pathway, has emerged as an effective alternative to surgical resection for many affected children. The decision between mTOR inhibitor therapy and surgical resection for a confirmed subependymal giant cell astrocytoma depends on factors including tumor size, growth rate, and the presence or absence of hydrocephalus at the time of diagnosis, and this specific treatment decision, like several others addressed throughout this book, is made collaboratively through multidisciplinary discussion rather than following a single, universally applicable algorithm.

Radial Migration Lines

Radial migration lines, linear bands of abnormal T2 signal extending from the ventricular margin toward the cortical surface, represent a further characteristic tuberous sclerosis complex brain finding, believed to reflect abnormal radial glial-guided neuronal migration analogous in embryologic mechanism to the migration disorders discussed in Chapter 7, though generally understood as a distinct, milder manifestation of the same underlying mTOR pathway dysregulation responsible for the cortical tubers and subependymal nodules discussed above rather than a separately named, distinct diagnostic entity; recognizing this specific linear pattern as an expected, characteristic finding in this syndrome, rather than a separate, concerning white matter abnormality, prevents unnecessary additional evaluation for an unrelated white matter disease process. These radial migration lines are most conspicuous on T2-weighted imaging in infancy and early childhood, and, similar to the cortical tuber signal evolution discussed above, tend to become less visually apparent as background myelination progresses, a further example of the age-specific interpretive framework from Chapter 2 applying directly to this syndrome's characteristic imaging findings.

Multisystem Manifestations Beyond the Brain

Tuberous sclerosis complex is a genuinely multisystem disorder, and comprehensive evaluation extends well beyond the brain imaging emphasized throughout this section to include renal ultrasound or MRI for angiomyolipoma, a characteristic benign renal tumor, cardiac echocardiography for rhabdomyoma, particularly important in the newborn period when cardiac rhabdomyoma is frequently the first identified manifestation prompting the diagnostic evaluation, and dermatologic examination for the characteristic facial angiofibromas and shagreen patch; a coordinated, multidisciplinary surveillance protocol addressing each of these organ systems, rather than a neurology-focused evaluation alone, reflects the genuinely multisystem nature of this diagnosis and its associated surveillance requirements.

Prenatal Detection Through Cardiac Rhabdomyoma

Because cardiac rhabdomyoma is frequently detectable on routine prenatal ultrasound, a substantial proportion of tuberous sclerosis complex diagnoses now originate prenatally, before any brain finding has been characterized, and identification of a fetal cardiac rhabdomyoma should prompt dedicated fetal or early postnatal brain MRI specifically to evaluate for the cortical tubers and subependymal nodules this chapter has developed, applying the same fetal MRI indication reasoning established in Chapter 1; this prenatal detection pathway allows earlier family counseling and earlier initiation of the structured surveillance protocol this chapter has emphasized, potentially before the child has developed any clinical symptom at all.

TAND: Tuberous Sclerosis-Associated Neuropsychiatric Disorders

Beyond the seizures and structural brain findings emphasized throughout this section, tuberous sclerosis complex carries a well-documented association with a broader spectrum of neuropsychiatric and neurodevelopmental manifestations, collectively termed TAND, including autism spectrum disorder, intellectual disability, and behavioral dysregulation, and proactive, structured neuropsychiatric screening, applying the same baseline-and-longitudinal-tracking principle developed in Chapter 11, is a standard, anticipated component of comprehensive care for this population regardless of seizure control status, since these neuropsychiatric manifestations can occur independently of, and do not necessarily correlate directly with, the specific severity of a child's epilepsy or structural imaging findings.

Genetic Testing and Family Screening

Tuberous sclerosis complex arises from mutation in either the TSC1 or TSC2 gene, both components of the same mTOR regulatory pathway, and while the diagnosis is frequently established clinically using defined major and minor diagnostic criteria analogous in structure to the neurofibromatosis type 1 criteria discussed earlier in this chapter, genetic confirmation carries direct value both for definitively establishing the diagnosis in an ambiguous clinical presentation and for enabling targeted prenatal or preimplantation testing for a family considering a future pregnancy; because a substantial proportion of cases arise from a de novo mutation rather than parental inheritance, careful parental clinical and, where indicated, genetic screening is warranted before assuming a sporadic, non-inherited pattern applies to a specific family. TSC2 mutations are generally associated with a more severe clinical phenotype than TSC1 mutations on average, though genuine variability exists within each genetic category, and this genotype-phenotype correlation, while imperfect, is worth incorporating into the family counseling conversation once genetic confirmation is available, alongside the appropriate caution that individual variability within either genetic category remains substantial and a specific genetic result does not by itself fully predict an individual child's eventual clinical course.

Figure 14.2: Cortical Tubers and Subependymal Nodules

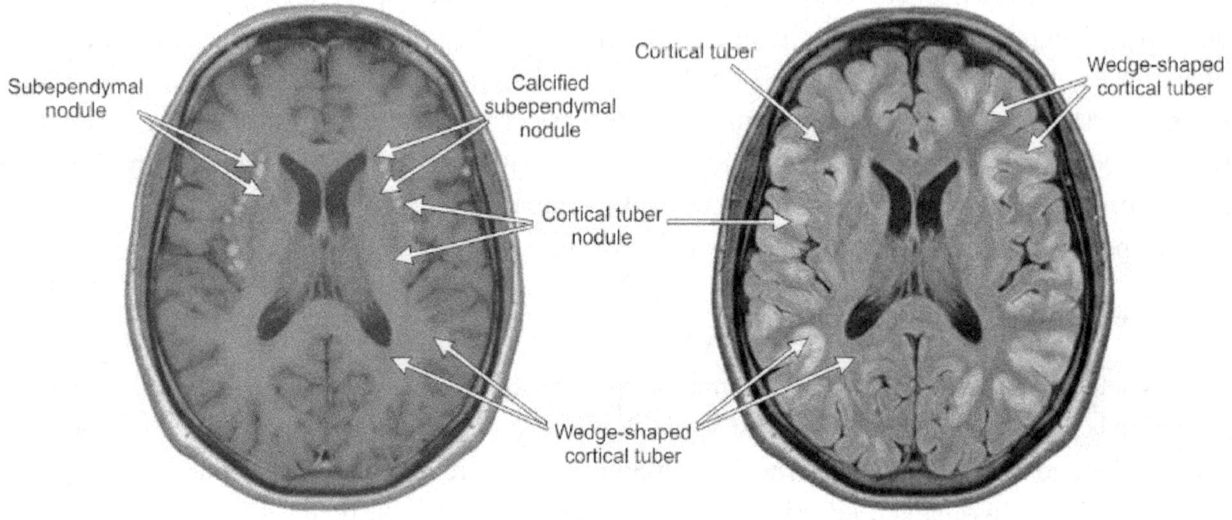

THE CLINICAL-IMAGING CROSSWALK SYSTEM — A Growing Subependymal Nodule Near the Foramen of Monro

The Crossing: A ten-year-old with known tuberous sclerosis complex undergoes routine surveillance MRI, which shows interval enlargement of a subependymal nodule near the right foramen of Monro compared to the study obtained eighteen months earlier.

Presentation Signature: A child with established tuberous sclerosis complex and a documented, quantitatively confirmed increase in size of a foramen-of-Monro-region subependymal nodule on serial surveillance imaging.

Imaging Correlate: The nodule is reclassified from a stable subependymal nodule to a subependymal giant cell astrocytoma given the demonstrated interval growth, and the ventricular system is carefully assessed for any early, accompanying size change suggesting early obstruction at the foramen of Monro.

Trap Logic: Evaluating this nodule at a single time point without reference to the prior comparison study would miss the growth that is the specific, defining criterion distinguishing a giant cell astrocytoma from a stable subependymal nodule, potentially delaying treatment until a more advanced, hydrocephalus-producing stage.

Crossing Anchor: A subependymal nodule near the foramen of Monro is reclassified as a giant cell astrocytoma based on demonstrated interval growth on serial, quantitatively compared surveillance imaging, not size or appearance at a single time point alone.

Sturge-Weber Syndrome

Sturge-Weber syndrome, a distinct neurocutaneous syndrome caused by a somatic, rather than germline, mutation in the GNAQ gene, presents with a characteristic combination of a facial capillary malformation (port-wine stain) and a leptomeningeal vascular malformation producing a specific, recognizable brain imaging pattern this section develops in detail. Unlike neurofibromatosis type 1, tuberous sclerosis complex, and von Hippel-Lindau disease, each caused by a germline mutation carrying a defined, calculable recurrence risk for future offspring, Sturge-Weber syndrome's somatic mutational mechanism means it is not inherited in the same predictable pattern, a distinction worth clarifying explicitly for a family who may otherwise assume every neurocutaneous syndrome discussed in this chapter shares the same germline, heritable mechanism.

The Facial Port-Wine Stain and Its Predictive Value

The facial capillary malformation characteristic of Sturge-Weber syndrome, most classically involving the ophthalmic (V1) division of the trigeminal nerve distribution, carries meaningful predictive value regarding the likelihood of associated intracranial involvement, with a port-wine stain involving the V1 distribution, particularly when bilateral, carrying a substantially higher risk of leptomeningeal involvement than a stain confined to other facial regions; this correlation between the specific cutaneous distribution and the intracranial risk directly informs the imaging-ordering decision for a newborn or infant with a facial port-wine stain, applying the evidence-based imaging threshold reasoning developed in Chapter 3 to this specific, well-characterized risk stratification. A port-wine stain confined entirely outside the V1 distribution carries a correspondingly low risk of intracranial involvement, and imaging is not routinely pursued for this lower-risk cutaneous distribution alone in an otherwise asymptomatic infant, reinforcing that precise anatomic mapping of the cutaneous finding itself, not merely its presence, directly determines the appropriate imaging pathway.

Leptomeningeal Angiomatosis

Leptomeningeal angiomatosis, the characteristic intracranial vascular malformation of Sturge-Weber syndrome, appears on postcontrast MRI as abnormal, serpentine leptomeningeal enhancement overlying the affected cerebral hemisphere, most commonly the parieto-occipital region, and is frequently accompanied by ipsilateral cortical atrophy and calcification that develops progressively over time as the underlying chronic venous congestion and resulting ischemia this vascular malformation produces takes its cumulative toll on the affected brain tissue; postcontrast imaging is essential for reliably detecting this specific finding, since the leptomeningeal enhancement pattern is frequently subtle or entirely inapparent on noncontrast sequences alone. Enlarged, abnormal choroid plexus ipsilateral to the leptomeningeal angiomatosis, reflecting an associated ipsilateral venous drainage anomaly, is a further, less universally recognized but characteristic accompanying finding worth actively searching for once the primary leptomeningeal finding has been identified, since its presence further supports the diagnosis and reflects the same underlying chronic venous congestion mechanism responsible for the syndrome's other structural findings.

Progressive Calcification and Atrophy Over Time

The gyriform, tram-track calcification pattern classically associated with Sturge-Weber syndrome, historically identified on skull radiography before the widespread availability of cross-sectional imaging and now more reliably characterized on CT or susceptibility-weighted MRI, develops progressively over childhood rather than being present from birth, meaning a young infant with confirmed leptomeningeal angiomatosis may show this classic calcification pattern only later, once the chronic venous congestion this malformation produces has had sufficient time to cause the underlying tissue injury this radiographic sign reflects; serial imaging tracking this progressive calcification and atrophy over time, rather than a single study at diagnosis, therefore provides the most complete picture of this syndrome's characteristic, evolving structural impact. A young infant's initial, normal-appearing noncontrast study, obtained before this progressive calcification has developed, should therefore not be interpreted as excluding the diagnosis in a child with a high-risk facial distribution port-wine stain, and the postcontrast leptomeningeal enhancement discussed above, rather than calcification, remains the more sensitive early finding in this specific young age group.

Seizures and Stroke-Like Episodes

Seizures, frequently the presenting neurologic symptom in Sturge-Weber syndrome, arise from the chronic cortical dysfunction the underlying leptomeningeal angiomatosis produces, and a distinctive, well-recognized additional clinical phenomenon, stroke-like episodes, in which a child develops an acute, transient neurologic deficit resembling stroke without a corresponding acute infarct on imaging, is believed to reflect acute, seizure- or migraine-related exacerbation of the chronic venous congestion and impaired perfusion already present in the affected hemisphere; recognizing this specific stroke-like episode phenomenon, rather than reflexively pursuing an acute stroke evaluation identical to that developed in Chapter 18 for a child without this specific underlying syndrome, appropriately calibrates the acute evaluation while still maintaining vigilance for a genuine, superimposed acute vascular event that this syndrome's baseline vascular fragility can also, less commonly, produce. Perfusion imaging obtained during an acute stroke-like episode characteristically shows a reversible, seizure-related perfusion pattern rather than the fixed, vascular-territory-based perfusion deficit characteristic of a true acute infarct, and this specific perfusion distinction, where obtained, offers a further, complementary tool supporting the correct classification of this specific, syndrome-associated acute presentation.

Neurodevelopmental Outcome and Early Intervention

Neurodevelopmental outcome in Sturge-Weber syndrome correlates broadly with the extent of leptomeningeal involvement and, particularly, with seizure control, since poorly controlled, frequent seizures appear to independently contribute to progressive cognitive decline beyond the syndrome's baseline structural impact alone; this correlation has motivated increasingly aggressive, early seizure control strategies in this specific population, including earlier consideration of the epilepsy surgical evaluation discussed in Chapter 11 for a child with Sturge-Weber syndrome and medically refractory seizures, reflecting a treatment philosophy that early, effective seizure control may itself be neuroprotective for this syndrome's long-term cognitive trajectory. Hemispherectomy or hemispherotomy, a more extensive surgical approach disconnecting or removing the severely affected hemisphere entirely, is reserved for the most severe, extensively affected, and medically refractory cases, and precise preoperative imaging characterization of the full extent of leptomeningeal involvement, applying the systematic anatomic mapping this chapter has emphasized throughout, directly informs whether this more extensive surgical approach, as opposed to a more limited, focal resection, is the appropriate recommendation for a specific child's extent of disease.

Ophthalmologic Surveillance for Glaucoma

Beyond the neurologic manifestations emphasized throughout this section, Sturge-Weber syndrome carries an independently elevated risk of glaucoma, particularly when the facial port-wine stain involves the periorbital region, and coordinated, proactive ophthalmologic surveillance for elevated intraocular pressure, initiated from infancy rather than deferred until a specific visual symptom emerges, is a standard, essential component of comprehensive care for this population, applying the same multisystem, anticipatory surveillance principle this book has emphasized for the other neurocutaneous syndromes discussed throughout this chapter.

Alternative Venous Drainage Pathways

As the normal superficial venous drainage pathways become progressively compromised by the chronic leptomeningeal venous congestion characteristic of Sturge-Weber syndrome, the brain increasingly relies on prominent, enlarged deep and transcerebral collateral venous channels to maintain adequate venous outflow, a compensatory pattern visible on venous-phase imaging that itself serves as a further, indirect marker of disease severity and chronicity; recognizing these enlarged collateral pathways as an expected, compensatory adaptation rather than an independent, separately concerning vascular abnormality reflects the same mechanistic, cause-and-effect imaging reasoning this book has applied throughout to distinguish a primary finding from its downstream physiologic consequences.

Skull and Soft Tissue Overgrowth

Ipsilateral calvarial and soft tissue overgrowth, including choroid plexus enlargement discussed above and, at times, mild facial or cranial asymmetry, can accompany the chronic vascular changes of Sturge-Weber syndrome, reflecting the trophic effects of the abnormal vascular malformation on adjacent bone and soft tissue growth over years of childhood development; recognizing this specific, syndrome-associated growth pattern prevents mistaking a mild, chronic facial or cranial asymmetry for an unrelated, separate craniofacial process requiring independent evaluation, distinct from the coordinated, syndrome-specific surveillance this chapter has emphasized throughout.

Figure 14.3: Leptomeningeal Angiomatosis With Progressive Calcification

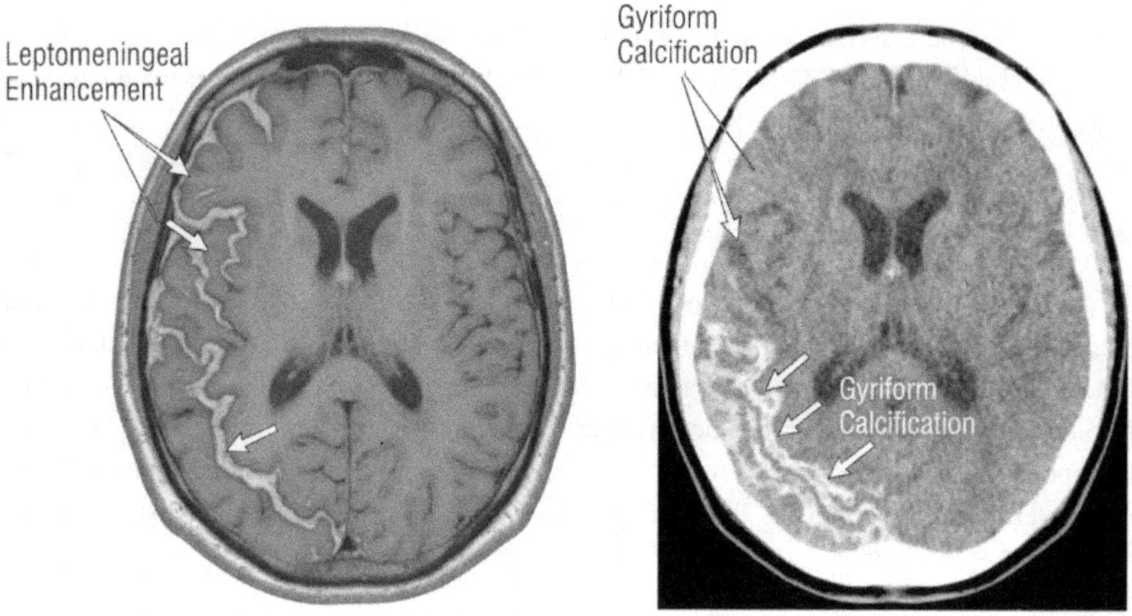

Von Hippel-Lindau Disease and Other Phakomatoses

This closing section addresses von Hippel-Lindau disease and briefly surveys several additional, less common phakomatoses, extending this chapter's syndrome-specific imaging framework to this final group of neurocutaneous disorders. As with the syndromes discussed earlier in this chapter, correct recognition of the specific underlying entity, rather than a generic label of vascular malformation syndrome, is what determines the specific, individualized surveillance program each of the entities in this closing section requires.

Central Nervous System Hemangioblastoma

Von Hippel-Lindau disease, caused by mutation in the VHL tumor suppressor gene, is characterized in the central nervous system by hemangioblastoma, a highly vascular tumor most commonly arising in the cerebellum and spinal cord, presenting on imaging as a well-circumscribed cystic mass with an intensely enhancing mural nodule, a morphology superficially similar to the pilocytic astrocytoma discussed in Chapters 12 and 13 but distinguished by its markedly greater vascularity, often producing flow voids on conventional sequences and requiring careful preoperative vascular imaging given the substantial intraoperative hemorrhage risk this tumor's rich vascularity carries if this vascular characterization is not obtained in advance. Spinal cord hemangioblastoma, in particular, is frequently accompanied by an extensive syrinx disproportionately large relative to the tumor itself, a finding that should prompt careful, deliberate search for the small, enhancing mural nodule responsible, since the syrinx alone, without identification of its causative nodule, would otherwise be mistaken for an isolated, idiopathic finding rather than correctly attributed to this specific, treatable underlying tumor.

Multiplicity as a Diagnostic Clue

Multiple hemangioblastomas, identified either synchronously at a single evaluation or metachronously across serial surveillance imaging, is a strong diagnostic clue supporting underlying von Hippel-Lindau disease over a sporadic, isolated hemangioblastoma, since sporadic hemangioblastoma, while it occurs, is considerably less likely to present with this specific multiplicity; a child or adolescent with more than one central nervous system hemangioblastoma identified on imaging warrants genetics referral and comprehensive multisystem screening for the syndrome's other characteristic manifestations, including retinal hemangioblastoma, renal cell carcinoma, and pheochromocytoma, applying the same systematic, syndrome-directed multisystem evaluation principle this chapter has emphasized throughout. Even a single hemangioblastoma identified in a young child or adolescent, an age at which sporadic hemangioblastoma is comparatively uncommon relative to its typical adult presentation, should prompt at least consideration of underlying von Hippel-Lindau disease, since age at presentation, independent of multiplicity alone, is itself a further relevant clue this chapter's diagnostic reasoning incorporates.

Retinal and Systemic Screening

Comprehensive von Hippel-Lindau disease surveillance extends well beyond the central nervous system imaging emphasized in this section to include regular dilated ophthalmologic examination for retinal hemangioblastoma, a frequently early and, if untreated, vision-threatening manifestation, and periodic abdominal imaging for renal cell carcinoma and pheochromocytoma, both of which carry their own distinct malignant or catecholamine-secreting risk requiring dedicated, syndrome-specific surveillance protocols; coordinating this multisystem surveillance across ophthalmology, urology, endocrinology, and neurosurgery, rather than a neurology-centered evaluation alone, reflects the genuinely multisystem nature of this diagnosis, consistent with the coordinated, anticipatory surveillance principle this chapter has developed for each of the neurocutaneous syndromes it addresses. A structured, written surveillance calendar specifying the recommended interval and specific modality for each organ system this syndrome affects, established at the time of initial diagnosis and shared explicitly with the family, supports adherence to this comprehensive, multiyear surveillance program in the same way this book has recommended for the other complex, longitudinal surveillance protocols addressed throughout its preceding chapters.

PHACE Syndrome

PHACE syndrome, an acronym denoting posterior fossa malformation, hemangioma, arterial anomalies, cardiac defects, and eye abnormalities, presents with a large, segmental facial infantile hemangioma together with a characteristic combination of the named associated findings, and dedicated neuroimaging, including intracranial and extracranial vascular imaging, is warranted in any infant with a large, segmental facial hemangioma specifically to evaluate for the arterial anomalies and posterior fossa malformation this syndrome can produce, since these specific structural and vascular findings carry direct implications for the timing and safety of hemangioma treatment, particularly propranolol therapy, given this medication's potential hemodynamic effects in a child with a coexisting significant arterial anomaly. The posterior fossa malformation component of this syndrome frequently overlaps with the Dandy-Walker spectrum discussed in Chapter 8, and recognizing PHACE syndrome as a specific, distinct diagnostic possibility when this overlapping posterior fossa finding co-occurs with a large facial hemangioma prompts the specific vascular imaging evaluation this syndrome requires, evaluation that would not otherwise be triggered by the posterior fossa finding in isolation.

Klippel-Trenaunay Syndrome and Related Vascular Malformation Syndromes

Klippel-Trenaunay syndrome and related capillary-venous-lymphatic malformation syndromes, while predominantly affecting the limbs and trunk rather than the central nervous system directly, are included in a comprehensive neurocutaneous syndrome discussion given their shared vascular malformation biology with several of the entities addressed throughout this chapter, and a minority of affected children show associated central nervous system vascular anomalies warranting the same coordinated, syndrome-directed imaging evaluation this chapter has applied throughout to its other named syndromes. The overlapping somatic mosaic genetic mechanisms increasingly identified across several of these vascular malformation syndromes, including PIK3CA-related overgrowth spectrum conditions sharing biological features with Klippel-Trenaunay syndrome, reflect a broader, evolving understanding that many phakomatoses previously classified as clinically distinct entities in fact share overlapping molecular pathway disruptions, a unifying biological theme worth holding alongside this chapter's syndrome-by-syndrome clinical organization.

The Value of Syndrome Recognition for Imaging Strategy

Across every neurocutaneous syndrome this chapter has addressed, the recurring, unifying lesson is that correctly recognizing the specific underlying syndrome, rather than characterizing each imaging finding in isolation, transforms the entire subsequent evaluation from a reactive, finding-by-finding workup into a proactive, comprehensive, syndrome-directed surveillance program addressing the full, predictable spectrum of manifestations a given genetic diagnosis carries; this chapter's cumulative emphasis on cutaneous findings as a direct gateway to a structured neuroimaging and multisystem evaluation protocol exemplifies, in perhaps its purest form, this book's broader Clinical-Imaging Crosswalk philosophy of using an accessible clinical sign to anchor a precise, evidence-based imaging pathway.

Imaging Protocol Considerations Across the Neurocutaneous Syndromes

While each neurocutaneous syndrome this chapter has addressed carries its own specific imaging protocol emphasis, hippocampal and hemispheric attention for Sturge-Weber syndrome, tuber-and-nodule-focused sequences for tuberous sclerosis complex, optic nerve and whole-body characterization for neurofibromatosis type 1, internal auditory canal detail for neurofibromatosis type 2, and vascular characterization for von Hippel-Lindau disease, all share the same underlying dedicated-protocol discipline established in Chapter 1, in which the specific clinical syndrome and its known manifestation spectrum directly determines the sequences obtained rather than a single, generic brain protocol applied uniformly regardless of the specific syndrome under evaluation. A referring clinician who communicates the specific suspected or confirmed syndrome clearly on the imaging order, rather than a generic indication such as rule out abnormality, gives the imaging department the essential information needed to select the correct, syndrome-specific protocol from the outset, avoiding the diagnostic delay and repeat-imaging burden a generic, non-specific order can otherwise produce.

Life-Course Transition of Neurocutaneous Syndrome Surveillance

Each of the neurocutaneous syndromes addressed in this chapter requires surveillance extending well beyond childhood into adulthood, and coordinating the transition of this structured, syndrome-specific surveillance program into adult-focused care, applying the same transition-of-care principles developed in Chapters 9 and 12, protects against a gap in monitoring at this vulnerable life-course transition point; providing the young adult and their receiving adult care team with a complete, organized summary of the specific surveillance protocol, imaging findings, and multisystem screening history this chapter has emphasized throughout ensures the lifelong, syndrome-appropriate vigilance these conditions require continues seamlessly across this transition. Because several of the tumors and vascular manifestations addressed throughout this chapter, plexiform neurofibroma malignant transformation, subependymal giant cell astrocytoma, and hemangioblastoma among them, can newly emerge or progress at any point across a person's lifespan, this transition summary is not a one-time historical document but the beginning of a continued, active surveillance relationship the receiving adult team must sustain indefinitely.

Figure 14.4: Cerebellar Hemangioblastoma in Von Hippel-Lindau Disease

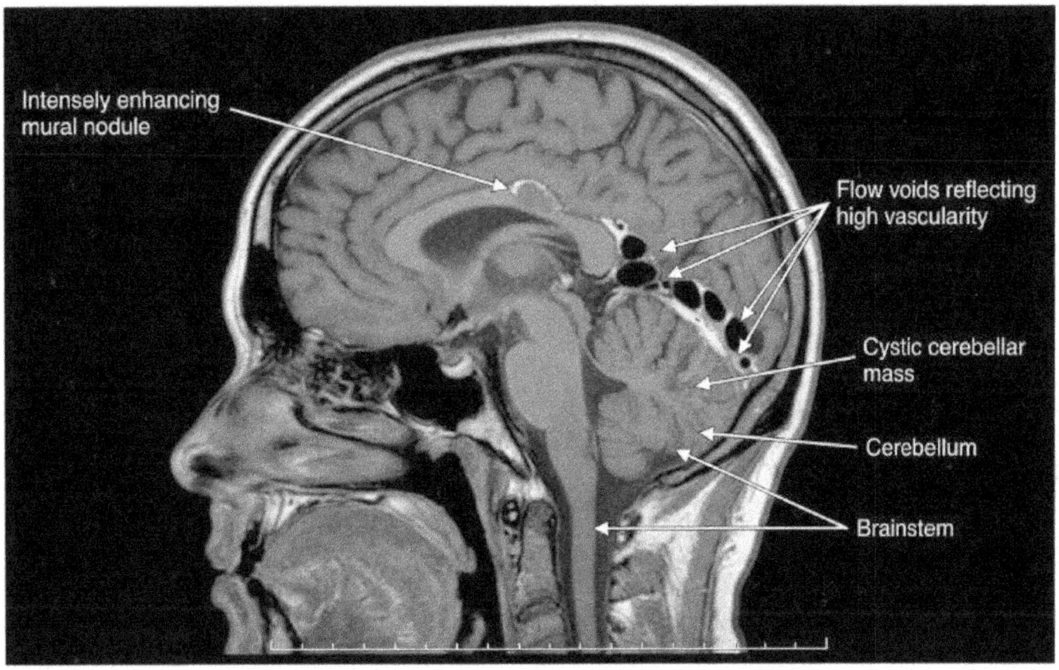

Case Presentation: Sturge-Weber Syndrome With Progressive Seizures

An infant with a facial port-wine stain involving the right V1 trigeminal distribution undergoes brain MRI given this specific, high-risk cutaneous distribution, applying the reasoning developed in this chapter, and postcontrast imaging demonstrates leptomeningeal enhancement overlying the right parieto-occipital region consistent with leptomeningeal angiomatosis. Applying the reasoning developed in this section, the family is counseled regarding the seizure risk this finding carries and the importance of aggressive seizure control given the documented association between seizure burden and cognitive outcome in this syndrome. The child subsequently develops seizures at eight months of age, and given rapid progression to medically refractory epilepsy over the following year, the family is referred for the epilepsy surgical evaluation discussed in Chapter 11 earlier than would typically be considered for many other pediatric epilepsy presentations, reflecting the neuroprotective, early-intervention philosophy this chapter has developed specifically for this syndrome. Ophthalmologic screening, initiated in parallel with the neurologic evaluation per this chapter's guidance, identifies early elevated intraocular pressure, allowing prompt glaucoma treatment before any vision loss has occurred, illustrating the coordinated, multisystem surveillance this syndrome requires from the earliest point of diagnosis.

Case Presentation: Multiple Hemangioblastomas Identifying Von Hippel-Lindau Disease

A sixteen-year-old presents with headache and ataxia, and brain MRI identifies a cystic cerebellar mass with an enhancing mural nodule, and, on careful review of the full study, a second, smaller similar lesion in the cervical spinal cord. Applying the multiplicity reasoning developed in this chapter, this finding of multiple hemangioblastomas prompts genetics referral rather than treating the cerebellar lesion as an isolated, sporadic pilocytic-astrocytoma-like tumor, and genetic testing confirms a germline VHL mutation. Comprehensive multisystem screening, applying the reasoning developed in this section, identifies an early, asymptomatic retinal hemangioblastoma on dilated ophthalmologic examination, allowing prompt treatment before vision-threatening progression, illustrating how the imaging-driven recognition of multiplicity in this chapter's final section directly triggered a comprehensive, multisystem diagnostic cascade that identified and addressed a second, independently significant manifestation of this same underlying genetic diagnosis. The family is further counseled regarding the autosomal dominant inheritance pattern this diagnosis carries and the availability of predictive genetic testing for at-risk first-degree relatives, extending this chapter's imaging-and-genetics integration into the broader family counseling context this book has emphasized throughout.

THE CLINICAL-IMAGING CROSSWALK SYSTEM — Neurocutaneous Syndrome Recognition

Crossing 1 Recap: A subependymal nodule near the foramen of Monro is reclassified as a giant cell astrocytoma based on demonstrated interval growth on serial, quantitatively compared surveillance imaging, not appearance at a single time point alone.

Chapter Anchor: Each neurocutaneous syndrome carries a specific, predictable central nervous system and multisystem manifestation spectrum; recognizing the syndrome from its cutaneous or clinical gateway finding transforms imaging from a reactive, isolated evaluation into a proactive, comprehensive, syndrome-directed surveillance program spanning the child's entire lifespan and requiring coordinated, multidisciplinary care beyond neurology alone.

Summary and Key Concepts

Neurofibromatosis type 1 and type 2 are genetically and clinically distinct despite their shared name; type 1 features optic pathway glioma, plexiform neurofibroma, and benign T2 hyperintensities, while type 2 is defined by bilateral vestibular schwannoma. Mosaic presentations and coordinated multidisciplinary clinic care apply to both.

Tuberous sclerosis complex produces cortical tubers, subependymal nodules, and radial migration lines from shared mTOR pathway dysregulation; subependymal giant cell astrocytoma is diagnosed by demonstrated growth near the foramen of Monro, and comprehensive care requires multisystem surveillance beyond the brain, including cardiac, renal, and neuropsychiatric (TAND) screening.

Sturge-Weber syndrome's facial port-wine stain distribution predicts intracranial risk; leptomeningeal angiomatosis produces progressive calcification and atrophy over time, and aggressive early seizure control is pursued given its association with cognitive outcome, alongside proactive glaucoma surveillance.

Von Hippel-Lindau disease produces highly vascular central nervous system hemangioblastoma, most reliably distinguished from pilocytic astrocytoma by its vascularity; multiplicity of hemangioblastomas is a strong clue to the underlying syndrome warranting comprehensive multisystem screening for retinal, renal, and adrenal manifestations.

PHACE and Klippel-Trenaunay syndromes exemplify further neurocutaneous entities requiring syndrome-specific vascular imaging; across this chapter, cutaneous or clinical syndrome recognition is the gateway to a comprehensive, proactive surveillance program rather than isolated, reactive imaging, and this surveillance must transition seamlessly into adult-focused care.

CHAPTER 15: INFECTIONS OF THE CENTRAL NERVOUS SYSTEM

Learning Objectives

1. Recognize the imaging findings of bacterial meningitis and its major complications, including subdural empyema and venous sinus thrombosis.
2. Distinguish the imaging patterns of the major pediatric viral encephalitides, including herpes simplex encephalitis.
3. Recognize the characteristic imaging findings of the major congenital TORCH infections and correlate them with timing of maternal infection.
4. Distinguish brain abscess from a mimicking tumor using diffusion-weighted imaging and describe the parameningeal infection pathways that produce it.

Bacterial Meningitis and Its Complications

Bacterial meningitis, a medical emergency requiring rapid clinical diagnosis and treatment, is primarily a clinical and cerebrospinal fluid diagnosis rather than an imaging one, and this section's central purpose is not to establish the primary diagnosis but to recognize the specific, actionable complications that imaging is uniquely positioned to identify once the diagnosis has already been made. This reframing, imaging as a complication-detection tool rather than a primary diagnostic tool, is the single most important conceptual orientation this section asks the reader to adopt, since it directly shapes both when imaging is appropriately obtained and how its findings, or the absence of findings, should be interpreted throughout the remainder of this section.

The Limited Role of Imaging in Uncomplicated Meningitis

Brain imaging in a child with suspected bacterial meningitis and no focal neurologic deficit, no papilledema, and no other sign of a mass lesion is generally not required before lumbar puncture, applying the same evidence-based imaging-ordering threshold this book has developed throughout, since imaging in this circumstance neither confirms nor excludes meningitis and, if pursued reflexively, delays the urgent lumbar puncture and antibiotic administration this diagnosis requires; imaging is instead reserved for the specific complications this section addresses, or for a child with a focal deficit, altered consciousness disproportionate to the clinical picture, or another specific finding raising concern for a mass effect or other structural process that would make lumbar puncture unsafe without prior imaging characterization. This specific, evidence-based threshold for pre-lumbar-puncture imaging, developed through extensive clinical research demonstrating the low yield of routine imaging in a child without these specific red-flag features, directly parallels the broader imaging-ordering discipline established in Chapter 3, applied here to one of the most time-sensitive clinical scenarios this book addresses.

Leptomeningeal Enhancement

When imaging is obtained in bacterial meningitis, characteristic findings include leptomeningeal enhancement on postcontrast sequences, reflecting inflammatory breakdown of the blood-brain barrier at the meningeal surface, a finding that can be subtle in early disease and, notably, is not required to establish the diagnosis given meningitis's fundamentally clinical and cerebrospinal-fluid basis; FLAIR sequences frequently show a complementary finding of sulcal hyperintensity from proteinaceous exudate within the subarachnoid space, and recognizing that a normal or near-normal imaging study does not exclude meningitis, given the primarily clinical basis of this diagnosis, prevents inappropriately deferring lumbar puncture pending a reassuring imaging result. This specific interpretive caution, that normal imaging never excludes meningitis, deserves particular emphasis given how easily a busy clinical team might otherwise be reassured by an unremarkable scan in a genuinely urgent clinical scenario where the lumbar puncture and empiric antibiotic administration this diagnosis requires should never be delayed pending or influenced by imaging findings alone.

Ventriculitis and Its Recognition

Ventriculitis, extension of the infectious and inflammatory process into the ventricular ependymal lining, appears on imaging as ependymal enhancement and, at times, debris or a fluid-fluid level within the ventricles on diffusion-weighted or FLAIR sequences, a finding carrying meaningful prognostic weight and, in some cases, direct treatment implications including the need for extended antibiotic duration or, for a child with an existing ventricular shunt, dedicated infection management for the device itself; recognizing this specific complication, rather than characterizing the infectious process as confined to the meninges alone, directly informs both prognosis and, where relevant, the specific treatment modifications this more extensive intraventricular involvement warrants. Ventriculitis carries a further, specific downstream risk of the loculated hydrocephalus discussed in Chapter 10, since inflammatory debris within the ventricular system can produce the same compartmentalizing adhesions responsible for that more complex hydrocephalus pattern, reinforcing why a child with confirmed ventriculitis warrants the same careful, compartment-by-compartment ventricular assessment this book has emphasized for that related condition.

Subdural Empyema and Effusion

Subdural empyema, a collection of frank pus within the subdural space, and the more common, generally benign sterile subdural effusion, a reactive fluid collection without true infection, must be carefully distinguished on imaging given their dramatically different management implications, surgical drainage for a true empyema versus observation alone for a simple, sterile effusion; diffusion-weighted imaging, applying the same restricted-diffusion-indicates-pus principle developed further in this chapter's abscess discussion, is the single most useful discriminating sequence, since a true empyema characteristically shows restricted diffusion from its purulent contents while a sterile effusion does not, a distinction of direct, immediate surgical planning consequence. A sterile effusion is a common, expected accompaniment of bacterial meningitis in infancy, related to the same inflammatory blood-brain barrier disruption responsible for the leptomeningeal enhancement discussed above, and this expected, benign accumulation should not by itself prompt neurosurgical referral in the absence of the specific diffusion-restricting, mass-effect-producing features that would instead indicate a true, surgically significant empyema.

Cerebral Venous Sinus Thrombosis as a Meningitis Complication

Cerebral venous sinus thrombosis, discussed in its broader context in Chapter 6, represents a recognized complication of bacterial meningitis, believed to arise from direct inflammatory extension to the adjacent dural venous sinuses or from the hypercoagulable state that severe systemic infection can produce, and a child with meningitis showing unexpected clinical deterioration, a new seizure, or a finding on imaging suggesting venous congestion or hemorrhagic venous infarction should prompt dedicated venous imaging applying the same venous imaging indications developed in Chapter 6, since this specific complication carries direct anticoagulation treatment implications distinct from the antibiotic-focused management of the underlying meningitis itself. The decision to anticoagulate a child with meningitis-associated venous sinus thrombosis requires careful, individualized weighing of thrombosis extent and clinical severity against the theoretical bleeding risk this treatment carries in a child with an active intracranial infection, a genuine area of clinical judgment best addressed through coordinated discussion between neurology, hematology, and infectious disease rather than a single, universally applied protocol.

Cerebral Infarction as a Meningitis Complication

Arterial infarction represents a further recognized, serious complication of bacterial meningitis, arising from vasculitis or vasospasm affecting the vessels traversing the inflamed subarachnoid space, most classically involving the vessels at the base of the brain given the typical basal predominance of the inflammatory exudate in this location; recognizing this specific complication, applying the acute stroke evaluation principles developed in Chapter 18 to this specific, infection-associated context, and distinguishing it from the venous thrombosis discussed above, since the two share some overlapping risk factors but require distinct evaluation and management approaches, is an essential component of comprehensive meningitis complication surveillance. Dedicated vascular imaging, whether MR angiography or, where more readily available given clinical urgency, CT angiography, characterizes the specific pattern and distribution of vessel narrowing this infectious vasculopathy produces, information that both confirms the mechanism responsible for a new focal deficit and helps distinguish this specific, infection-associated vasculopathy from an unrelated, coincidental vascular process.

Long-Term Hearing Screening After Bacterial Meningitis

Sensorineural hearing loss, arising from direct cochlear inflammatory involvement, is among the most common long-term complications of bacterial meningitis, particularly pneumococcal meningitis, and universal, structured audiologic screening before hospital discharge and at defined follow-up intervals is a standard, essential component of comprehensive post-meningitis care, applying the same proactive, structured surveillance principle this book has emphasized throughout; dedicated temporal bone imaging, evaluating for the labyrinthitis ossificans discussed further in this chapter's imaging correlate discussion, is pursued when hearing loss is confirmed, since early identification of ossification, which can progress within weeks of the acute infection, directly informs the urgency of cochlear implantation candidacy evaluation before this ossification process might otherwise preclude successful implantation.

Pathogen-Specific Considerations by Age

The likely causative pathogen in bacterial meningitis varies substantially by age, with group B streptococcus and Escherichia coli predominating in the neonate, and Streptococcus pneumoniae and Neisseria meningitidis predominating in the older infant and child, a distinction with direct implications for both empiric antibiotic selection and the specific complication profile each pathogen carries, since pneumococcal meningitis in particular carries a disproportionate hearing loss and cerebral infarction risk relative to some other pathogens; while pathogen identification ultimately depends on cerebrospinal fluid culture rather than imaging, this age-and-pathogen association is worth holding in mind when interpreting the specific complication pattern imaging identifies in a given child, since it shapes the anticipated complication profile even before culture results return. Group B streptococcal meningitis in the neonate, in particular, carries a disproportionately high risk of the ventriculitis and abscess formation discussed throughout this chapter relative to the pneumococcal and meningococcal disease more typical of the older child, reinforcing why age-appropriate anticipation of the specific complication spectrum, rather than a uniform expectation applied across every age group, should guide the imaging surveillance intensity pursued in a given case.

Repeat Imaging for Persistent or Recurrent Fever

A child with bacterial meningitis showing persistent or recurrent fever despite appropriate antibiotic therapy warrants repeat imaging to actively search for an evolving or previously subclinical complication, including the subdural empyema, ventriculitis, or venous thrombosis discussed throughout this section, rather than assuming inadequate antibiotic dosing or an expected, self-limited fever pattern alone; this specific clinical trigger for repeat imaging, persistent fever despite appropriate treatment, exemplifies the broader principle this book has emphasized throughout that an unexpected clinical trajectory should prompt active reconsideration and, where appropriate, repeat imaging rather than a passive assumption that the original diagnosis and management plan remain fully adequate.

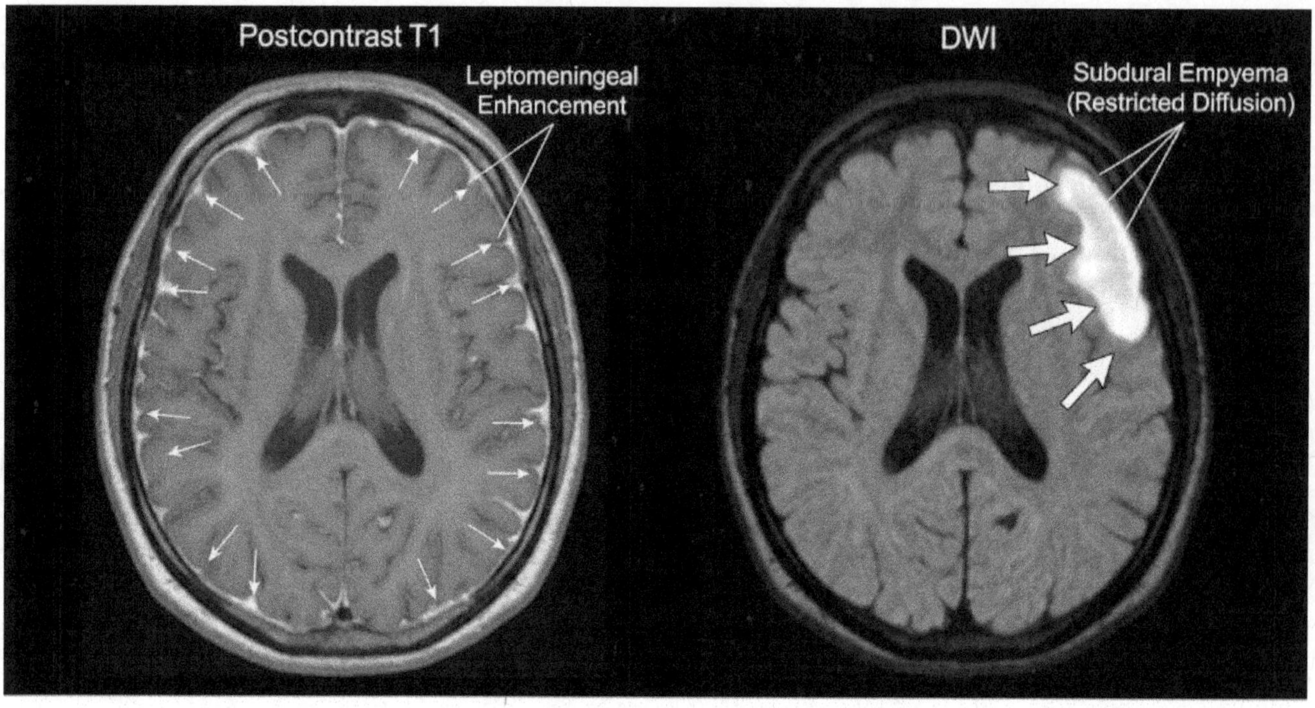

Figure 15.1: Leptomeningeal **Enhancement and Subdural Empyema**

Complication	Key Imaging Finding	Management Implication
Ventriculitis	Ependymal enhancement, intraventricular debris	Extended antibiotic duration
Subdural empyema	Restricted diffusion within subdural collection	Surgical drainage
Venous sinus thrombosis	Absent flow signal, venous infarction	Anticoagulation
Arterial infarction	Restricted diffusion in arterial territory	Stroke-specific management

Viral Encephalitis

Viral encephalitis encompasses a heterogeneous group of pathogens producing overlapping but, at times, distinctively patterned imaging findings, and this section develops the specific imaging recognition that distinguishes the most urgent, treatable presentation, herpes simplex encephalitis, from the broader, more heterogeneous viral encephalitis differential. Where the preceding section on bacterial meningitis emphasized imaging's complication-detection role, this section instead emphasizes imaging's positive, pattern-recognition role, since a confidently recognized distributional pattern can meaningfully narrow an otherwise broad infectious differential even before pathogen-specific laboratory confirmation becomes available.

Herpes Simplex Encephalitis: The Diagnostic Emergency

Herpes simplex encephalitis, the most common identifiable cause of sporadic viral encephalitis and a true diagnostic and treatment emergency given the availability of effective antiviral therapy that dramatically improves outcome when initiated promptly, classically produces asymmetric T2/FLAIR signal abnormality and swelling involving the temporal lobes, insula, and inferior frontal lobes, characteristically sparing the basal ganglia, a specific distributional pattern that helps distinguish it from several of the mimicking entities discussed elsewhere in this book; empiric acyclovir therapy is initiated immediately upon clinical suspicion, before imaging or cerebrospinal fluid confirmation is available, reflecting this diagnosis's time-sensitive, treat-first-confirm-second management philosophy given the severe, often irreversible consequences of treatment delay. This basal-ganglia-sparing pattern specifically distinguishes herpes simplex encephalitis from several vascular and metabolic mimics that instead preferentially involve the basal ganglia, making this single distributional detail one of the most clinically consequential individual observations addressed anywhere in this chapter.

Early Versus Established Herpes Simplex Encephalitis Imaging

Early in the disease course, conventional T2 and FLAIR sequences can appear deceptively normal or only subtly abnormal, and diffusion-weighted imaging, showing restricted diffusion in the affected temporal and insular regions reflecting early cytotoxic injury, is frequently the most sensitive sequence for detecting this diagnosis at its earliest, most treatable stage; a normal conventional MRI in a child with a clinical presentation concerning for herpes simplex encephalitis should not defer empiric antiviral treatment, and dedicated diffusion-weighted sequences, together with cerebrospinal fluid PCR testing, remain the most reliable early diagnostic tools when conventional imaging has not yet demonstrated the more established, later-stage signal abnormality this section has described. Cerebrospinal fluid PCR itself carries a recognized false-negative rate particularly early in the disease course, before viral replication has reached a level reliably detectable by this specific assay, meaning a single negative PCR result obtained very early in the presentation should not, by itself, prompt discontinuation of empiric antiviral therapy, and repeat testing after several days, once viral replication has had time to increase, is appropriate when the clinical suspicion for this diagnosis remains genuinely high despite an initially negative result.

Hemorrhagic Transformation in Herpes Simplex Encephalitis

As herpes simplex encephalitis progresses, particularly in inadequately or belatedly treated disease, hemorrhagic transformation within the affected temporal and insular regions can develop, visible as susceptibility artifact on gradient-echo or susceptibility-weighted sequences, reflecting the severe, necrotizing nature of this specific viral infection's tissue injury; recognizing this hemorrhagic evolution as an expected feature of more advanced or inadequately treated disease, rather than an unrelated, separate hemorrhagic process, reinforces the urgency of prompt treatment initiation this section has emphasized throughout, since this specific complication reflects a more severe, established stage of injury that earlier, prompt antiviral treatment aims specifically to prevent. The specific mechanism underlying this necrotizing, hemorrhagic pattern relates to the virus's direct cytopathic effect on temporal and insular cortical tissue combined with the intense secondary inflammatory response this infection provokes, together producing a degree of tissue destruction more severe than most other pediatric viral encephalitides this chapter addresses, a mechanistic distinction worth holding in mind when counseling a family regarding this specific diagnosis's generally more guarded long-term prognosis relative to several of the other viral entities this section discusses.

Other Viral Encephalitides

Beyond herpes simplex, a broad range of additional viral pathogens, including enterovirus, particularly enterovirus-associated rhombencephalitis producing a distinctive brainstem-predominant signal abnormality pattern, arboviruses transmitted by mosquito or tick vectors with variable, often nonspecific imaging appearances, and, less commonly in the era of widespread vaccination, measles and other vaccine-preventable pathogens, produce a more heterogeneous, less consistently patterned imaging appearance than the relatively distinctive herpes simplex pattern discussed above; correlating the specific imaging pattern with the child's epidemiologic history, including season, geographic exposure, and vaccination status, narrows this broader differential even when the imaging pattern alone does not point definitively to a single specific pathogen. Enterovirus-associated rhombencephalitis in particular carries specific epidemiologic significance given its association with recognized outbreak clusters and its characteristic dorsal brainstem signal abnormality pattern, worth distinguishing explicitly from the more common, generally milder aseptic meningitis presentation enterovirus more typically produces, since this specific rhombencephalitis presentation carries a meaningfully more severe clinical course and, at times, associated cardiopulmonary complications requiring intensive supportive care beyond the neurologic manifestations this section's imaging discussion primarily addresses.

Autoimmune Encephalitis as a Critical Mimic

Autoimmune encephalitis, discussed further in Chapter 16, represents a critical mimic of infectious viral encephalitis, at times producing overlapping clinical presentation and, less consistently, overlapping imaging findings, and distinguishing these two categories carries direct treatment implications, since autoimmune encephalitis requires immunotherapy rather than antimicrobial treatment; a child with an encephalitis presentation not responding as expected to empiric antiviral therapy, or with a specific clinical feature such as prominent psychiatric symptoms or movement abnormality atypical for a straightforward infectious process, should prompt active consideration of this alternative, immunologically mediated diagnosis rather than assuming treatment failure of a presumed infectious process alone. A recognized, well-documented clinical scenario worth actively anticipating is autoimmune encephalitis emerging as a delayed, post-infectious complication following confirmed herpes simplex encephalitis itself, in which a child who has completed appropriate antiviral treatment and shown initial improvement subsequently deteriorates again days to weeks later, a biphasic clinical course that should prompt specific consideration of this post-herpetic autoimmune phenomenon rather than presumed antiviral treatment failure or recurrent herpes simplex infection.

Cerebrospinal Fluid and Serologic Correlation

While imaging provides essential structural information regarding the pattern and severity of viral encephalitis, definitive pathogen identification depends on cerebrospinal fluid PCR testing and, for certain pathogens, serologic studies, and imaging findings should be interpreted in active correlation with these laboratory results rather than in isolation, since the same general encephalitis imaging pattern, T2/FLAIR signal abnormality with variable enhancement and diffusion restriction, can be produced by multiple different pathogens with distinct treatment implications; this correlation-dependent diagnostic approach exemplifies the broader clinical-imaging integration principle this book's Crosswalk System embodies throughout, applied here to the specific context of infectious disease diagnosis.

Long-Term Sequelae and Epilepsy Risk

Viral encephalitis, particularly herpes simplex encephalitis given the severity and characteristic temporal lobe location of its typical injury pattern, carries a substantial risk of long-term neurologic sequelae including cognitive impairment, focal neurologic deficit, and epilepsy, and structured, longitudinal neurodevelopmental and neurologic surveillance, applying the same baseline-and-longitudinal-tracking principle developed in Chapter 11, is a standard, anticipated component of long-term post-encephalitis care; a child with residual temporal lobe injury from herpes simplex encephalitis is at particular risk for the temporal lobe epilepsy discussed in Chapter 11, and this specific, mechanistically explicable risk connection is worth communicating proactively to the family rather than only addressed reactively if and when seizures eventually develop.

Imaging Follow-Up After Herpes Simplex Encephalitis

Following acute treatment of herpes simplex encephalitis, follow-up imaging typically demonstrates progressive volume loss and gliotic signal change within the originally affected temporal and insular regions, reflecting the destructive nature of this infection's tissue injury even with prompt, appropriate antiviral treatment, and documenting this expected evolution on interval imaging provides both a structural correlate for any residual clinical deficit and a baseline against which any subsequent, unexpected change, including the epilepsy-related findings discussed above, can be meaningfully compared over the child's subsequent long-term follow-up.

Figure 15.2: Herpes Simplex Encephalitis: Temporal and Insular Involvement

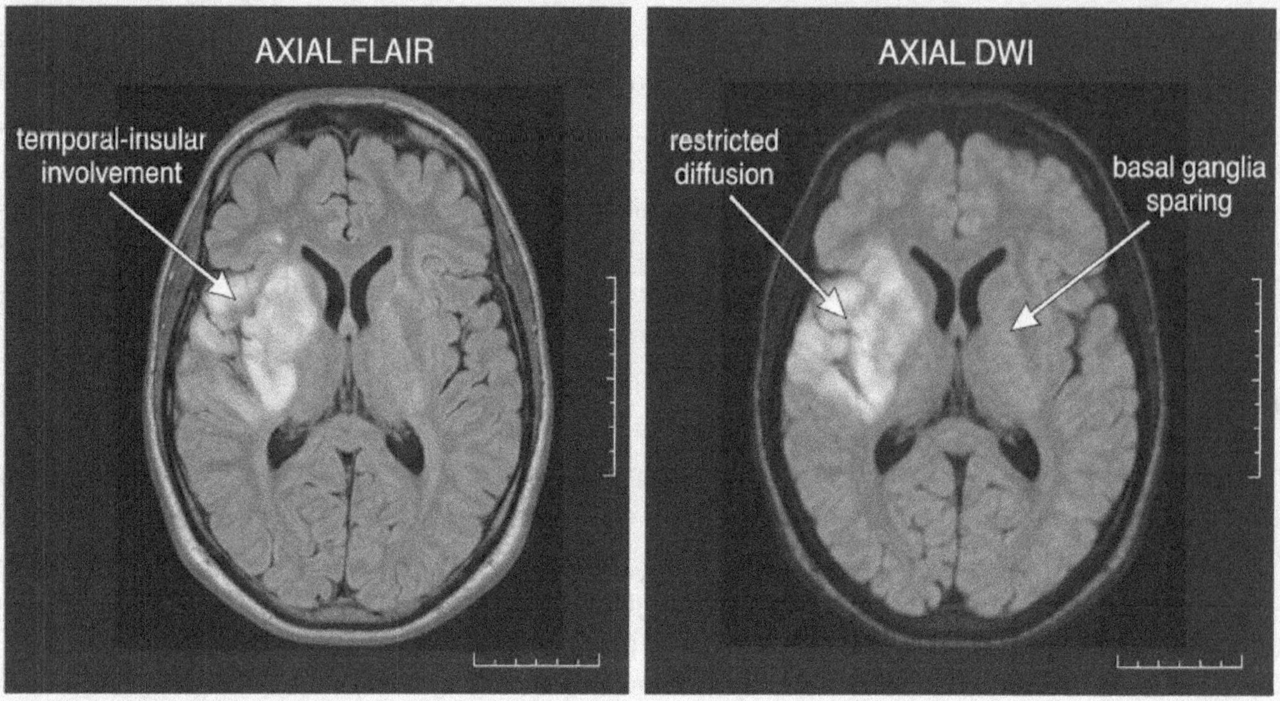

THE CLINICAL-IMAGING CROSSWALK SYSTEM — Normal Early MRI in Suspected Herpes Simplex Encephalitis

The Crossing: A four-year-old presents with fever, altered mental status, and new focal seizures, and conventional T2 and FLAIR brain MRI obtained within twelve hours of symptom onset appears grossly unremarkable.

Presentation Signature: A child with a clinical presentation strongly concerning for herpes simplex encephalitis but a deceptively normal-appearing conventional MRI obtained very early in the disease course.

Imaging Correlate: Diffusion-weighted sequences are specifically reviewed and demonstrate subtle restricted diffusion within the right temporal lobe and insula not appreciated on the conventional T2 and FLAIR sequences, and empiric acyclovir, already initiated based on clinical suspicion alone, is continued while cerebrospinal fluid PCR confirmation is pending.

Trap Logic: Interpreting a normal-appearing conventional MRI as evidence against herpes simplex encephalitis, and withholding or discontinuing empiric antiviral therapy on this basis, risks a severe, potentially preventable outcome given this diagnosis's time-sensitive treatment window and the well-recognized insensitivity of conventional sequences in the earliest disease stage.

Crossing Anchor: A normal conventional MRI does not exclude early herpes simplex encephalitis; diffusion-weighted imaging is the most sensitive early sequence, and empiric antiviral treatment, once clinically initiated, continues pending cerebrospinal fluid confirmation regardless of an equivocal or falsely reassuring imaging appearance.

Congenital and TORCH Infections

This section addresses the congenital infections collectively, though somewhat imprecisely, grouped under the TORCH acronym, Toxoplasmosis, Other (including syphilis and Zika virus), Rubella, Cytomegalovirus, and Herpes simplex, each producing distinct, timing-dependent patterns of fetal brain injury this section develops in turn. Though grouped together under this shared historical acronym, these pathogens differ substantially in transmission mechanism, current epidemiologic prevalence, and specific resulting imaging pattern, and this section's organization by individual pathogen, rather than as a single undifferentiated category, reflects the same precision-over-generality principle this book has applied consistently to every other constellation of related entities it has addressed.

The Principle of Gestational Timing

Across every congenital infection this section addresses, the gestational timing of maternal infection is the single most important determinant of the resulting fetal brain injury pattern, since infection during the period of active neuronal migration, discussed in Chapter 7, produces a fundamentally different injury pattern, malformation of cortical development, than infection occurring later in gestation, which instead produces destructive, encephaloclastic injury superimposed on an otherwise normally formed brain; holding this timing-dependent framework in mind while evaluating a suspected congenital infection allows the reader to interpret the specific imaging pattern observed as a clue to the likely gestational timing of the maternal infection, complementing rather than replacing the serologic and clinical history that ultimately establishes the specific pathogen involved. This same principle, that the developmental stage at which an insult occurs determines its resulting imaging pattern as much as the insult's specific nature, echoes the recurring embryologic-timing theme this book has developed since Chapter 2, now applied specifically to the infectious, rather than purely genetic or malformative, category of prenatal brain injury this chapter addresses.

Congenital Cytomegalovirus

Congenital cytomegalovirus, the most common congenital infection overall and a leading cause of non-genetic sensorineural hearing loss, produces a spectrum of findings depending on gestational timing, including periventricular calcification, the most classic and frequently cited finding, polymicrogyria and other migrational abnormalities when infection occurs early enough to disrupt active neuronal migration, discussed in Chapter 7, cerebellar hypoplasia, and, on T2/FLAIR sequences, characteristic temporal lobe white matter cysts and periventricular signal abnormality; recognizing this specific combination of calcification pattern, migrational abnormality where present, and temporal lobe cystic change, rather than any single finding in isolation, supports this specific diagnosis and directs confirmatory testing, most reliably urine or saliva PCR obtained within the first three weeks of life given the diagnostic ambiguity a later-obtained test introduces regarding congenital versus postnatally acquired infection. The severity spectrum of congenital cytomegalovirus is broad, ranging from an entirely asymptomatic infection detected only through targeted or, where implemented, universal newborn screening, to the severe, multi-finding pattern this section has described, and even an asymptomatic infection at birth carries a meaningful risk of delayed-onset sensorineural hearing loss, underscoring why structured, longitudinal audiologic surveillance, rather than a single newborn screening test alone, is warranted across early childhood for every confirmed case regardless of initial severity.

Congenital Toxoplasmosis

Congenital toxoplasmosis classically produces a triad of hydrocephalus, intracranial calcification, most characteristically diffusely scattered throughout the brain parenchyma rather than the more periventricular-predominant pattern of cytomegalovirus, and chorioretinitis, and this classic triad, when present in combination, strongly supports this specific diagnosis over the other TORCH entities this section addresses; the hydrocephalus characteristic of congenital toxoplasmosis most commonly reflects aqueductal obstruction from the inflammatory process, applying the obstructive hydrocephalus reasoning developed in Chapter 10, and recognizing this specific mechanism directs appropriate neurosurgical evaluation alongside the antimicrobial treatment this specific congenital infection requires. Maternal toxoplasmosis infection acquired earlier in gestation generally produces more severe fetal disease than infection acquired later, an inverse relationship between transmission likelihood and disease severity worth noting, since transmission itself is actually more likely with later maternal infection even though the resulting fetal disease, when transmission does occur, tends to be less severe than the less common but more devastating early-gestation transmission this section's severity discussion primarily reflects.

Congenital Zika Virus Infection

Congenital Zika virus infection, recognized as a significant cause of congenital microcephaly following outbreaks in the Americas beginning in 2015, produces a characteristic and severe pattern of destructive brain injury including marked cortical thinning, ventriculomegaly, extensive calcification at the gray-white junction rather than the more periventricular pattern of cytomegalovirus, and a collapsed, disorganized skull shape reflecting severe, early brain volume loss disproportionate to skull growth; recognizing this specific, severe destructive pattern and its distinctive gray-white junction calcification distribution, combined with an appropriate travel or exposure history, supports this diagnosis and directs the family toward the specific, comprehensive multidisciplinary developmental support this severe presentation typically requires. The severity of congenital Zika syndrome, generally more severe on average than the other TORCH entities addressed in this section, reflects the virus's particular tropism for neural progenitor cells during the critical early period of cortical development discussed in Chapter 7, explaining both the profound cortical thinning and the disorganized, collapsed skull shape this section has described as this syndrome's most characteristic and severe imaging features.

Congenital Rubella and Congenital Syphilis

Congenital rubella, now rare in regions with robust maternal vaccination programs but still encountered where vaccination coverage remains incomplete, produces findings including microcephaly, cerebral calcification, and, characteristically, an associated vasculopathy, while congenital syphilis, experiencing a concerning epidemiologic resurgence in several regions in recent years, produces findings that can range from subtle to a more severe meningoencephalitis pattern, underscoring why a broad, systematic congenital infection screening panel, rather than testing for only the more commonly considered entities, remains clinically relevant in a child presenting with findings suggestive of this broader category regardless of which specific pathogen initially seems most likely based on epidemiologic factors alone. The recent resurgence of congenital syphilis specifically reinforces this book's broader theme that established patterns of disease prevalence can shift meaningfully over time, and a clinician's mental differential diagnosis should be actively updated to reflect current epidemiologic trends rather than remaining anchored to an outdated understanding of which congenital infections are common versus rare in contemporary practice.

Distinguishing Congenital Infection From a Primary Malformation

A destructive, encephaloclastic pattern of injury superimposed on an otherwise appropriately formed brain, as opposed to a primary malformation of cortical development discussed in Chapter 7 arising from a genetic or non-infectious embryologic disruption, is an important distinguishing clue supporting a congenital infectious rather than primary genetic etiology, since the two categories, while sharing some overlapping imaging features including polymicrogyria in particular, carry substantially different family counseling and recurrence risk implications; correlating the specific imaging pattern against maternal infection history, serologic testing, and, where the distinction remains genuinely ambiguous, targeted genetic testing to exclude a primary malformation syndrome, applies the same evidence-integration principle this chapter's viral encephalitis section has emphasized to this related, congenital infection context.

Maternal Screening and Prevention Counseling

Beyond the postnatal diagnostic imaging emphasized throughout this section, maternal counseling regarding congenital infection prevention, including cytomegalovirus-specific hygiene precautions given this pathogen's transmission through bodily fluids commonly encountered in caregiving for young children, and toxoplasmosis-specific dietary and exposure precautions, represents an important preventive component of comprehensive prenatal and interpregnancy care extending beyond this chapter's primarily diagnostic imaging focus; a family who has experienced one congenital infection affected pregnancy benefits from explicit counseling regarding these specific prevention strategies for any future pregnancy, given the generally modifiable nature of the exposure risk factors underlying several of the pathogens this section addresses.

Postnatal Versus Congenital Infection Timing Distinction

For cytomegalovirus in particular, distinguishing a truly congenital infection, acquired in utero, from a postnatally acquired infection, which can occur through breast milk or other postnatal exposure and generally carries a substantially more favorable prognosis in the term infant, depends critically on the specific timing of confirmatory testing discussed above, since a positive test obtained beyond the first three postnatal weeks cannot reliably distinguish between these two categories; this timing-dependent diagnostic window is a further, specific illustration of this chapter's recurring theme that the precise timing of both the underlying infectious exposure and the confirmatory testing itself directly shapes both diagnostic certainty and prognostic counseling.

Figure 15.3: Periventricular Calcification in Congenital Cytomegalovirus

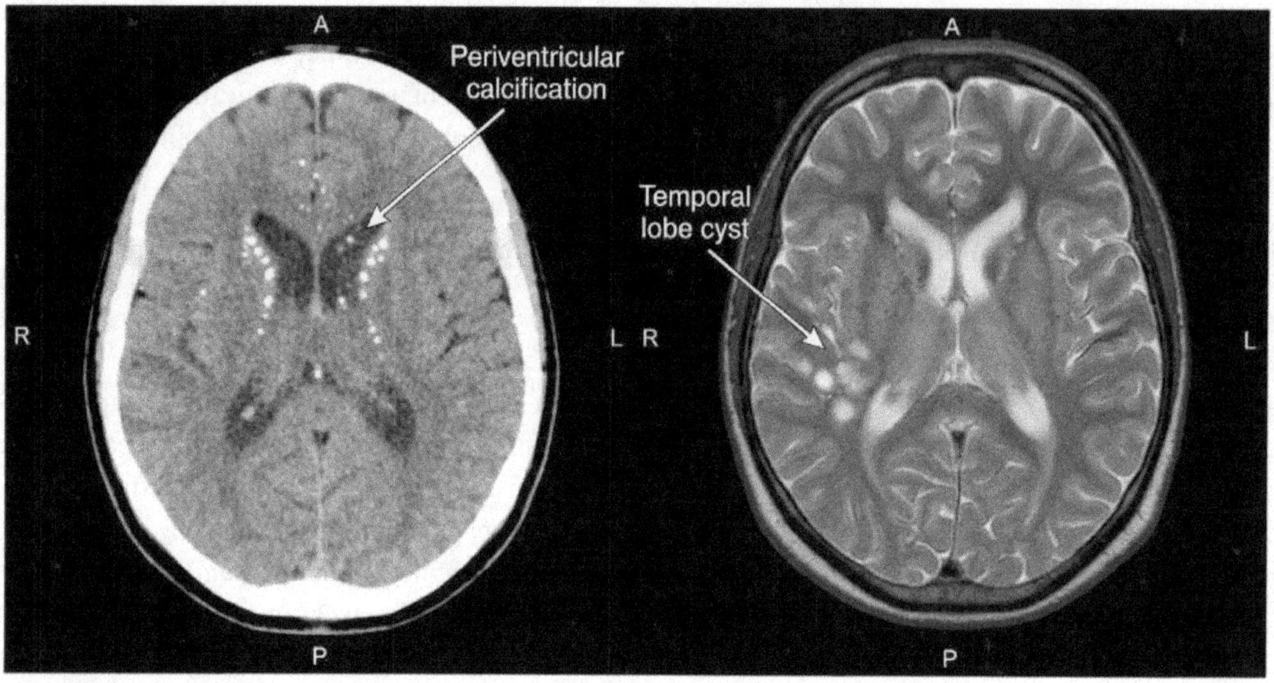

Brain Abscess and Parameningeal Infection

This closing section addresses brain abscess, its critical distinction from a mimicking neoplasm, and the specific parameningeal infection pathways, sinusitis, otitis, and dental infection, that most commonly produce it in the pediatric population. This closing focus on source identification, rather than the abscess itself in isolation, reflects this chapter's cumulative theme that a complete CNS infection evaluation extends beyond characterizing the immediate finding to actively identifying and addressing its underlying cause, whether that cause is a parameningeal infectious source, as in this section, or the specific maternal infection timing addressed in the preceding section on congenital infection.

Diffusion-Weighted Imaging: The Critical Discriminator

Brain abscess characteristically shows a well-defined, ring-enhancing lesion with pronounced restricted diffusion within the central, purulent cavity, a finding that provides the single most reliable discriminator between abscess and a ring-enhancing tumor, most notably the high-grade glioma discussed in Chapter 12, which characteristically does not show this same degree of central diffusion restriction given its predominantly necrotic, rather than purulent, cavity contents; applying this diffusion-based distinction with confidence, rather than relying on the ring-enhancement pattern alone, which both entities can share, resolves what would otherwise be one of the most consequential differential diagnostic challenges in pediatric neuroimaging, given the dramatically different management pathways, urgent surgical drainage and antibiotics for abscess versus the oncologic evaluation discussed in Chapter 12 for tumor, that these two entities require. The high cellular viscosity and inflammatory cellular debris within a purulent abscess cavity mechanically restrict water molecule diffusion far more effectively than the more liquid, less viscous necrotic contents of a tumor cavity, providing the underlying biophysical basis for this reliable, high-yield imaging distinction the reader should understand at a mechanistic, not merely pattern-recognition, level.

The Capsule and Its Maturation Stages

A maturing brain abscess develops a characteristic, relatively thin, smooth enhancing capsule, generally thinner along its medial, deep margin than its lateral, more superficial margin, reflecting differential vascularity across the capsule related to the underlying cerebral blood supply pattern, a subtle but recognized asymmetry worth noting when present as further supportive evidence for abscess over tumor, whose capsule, when present, tends to be more irregular and variably thick; recognizing the specific stage of abscess maturation, from an early, poorly organized cerebritis without a discrete capsule through a fully mature, well-organized abscess with a defined capsule, also carries direct treatment timing implications, since surgical drainage is generally more technically favorable and more definitively curative once a mature, well-defined capsule has formed. Early cerebritis, occurring before this capsule has organized, may respond to antibiotic therapy alone without surgical drainage in a carefully selected, closely monitored child, and serial imaging demonstrating the expected evolution, or lack thereof, from this early cerebritis stage directly informs the ongoing decision between continued medical management and surgical intervention as the infection's natural stage-by-stage progression unfolds.

Sinogenic and Otogenic Parameningeal Infection

Sinusitis, particularly frontal sinusitis given its direct anatomic proximity to the frontal lobes, and otitis media or mastoiditis, given proximity to the temporal lobe and posterior fossa, represent the most common parameningeal sources of pediatric brain abscess, spreading intracranially either through direct extension across the adjacent bone or through retrograde spread along the valveless emissary veins connecting the sinus or mastoid venous system to the intracranial venous system; recognizing this specific anatomic and pathophysiologic connection directs the imaging evaluation to actively include and carefully characterize the adjacent sinuses or mastoid air cells whenever a frontal or temporal lobe abscess is identified, since identifying and definitively treating the primary parameningeal source is essential to preventing recurrence even after successful drainage of the resulting intracranial abscess itself. Because this valveless emissary vein pathway allows infection to spread intracranially without necessarily producing the bony erosion visible on CT that would otherwise serve as a more obvious anatomic clue, the absence of visible bony erosion adjacent to a sinus or mastoid infection does not, by itself, exclude this specific route of intracranial spread, and a temporal or frontal lobe finding concerning for abscess in a child with a coexisting sinus or ear infection warrants this specific correlation regardless of whether bony erosion is separately identified.

Odontogenic Sources of Intracranial Infection

Dental infection, a less commonly recognized but well-documented source of intracranial abscess, particularly in the older child or adolescent, spreads intracranially through a mechanism analogous to the sinogenic and otogenic pathways discussed above, and a careful dental history and, where clinically indicated, dedicated dental imaging should be incorporated into the evaluation of a brain abscess without an obvious sinus or ear source identified on the standard cranial imaging this section otherwise emphasizes, applying the same principle of actively searching for an underlying, treatable source rather than accepting cryptogenic as a final, unexplored explanation. A history of a recent dental procedure or a known, untreated dental abscess in an adolescent presenting with a frontal or temporal lobe brain abscess without an identified sinus or ear source should prompt specific, targeted questioning about dental symptoms and, where warranted, coordinated evaluation with oral and maxillofacial specialists to identify and definitively treat this less commonly considered but clinically important source.

Epidural Abscess and Subdural Empyema From Parameningeal Spread

Beyond the intraparenchymal abscess emphasized throughout this section, the same sinogenic, otogenic, and odontogenic infectious pathways can produce epidural abscess and subdural empyema, discussed earlier in this chapter's meningitis complications section, without necessarily producing a coexisting intraparenchymal abscess, and systematically evaluating each of the extra-axial spaces, epidural, subdural, and intraparenchymal, whenever a parameningeal infectious source is identified, rather than assuming a single compartment is involved to the exclusion of others, ensures a complete, rather than partial, characterization of the infection's full intracranial extent. Multiple, coexisting compartments of infection, epidural, subdural, and intraparenchymal simultaneously, can occur in a single child with a particularly aggressive parameningeal source, and this specific, multi-compartment presentation warrants a correspondingly comprehensive surgical approach addressing each identified collection rather than a single, isolated drainage procedure targeting only the most clinically apparent compartment.

Immunocompromised Host Considerations

An immunocompromised child, whether from an underlying primary immunodeficiency, oncologic treatment, or another cause of immune suppression, presents with a broader, atypical brain abscess pathogen spectrum, including fungal organisms such as Aspergillus, which can produce a distinct, often less well-organized and less diffusion-restricting imaging appearance than the classic bacterial abscess pattern this section has otherwise emphasized; maintaining a lower threshold for early biopsy or aspiration in this specific, higher-risk population, rather than relying on imaging characterization alone to the same degree appropriate in an immunocompetent child, reflects this population's distinct diagnostic and management needs given both the broader pathogen differential and this population's generally more limited capacity to mount the organized inflammatory response the classic imaging findings this section has described actually depend upon.

Serial Imaging During Antibiotic Treatment

Following surgical drainage and initiation of targeted antibiotic therapy, serial imaging surveillance tracking abscess cavity size and enhancement pattern over the treatment course provides objective, quantitative evidence of treatment response, complementing the clinical improvement a treating team otherwise relies upon, and a cavity failing to demonstrate the expected progressive size reduction over serial studies should prompt reconsideration of the antibiotic regimen, the possibility of a resistant or atypical organism, or an inadequately drained residual collection requiring further surgical intervention; this serial, quantitative comparison approach mirrors the same structured surveillance discipline this book has applied throughout to numerous other conditions requiring longitudinal imaging tracking of treatment response.

Multiloculated and Satellite Abscesses

A subset of brain abscesses present as multiloculated collections with internal septations, or with one or more smaller satellite abscesses adjacent to a dominant, larger lesion, patterns that carry direct implications for surgical planning, since a simple aspiration approach adequate for a single, unilocular abscess may inadequately address a multiloculated or multifocal collection requiring a more extensive surgical approach or, at times, multiple separate drainage procedures; systematically searching the entire brain, rather than concluding the evaluation upon identifying a single, obvious dominant lesion, applies the same complete, thorough search discipline this book has emphasized throughout for other conditions in which a second, less obvious finding carries independent management significance.

Figure 15.4: Brain Abscess Versus Ring-Enhancing Tumor

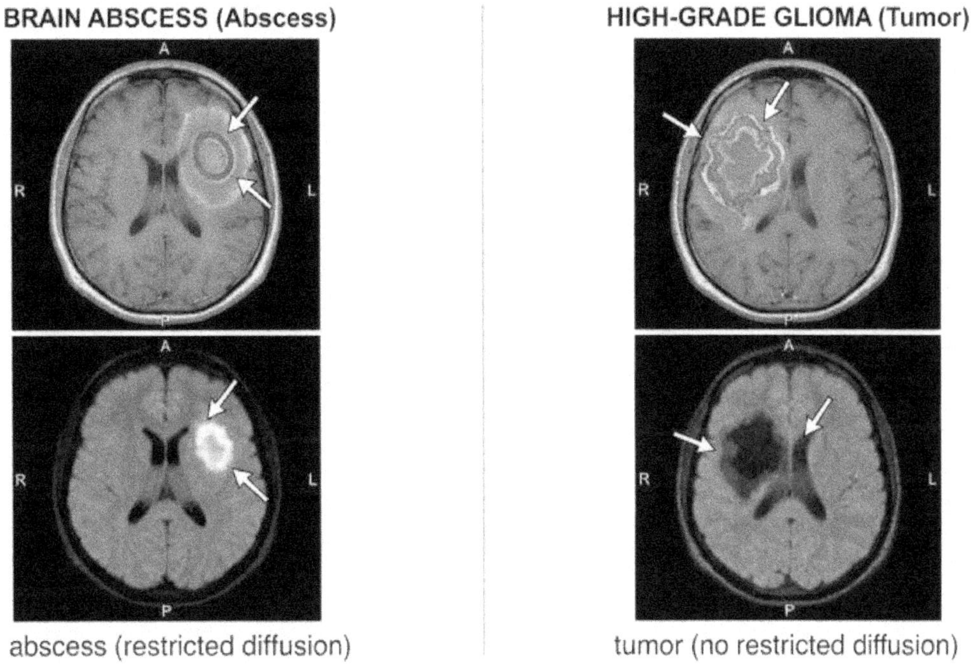

Case Presentation: Frontal Sinusitis Complicated by Epidural and Intraparenchymal Abscess

A fourteen-year-old presents with headache, fever, and frontal swelling, and CT demonstrates opacified frontal sinuses with erosion of the posterior sinus wall. Applying the reasoning developed in this chapter, dedicated brain MRI is obtained given this specific finding of bony erosion suggesting intracranial extension, and the study demonstrates a small epidural abscess adjacent to the eroded bone together with a separate, ring-enhancing frontal lobe intraparenchymal abscess showing pronounced central restricted diffusion. Applying the diffusion-based discrimination developed in this chapter, the intraparenchymal lesion is confidently characterized as abscess rather than tumor, and the neurosurgical and otolaryngology teams coordinate combined surgical drainage of both the epidural and intraparenchymal collections alongside definitive treatment of the underlying frontal sinusitis, illustrating the complete source-to-complication evaluation this chapter's parameningeal infection framework has developed. Serial postoperative imaging over the following weeks confirms progressive resolution of both collections without evidence of a residual or satellite abscess, and the patient is transitioned to oral antibiotic therapy to complete a total treatment course guided by this documented radiographic response.

Case Presentation: Congenital Cytomegalovirus Identified Through Failed Newborn Hearing Screen

A newborn fails the standard newborn hearing screen, and, applying the reasoning developed in this chapter, urine cytomegalovirus PCR is obtained within the first three weeks of life given the diagnostic importance of testing within this specific early window, returning positive and confirming congenital cytomegalovirus infection. Brain MRI demonstrates periventricular calcification and bilateral temporal lobe white matter cysts without an associated migrational abnormality, suggesting infection occurred later in gestation, after the period of active neuronal migration discussed in Chapter 7 had largely concluded. Applying the reasoning developed in this section, the family is counseled regarding the specific pattern identified and its implications, and antiviral treatment, coordinated ophthalmologic and audiologic follow-up, and structured developmental surveillance are initiated, illustrating the complete diagnostic-to-management pathway this chapter's congenital infection framework establishes from an initial, seemingly unrelated newborn hearing screen finding. The family is further counseled regarding the future pregnancy prevention strategies discussed in this chapter, since this specific pathogen's transmission risk from close contact with young children carries direct, actionable implications for the family's planning around any subsequent pregnancy.

THE CLINICAL-IMAGING CROSSWALK SYSTEM — CNS Infection Recognition Across Meningitis, Encephalitis, Congenital Infection, and Abscess

Crossing 1 Recap: A normal conventional MRI does not exclude early herpes simplex encephalitis; diffusion-weighted imaging is the most sensitive early sequence, and empiric antiviral treatment continues pending cerebrospinal fluid confirmation regardless of an equivocal imaging appearance.

Chapter Anchor: CNS infection imaging serves a fundamentally complication-and-confirmation role rather than a primary diagnostic one for meningitis, a distributional-pattern role for encephalitis, a timing-inference role for congenital infection, and a diffusion-based discrimination role for abscess versus tumor; each context requires its own specific imaging reasoning integrated tightly with the clinical and laboratory picture.

Summary and Key Concepts

Imaging in bacterial meningitis serves primarily to identify complications, ventriculitis, subdural empyema (distinguished from sterile effusion by restricted diffusion), venous sinus thrombosis, and arterial infarction, rather than to establish the primary clinical and cerebrospinal-fluid diagnosis; audiologic screening is essential given the sensorineural hearing loss risk.

Herpes simplex encephalitis produces asymmetric temporal-insular signal abnormality with basal ganglia sparing; diffusion-weighted imaging is the most sensitive early sequence, and empiric antiviral treatment is never withheld pending imaging or laboratory confirmation given this diagnosis's severe, time-sensitive consequences.

Congenital TORCH infections produce timing-dependent injury patterns; congenital cytomegalovirus shows periventricular calcification and temporal lobe cysts, toxoplasmosis shows diffuse calcification with hydrocephalus and chorioretinitis, and Zika virus produces severe destructive injury with gray-white junction calcification.

Brain abscess is distinguished from a ring-enhancing tumor by pronounced central restricted diffusion on diffusion-weighted imaging; sinogenic, otogenic, and odontogenic parameningeal sources should be actively identified and treated to prevent recurrence, with immunocompromised children warranting a broader pathogen differential and lower biopsy threshold.

Across this chapter, imaging is integrated tightly with clinical presentation, cerebrospinal fluid findings, and epidemiologic history rather than interpreted in isolation, reflecting the fundamentally multimodal nature of pediatric CNS infection diagnosis.

CHAPTER 16: INFLAMMATORY, DEMYELINATING, AND AUTOIMMUNE DISORDERS

Learning Objectives

1. Distinguish acute disseminated encephalomyelitis from pediatric multiple sclerosis based on clinical course and imaging evolution over time, including the diagnostic role of follow-up imaging.
2. Recognize the imaging findings distinguishing MOG antibody-associated disease and NMOSD from multiple sclerosis, including area postrema syndrome and longitudinally extensive lesion patterns.
3. Describe the imaging approach to suspected autoimmune and paraneoplastic encephalitis, including anti-NMDA receptor encephalitis and its ovarian teratoma association.
4. Recognize the imaging findings of primary and secondary CNS vasculitis in children, including the angiography-negative small-vessel variant.

Acute Disseminated Encephalomyelitis and Pediatric Multiple Sclerosis

Acute disseminated encephalomyelitis and pediatric multiple sclerosis represent opposite ends of a clinical and imaging spectrum, monophasic versus relapsing demyelinating disease, and this section develops the specific distinguishing features that separate these two fundamentally different diagnostic and prognostic categories, both of which can present with an initial episode of overlapping clinical and imaging appearance. Because the correct classification of a first demyelinating episode directly determines whether a child receives ongoing disease-modifying therapy for a lifelong relapsing condition or no ongoing treatment for a resolved, monophasic illness, the diagnostic discipline this section develops carries consequences extending across a child's entire subsequent medical course, not merely the acute presenting episode itself.

Acute Disseminated Encephalomyelitis: Clinical and Imaging Pattern

Acute disseminated encephalomyelitis, a monophasic, immune-mediated demyelinating disorder frequently following a preceding viral infection or, less commonly, vaccination, presents with multifocal, bilateral, poorly demarcated white matter lesions on T2/FLAIR imaging, frequently involving the deep gray matter structures, thalami and basal ganglia, a pattern of gray matter involvement distinctly less typical of the multiple sclerosis discussed later in this section; the clinical presentation characteristically includes encephalopathy, altered mental status or behavioral change, as a defining feature distinguishing this diagnosis from multiple sclerosis, in which encephalopathy is distinctly uncommon at any point in the disease course, making this single clinical feature among the most useful individual discriminators this section addresses. Spinal cord involvement, when present, tends to be longitudinally extensive and diffuse rather than the shorter, more discrete segmental lesions characteristic of multiple sclerosis, providing a further, complementary spinal cord imaging feature that parallels the brain imaging distinctions this section has already emphasized between these two entities.

The Monophasic Course and Diagnostic Uncertainty at Presentation

By definition, acute disseminated encephalomyelitis is a monophasic illness, meaning a definitive diagnosis technically cannot be made with full confidence at the time of initial presentation, since the diagnosis depends partly on the absence of subsequent relapse, a determination only possible in retrospect after adequate follow-up time has elapsed; this diagnostic uncertainty at first presentation is worth communicating honestly to a family, consistent with the honest, proportionate communication principle this book has emphasized throughout, while still applying the specific clinical and imaging features this section develops to generate the most probable initial working diagnosis and appropriate initial treatment approach, typically high-dose corticosteroids, pending this longer-term clinical confirmation.

Pediatric Multiple Sclerosis: Diagnostic Criteria

Pediatric multiple sclerosis, a relapsing-remitting demyelinating disease, is diagnosed using the same core McDonald criteria applied in adult multiple sclerosis, requiring dissemination of demyelinating lesions in both space, more than one anatomic location, and time, either through a new clinical relapse or new lesions on follow-up imaging, though these criteria require particular caution in application to a child younger than eleven years, given the greater diagnostic overlap with acute disseminated encephalomyelitis in this younger age group and the correspondingly higher risk of a premature, ultimately incorrect multiple sclerosis diagnosis in a child whose presentation may still evolve into a monophasic, rather than relapsing, course. A single clinical event without evidence of dissemination in time, termed a clinically isolated syndrome, is managed with the same watchful, structured follow-up imaging approach this section develops for the broader diagnostic ambiguity between ADEM and multiple sclerosis, since a clinically isolated syndrome may represent the first attack of eventual multiple sclerosis, an isolated monophasic event, or, less commonly, the presenting attack of one of the other demyelinating entities discussed later in this chapter.

Characteristic Lesion Morphology in Multiple Sclerosis

Multiple sclerosis lesions characteristically appear as well-demarcated, ovoid white matter lesions oriented perpendicular to the ventricular surface, a pattern termed Dawson fingers reflecting the perivenular distribution of the underlying demyelinating process, and periventricular, juxtacortical, infratentorial, and spinal cord locations are each considered separately in applying the dissemination-in-space criterion, meaning lesions confined entirely to a single one of these anatomic categories do not, by themselves, satisfy this specific diagnostic requirement regardless of how numerous the lesions within that single category might be; this well-demarcated, ovoid, perpendicular-oriented morphology, in contrast to the poorly demarcated, larger, more confluent lesions characteristic of acute disseminated encephalomyelitis discussed above, provides a further, complementary morphologic distinguishing feature beyond the clinical encephalopathy criterion already discussed. A black hole, a chronic, T1-

hypointense lesion reflecting more severe, irreversible axonal loss within an area of prior demyelination, represents a further, specific imaging finding worth recognizing on follow-up imaging, since its presence indicates a degree of permanent tissue injury beyond the fully reversible edema and demyelination characteristic of an acute, actively inflamed lesion, carrying independent prognostic significance regarding a child's likely accumulated long-term disability.

The Critical Role of Follow-Up Imaging

Given the genuine diagnostic overlap between acute disseminated encephalomyelitis and a first multiple sclerosis attack at the time of initial presentation, scheduled follow-up imaging, typically at three to six months, is an essential, structured component of the diagnostic pathway this section has developed, since resolution of the initial lesions without new lesion development supports the monophasic acute disseminated encephalomyelitis diagnosis, while new, clinically silent lesions on this follow-up study, even without a corresponding new clinical relapse, can independently satisfy the dissemination-in-time criterion supporting a multiple sclerosis diagnosis; this follow-up imaging is not merely confirmatory but genuinely diagnostic in its own right, directly determining which of these two fundamentally different long-term management pathways, no ongoing disease-modifying treatment for monophasic acute disseminated encephalomyelitis versus initiation of disease-modifying therapy for confirmed multiple sclerosis, is appropriate for a specific child. Communicating the specific purpose and diagnostic weight of this follow-up study clearly to the family at the time it is scheduled, rather than presenting it as a routine, lower-stakes check-in, helps the family understand why attendance at this particular study carries genuine, decision-determining significance rather than being treated as an optional or lower-priority component of the child's overall care.

Oligoclonal Bands and Cerebrospinal Fluid Correlation

Cerebrospinal fluid oligoclonal bands, reflecting intrathecal immunoglobulin synthesis, are present in a substantial majority of pediatric multiple sclerosis cases but distinctly less common in acute disseminated encephalomyelitis, making this laboratory finding a further, complementary piece of evidence supporting the multiple sclerosis diagnosis when the clinical and imaging picture remains genuinely ambiguous; integrating this cerebrospinal fluid finding alongside the imaging and clinical criteria this section has developed exemplifies the same multimodal, converging-evidence diagnostic approach this book has applied consistently throughout, rather than relying on any single data source, imaging, clinical course, or laboratory testing, in isolation.

Disease-Modifying Therapy Considerations in Pediatric Multiple Sclerosis

Once pediatric multiple sclerosis is confirmed through the criteria this section has developed, prompt initiation of disease-modifying therapy is standard practice given accumulating evidence that early treatment meaningfully reduces relapse frequency and long-term disability accrual, and structured, longitudinal surveillance imaging, typically annually or following any new clinical symptom, monitors both ongoing disease activity and treatment response over the child's subsequent, often decades-long disease course; this early-treatment philosophy reflects a broader shift in the field toward proactive, rather than purely reactive, management once a confirmed relapsing diagnosis has been established, applying the same early-intervention principle this book has emphasized for several other chronic, longitudinally managed pediatric neurologic conditions. A new, clinically silent lesion identified on this routine surveillance imaging, even without a corresponding clinical relapse, is generally interpreted as evidence of breakthrough disease activity warranting treatment escalation, applying the same treat-to-no-evidence-of-disease-activity philosophy increasingly standard in contemporary multiple sclerosis management across both the pediatric and adult populations.

Neuropsychological Impact of Pediatric Multiple Sclerosis

Beyond the physical and sensory manifestations more classically associated with multiple sclerosis, pediatric-onset disease carries a documented risk of cognitive impact, particularly affecting processing speed and attention, given the disease's onset during a period of active, ongoing brain development, and structured neuropsychological baseline assessment and longitudinal monitoring, applying the same baseline-and-longitudinal-tracking principle developed in Chapter 11, is an increasingly recognized, essential component of comprehensive pediatric multiple sclerosis care extending beyond the disease-modifying therapy and relapse-focused surveillance this section has otherwise emphasized.

Figure 16.1: Acute Disseminated Encephalomyelitis Versus Multiple Sclerosis Lesion Morphology

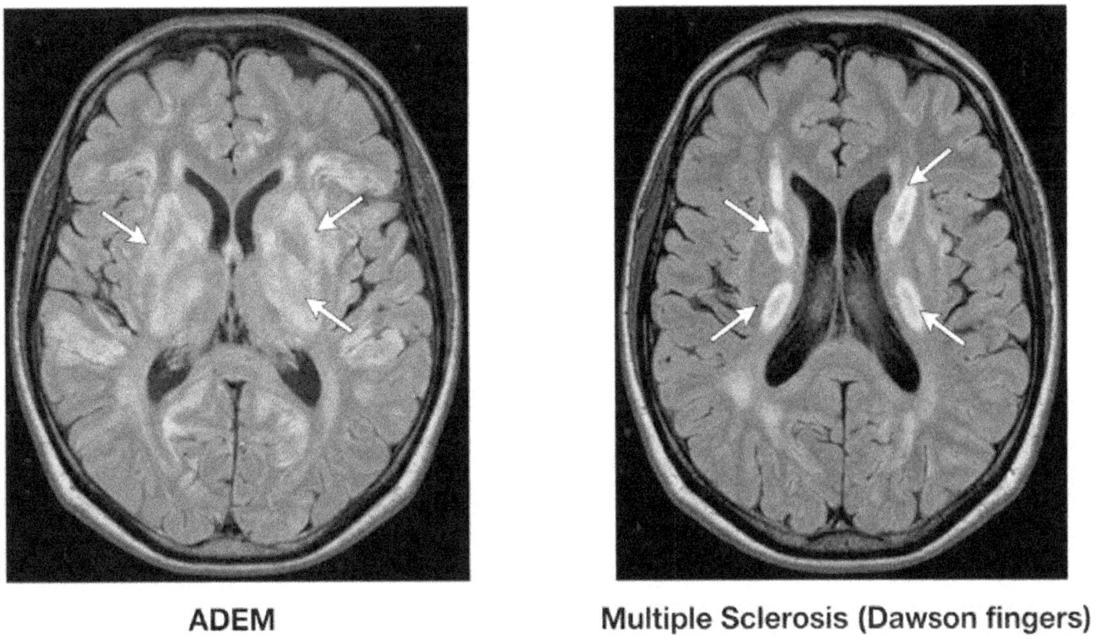

Feature	ADEM	Pediatric Multiple Sclerosis
Clinical course	Monophasic	Relapsing-remitting
Encephalopathy	Characteristic, defining feature	Distinctly uncommon

Lesion margins	Poorly demarcated, large	Well-demarcated, ovoid
Gray matter (thalamic/basal ganglia) involvement	Common	Uncommon
Oligoclonal bands	Uncommon	Present in majority

MOG Antibody-Associated Disease and NMOSD

MOG antibody-associated disease and neuromyelitis optica spectrum disorder, both antibody-mediated demyelinating conditions distinct from multiple sclerosis, are addressed together in this section given their overlapping clinical presentations, optic neuritis and transverse myelitis prominent in both, while this section develops the specific serologic and imaging features that distinguish them from each other and from the multiple sclerosis spectrum discussed in the preceding section. The recognition that these two conditions, once frequently conflated with multiple sclerosis or with each other under the older term neuromyelitis optica, are now understood as distinct, antibody-defined entities each requiring a specific, correspondingly distinct treatment approach exemplifies how rapidly evolving serologic testing has reshaped this entire diagnostic category within a relatively short span of medical practice.

MOG Antibody-Associated Disease: Clinical Spectrum

MOG antibody-associated disease, defined by the presence of serum antibodies against myelin oligodendrocyte glycoprotein, produces a clinical spectrum spanning optic neuritis, frequently bilateral and simultaneous in the pediatric population, transverse myelitis, and, in younger children particularly, an acute disseminated encephalomyelitis-like presentation, meaning MOG antibody testing is an appropriate component of the initial evaluation for a child presenting with a first acute disseminated encephalomyelitis-like episode given the potential for this specific, antibody-defined entity to explain and reclassify what might otherwise be labeled idiopathic acute disseminated encephalomyelitis. This age-dependent clinical presentation pattern, ADEM-like disease more typical of the younger child and optic neuritis or myelitis more typical of the older child and adolescent, mirrors the age-dependent clinical presentation variability this chapter has already noted for both anti-NMDA receptor encephalitis and NMOSD, reinforcing age as a further, recurring dimension of clinical variability the reader should actively incorporate when constructing a differential diagnosis for any of the entities this chapter addresses.

Optic Nerve Involvement in MOG-Associated Disease

Optic neuritis in MOG antibody-associated disease characteristically shows longitudinally extensive optic nerve involvement with perineural enhancement extending along the optic nerve sheath, a pattern distinguishing it from the more focal, typically unilateral optic neuritis characteristic of multiple sclerosis, and this specific perineural enhancement pattern, together with the bilateral, simultaneous presentation more characteristic of MOG-associated disease, should prompt MOG antibody testing even before serologic confirmation is available, since this distinct imaging pattern itself provides meaningful diagnostic direction pending laboratory results. Optic disc swelling on funduscopic examination is frequently more pronounced in MOG antibody-associated optic neuritis than in the optic neuritis of multiple sclerosis, a further clinical, examination-based clue worth correlating alongside the imaging findings this section has emphasized, reinforcing the same multimodal, converging-evidence diagnostic approach this chapter applies consistently across each of its constituent entities.

NMOSD and Aquaporin-4 Antibodies

Neuromyelitis optica spectrum disorder, most commonly associated with antibodies against aquaporin-4, a water channel protein densely expressed in astrocytic foot processes, classically produces longitudinally extensive transverse myelitis, spanning three or more vertebral segments, a pattern distinctly different from the shorter-segment lesions typical of multiple sclerosis, and area postrema syndrome, a distinctive presentation of intractable nausea, vomiting, and hiccups reflecting involvement of this specific dorsal medullary structure rich in aquaporin-4 expression; recognizing this specific clinical syndrome, easily mistaken for a primary gastrointestinal process if the underlying neurologic mechanism is not actively considered, exemplifies this book's broader emphasis on recognizing an unusual clinical presentation as a potential clue to an underlying, mechanistically explicable neurologic process. Severe, bilateral, simultaneous optic neuritis with poor visual recovery is a further, characteristic NMOSD presentation, generally more visually devastating on average than the optic neuritis of multiple sclerosis, reflecting the astrocytopathic, rather than purely demyelinating, mechanism underlying aquaporin-4-mediated tissue injury in this specific condition.

Distinguishing NMOSD From Multiple Sclerosis on Brain Imaging

Beyond the spinal cord and optic nerve findings emphasized above, NMOSD produces characteristic brain lesions in regions of high aquaporin-4 expression, including the periependymal region surrounding the third and fourth ventricles, the area postrema itself, and the hypothalamus, a distribution pattern distinct from the periventricular, Dawson-finger pattern of multiple sclerosis discussed in the preceding section; recognizing this specific, aquaporin-4-expression-guided distribution provides a further, brain-imaging-based discriminator between these two entities beyond the spinal cord and clinical features already discussed, reinforcing that the underlying molecular target, aquaporin-4 in NMOSD versus the more heterogeneous target antigens of multiple sclerosis, directly explains the resulting anatomic distribution pattern each disease produces. Diencephalic and hypothalamic involvement in NMOSD can produce a distinctive clinical syndrome of narcolepsy-like hypersomnolence or endocrine dysfunction reflecting direct hypothalamic injury, a further, clinically recognizable manifestation worth correlating against the specific periependymal and hypothalamic imaging distribution this paragraph has described, extending the clinical-imaging correlation reasoning this book has applied throughout to this specific demyelinating disease category.

Treatment Implications of Correct Serologic Classification

Correctly distinguishing multiple sclerosis, MOG antibody-associated disease, and NMOSD carries direct, consequential treatment implications, since several disease-modifying therapies effective for multiple sclerosis are ineffective or, in the case of NMOSD specifically, can paradoxically worsen disease activity, making accurate serologic and imaging-based classification a genuine treatment-safety issue rather than a purely academic nosologic distinction; a child initially treated empirically for presumed multiple sclerosis who is subsequently found to have NMOSD or MOG antibody-associated disease requires prompt treatment reassessment and transition to the antibody-specific therapy appropriate to their actual, now correctly identified diagnosis. This treatment-safety consideration is worth communicating explicitly to a family whenever a diagnosis remains genuinely provisional pending serologic confirmation, since it directly explains why a treating team may recommend withholding a specific disease-modifying therapy until this confirmatory testing returns, rather than proceeding empirically with a treatment that could, if the underlying diagnosis proves to be NMOSD rather than multiple sclerosis, actively worsen the child's condition.

Relapsing MOG-Associated Disease and Antibody Titer Monitoring

While MOG antibody-associated disease can present as a monophasic illness similar in course to idiopathic acute disseminated encephalomyelitis, a substantial proportion of children experience a relapsing course, and persistently elevated MOG antibody titers on serial testing are associated with a higher relapse risk than titers that decline or clear over time, informing both the duration of maintenance immunotherapy considered and the intensity of ongoing clinical and imaging surveillance a specific child's titer trajectory warrants.

Pediatric-Specific Features of NMOSD

NMOSD in the pediatric population shows several distinct features relative to its more extensively characterized adult presentation, including a higher relative frequency of the ADEM-like and brain-involvement presentations discussed above relative to the more classically described optic-spinal presentation emphasized in adult NMOSD literature, and recognizing that pediatric NMOSD does not always conform precisely to adult-derived diagnostic criteria and typical presentation patterns is essential to avoiding diagnostic delay in a child whose presentation, while genuinely reflecting this same underlying aquaporin-4-mediated disease process, differs meaningfully from the textbook adult presentation a clinician might otherwise expect. This pediatric-adult presentation divergence has motivated ongoing refinement of diagnostic criteria specifically validated in the pediatric population, rather than a simple, unmodified application of adult-derived criteria, reflecting the broader theme this book has emphasized throughout that pediatric neurologic disease frequently requires its own, age-specific diagnostic framework rather than a downward extrapolation from adult medicine.

Acute Treatment and Attack Severity

Acute attacks of NMOSD and MOG antibody-associated disease are generally treated more aggressively than a typical multiple sclerosis relapse, often incorporating high-dose corticosteroids combined with plasma exchange or intravenous immunoglobulin from the outset given these conditions' generally more severe attack-related tissue injury and correspondingly higher risk of incomplete recovery if treatment is delayed or under-intensified; this more aggressive acute treatment approach, distinct from the treatment intensity more typical of a straightforward multiple sclerosis relapse, further underscores why the correct serologic classification this section has emphasized throughout carries direct, immediate treatment intensity implications from the very first acute attack, not only for longer-term disease-modifying therapy selection. Delayed recognition of NMOSD, mistaking an initial attack for a milder multiple sclerosis relapse and consequently under-treating it, risks a degree of permanent tissue injury and disability that more aggressive, appropriately intensive initial treatment could otherwise have substantially mitigated, reinforcing the genuine clinical urgency underlying the correct diagnostic classification this section has developed throughout.

Figure 16.2: Longitudinally Extensive Transverse Myelitis in NMOSD

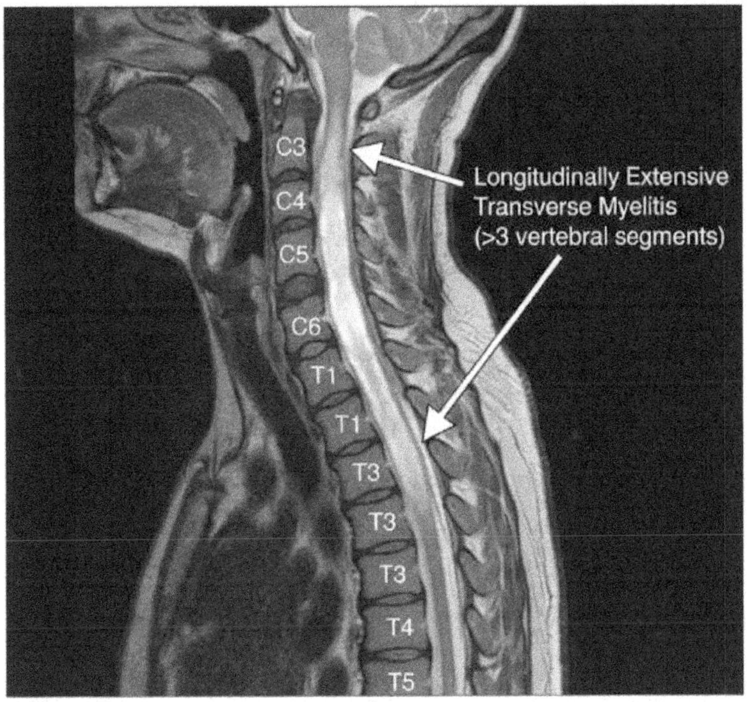

THE CLINICAL-IMAGING CROSSWALK SYSTEM — Intractable Vomiting as a Neurologic, Not Gastrointestinal, Presentation

The Crossing: A twelve-year-old girl presents with two weeks of intractable nausea, vomiting, and hiccups, having undergone an extensive gastroenterology evaluation without an identified cause before neurology is finally consulted.

Presentation Signature: A school-age or adolescent child with prolonged, otherwise unexplained intractable vomiting and hiccups without a clear gastrointestinal cause identified on standard evaluation.

Imaging Correlate: Dedicated brain MRI centered on the dorsal medulla identifies a small area postrema lesion, and serum aquaporin-4 antibody testing, prompted by this specific imaging finding and clinical syndrome recognition, returns positive, confirming NMOSD.

Trap Logic: Pursuing an exclusively gastroenterology-focused evaluation for intractable vomiting and hiccups without considering this specific neurologic syndrome risks a substantial, harmful delay in recognizing and treating NMOSD, a diagnosis for which prompt immunotherapy meaningfully affects long-term outcome.

Crossing Anchor: Intractable vomiting and hiccups without an identified gastrointestinal cause should prompt consideration of area postrema syndrome and dedicated dorsal medullary imaging, particularly in a child or adolescent, rather than an exclusively gastrointestinal diagnostic pathway.

Autoimmune and Paraneoplastic Encephalitis

This section addresses autoimmune encephalitis, a category of antibody-mediated neurologic disease targeting neuronal surface or synaptic proteins rather than the myelin-directed targets of the demyelinating diseases discussed earlier in this chapter, with particular attention to anti-NMDA receptor encephalitis, the most common and best-characterized pediatric autoimmune encephalitis. This shift in target, neuronal surface and synaptic proteins rather than myelin, explains why this section's imaging findings differ so substantially from the demyelinating entities discussed earlier in this chapter, since a fundamentally different underlying pathophysiologic mechanism, one that need not necessarily produce visible structural or signal change on conventional imaging at all, is at work in this section's diagnostic category.

Anti-NMDA Receptor Encephalitis: Clinical Presentation

Anti-NMDA receptor encephalitis, caused by antibodies targeting the NR1 subunit of the N-methyl-D-aspartate receptor, classically presents with a characteristic, staged clinical evolution beginning with a nonspecific prodrome, followed by prominent psychiatric symptoms, behavioral change, hallucinations, and agitation, that can initially be mistaken for a primary psychiatric illness, before progressing to movement abnormalities, most classically orofacial dyskinesias, autonomic instability, and, in more severe cases, decreased consciousness; recognizing this specific, staged clinical evolution, particularly the movement abnormality and autonomic features that emerge as the illness progresses beyond its initial, potentially misleading psychiatric presentation, should prompt active consideration of this diagnosis in a child or adolescent presenting with new-onset psychiatric symptoms accompanied by any of these additional neurologic features. Younger children, particularly those below school age, more often present with seizures and movement abnormalities as prominent early features rather than the more classic psychiatric prodrome emphasized in the adolescent and young adult literature, a further age-dependent presentation variation worth holding alongside the pediatric-specific NMOSD presentation variability discussed elsewhere in this chapter.

The Frequently Normal or Nonspecific Imaging Appearance

A substantial proportion of children with confirmed anti-NMDA receptor encephalitis show a normal or only subtly, nonspecifically abnormal brain MRI, meaning imaging in this specific diagnosis serves primarily to exclude alternative structural or infectious causes rather than to positively establish the diagnosis, a role parallel to the exclusionary imaging function developed in Chapter 10 for idiopathic intracranial hypertension; when present, imaging abnormalities in anti-NMDA receptor encephalitis are frequently nonspecific T2/FLAIR signal change in the medial temporal lobes, cortex, or basal ganglia, and this nonspecific appearance should not be interpreted as evidence against the diagnosis in a child with a compatible, staged clinical presentation. Advanced imaging techniques, including FDG-PET, which frequently shows a characteristic pattern of frontal and temporal hypermetabolism with parieto-occipital hypometabolism even when conventional structural MRI appears entirely normal, offer a complementary tool that can support this diagnosis when conventional imaging alone leaves genuine diagnostic uncertainty, though this specific technique remains available primarily at specialized centers rather than as a routine, universally accessible diagnostic tool.

Cerebrospinal Fluid and Serum Antibody Testing

Definitive diagnosis of anti-NMDA receptor encephalitis depends on cerebrospinal fluid antibody testing, generally more sensitive than serum testing alone for this specific diagnosis, and a child with a compatible clinical presentation and negative serum testing alone should still undergo cerebrospinal fluid testing before this diagnosis is excluded, given this specific, well-documented sensitivity difference between the two testing compartments; this compartment-specific testing sensitivity consideration parallels, in a different laboratory testing context, the same location-and-timing-dependent diagnostic sensitivity themes this book has emphasized throughout, applied here to the specific choice between cerebrospinal fluid and serum sampling for this particular antibody. Routine cerebrospinal fluid studies, beyond the specific antibody testing this section emphasizes, frequently show a mild lymphocytic pleocytosis and, at times, oligoclonal bands in anti-NMDA receptor encephalitis, findings that, while nonspecific individually, support the overall inflammatory, autoimmune nature of the presentation and help distinguish it from a purely primary psychiatric illness without an underlying inflammatory process, a distinction of genuine diagnostic value particularly at the earliest, most clinically ambiguous stage of presentation.

The Ovarian Teratoma Association

Anti-NMDA receptor encephalitis carries a well-documented association with ovarian teratoma in the adolescent and young adult female population, believed to arise from an immune response initially directed against NMDA receptor-expressing neural tissue within the teratoma that subsequently cross-reacts with the patient's own central nervous system NMDA receptors, and pelvic imaging, most commonly ultrasound given its ready availability and lack of radiation or sedation requirement, is a standard, essential component of the evaluation for any adolescent or young adult female with confirmed or strongly suspected anti-NMDA receptor encephalitis, since identification and surgical removal of an underlying teratoma, where present, is directly therapeutic and meaningfully improves the likelihood of treatment response. A single, normal pelvic ultrasound at initial presentation does not permanently exclude an underlying teratoma given the possibility of a small lesion below this modality's detection threshold, and repeat imaging, at times with the more detailed anatomic resolution of MRI, is reasonable in a child with confirmed antibody-positive disease showing an inadequate response to immunotherapy despite an initially unremarkable pelvic ultrasound, since a still-undetected teratoma may be driving ongoing, treatment-resistant disease activity.

Other Autoimmune Encephalitis Antibody Targets

Beyond anti-NMDA receptor encephalitis, a growing number of additional autoimmune encephalitis antibody targets have been characterized, including antibodies against the GABA-B receptor, associated with a distinctive seizure-predominant presentation, and antibodies against the LGI1 protein, more classically an adult presentation but occasionally encountered in adolescence, each carrying its own somewhat distinct clinical presentation pattern; a broad autoimmune encephalitis antibody panel, rather than testing for anti-NMDA receptor antibodies alone, is appropriately pursued when the clinical presentation is compatible with autoimmune encephalitis generally but does not fit the specific, classic staged presentation of anti-NMDA receptor encephalitis this section has emphasized as the most common pediatric presentation. Antibody-negative autoimmune encephalitis, in which a clinical and cerebrospinal fluid picture strongly consistent with an autoimmune process is present despite negative testing across the currently available antibody panel, is a further, recognized clinical scenario, reflecting either a still-uncharacterized antibody target or a cell-mediated, rather than antibody-mediated, autoimmune mechanism, and empiric immunotherapy is reasonably pursued in this specific circumstance based on the compatible clinical and cerebrospinal fluid picture despite the absence of a positive, specific antibody result.

Treatment Response Monitoring

Given the frequently normal or nonspecific baseline imaging discussed above, treatment response monitoring in autoimmune encephalitis relies substantially more heavily on serial clinical assessment than on serial imaging comparison, in contrast to several of the other conditions addressed throughout this book in which imaging serves as a primary, objective treatment response metric; this shift toward clinical, rather than imaging-based, treatment response monitoring is a further, specific illustration of this chapter's broader theme that autoimmune encephalitis occupies a genuinely distinct diagnostic and monitoring paradigm relative to the more structurally evident conditions addressed elsewhere in this book.

First-Line and Second-Line Immunotherapy

Treatment of confirmed autoimmune encephalitis typically follows a structured, escalating approach, beginning with first-line immunotherapy, high-dose corticosteroids, intravenous immunoglobulin, or plasma exchange, and progressing to second-line agents, including rituximab or cyclophosphamide, for a child showing inadequate response to first-line treatment, and this structured treatment escalation, together with the tumor removal discussed above when a teratoma is identified, together constitute the multimodal treatment approach this specific diagnostic category requires; the pace of this escalation, and the specific threshold for transitioning to second-line therapy, is guided predominantly by clinical response given the imaging limitations this section has discussed throughout, reinforcing the clinical, rather than imaging-centered, monitoring paradigm this section has emphasized. Earlier initiation of second-line therapy in a child showing an inadequate or delayed response to first-line treatment, rather than prolonged, repeated cycles of first-line treatment alone, has been associated with improved long-term outcomes in published cohort data, informing a generally more assertive, earlier escalation philosophy in contemporary practice than was more typical in earlier eras of this diagnosis's management.

Post-Infectious Autoimmune Encephalitis After Herpes Simplex

As introduced in Chapter 15, a recognized and clinically important phenomenon involves anti-NMDA receptor encephalitis emerging as a delayed, post-infectious complication following confirmed herpes simplex encephalitis, in which a child who has completed appropriate antiviral treatment and shown initial improvement subsequently deteriorates again days to weeks later with a new, distinct clinical picture more consistent with autoimmune, rather than infectious, encephalitis; recognizing this specific biphasic pattern and pursuing autoimmune encephalitis antibody testing in this specific clinical scenario, rather than presuming herpes simplex treatment failure or viral recurrence, prevents a diagnostic delay that would otherwise leave this distinct, treatable second process unaddressed.

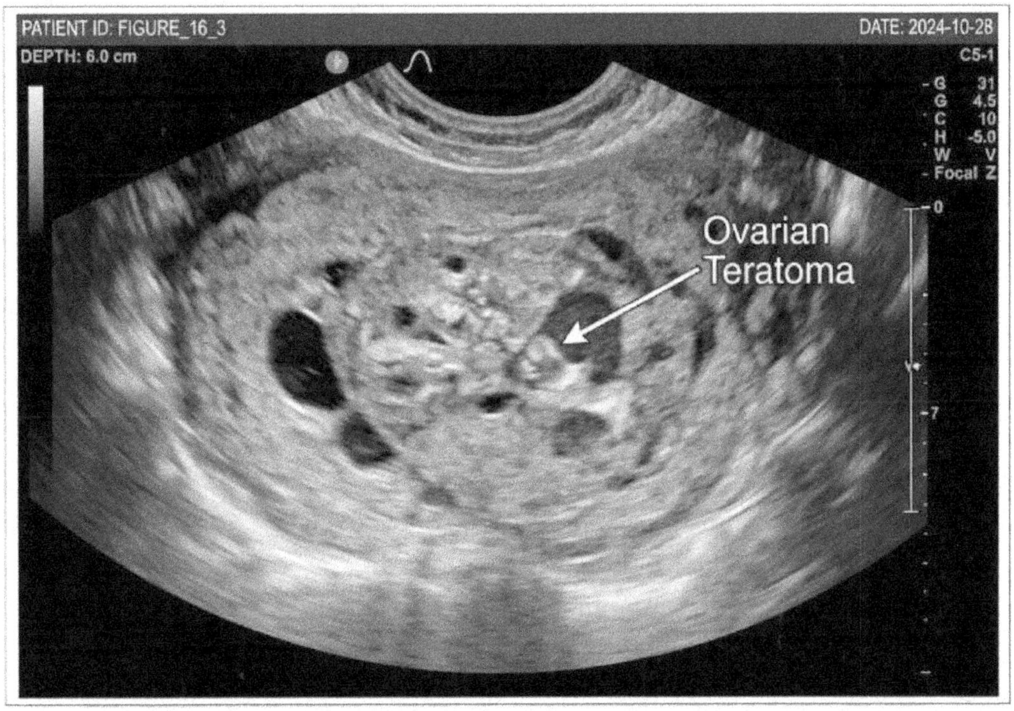

Figure 16.3: Ovarian Teratoma Associated With Anti-NMDA Receptor Encephalitis

Vasculitis and Other Inflammatory CNS Disorders

This closing section addresses primary and secondary central nervous system vasculitis in children, along with several additional inflammatory disorders not captured by the demyelinating and autoimmune encephalitis categories addressed earlier in this chapter, closing this chapter's survey of the acquired and inflammatory disease spectrum. Where the preceding sections addressed conditions targeting myelin or neuronal surface proteins, this closing section returns the reader's attention to the vasculature itself as a direct target of inflammatory disease, completing this chapter's coverage of the full range of tissue compartments, myelin, neurons, and blood vessels, that pediatric inflammatory CNS disease can primarily affect.

Primary Angiitis of the Childhood Central Nervous System

Primary angiitis of the childhood central nervous system, an inflammatory vasculopathy confined to the central nervous system without an identifiable systemic cause, is classified into an angiography-positive form, showing focal or multifocal arterial narrowing on dedicated vascular imaging, and, less commonly recognized, an angiography-negative, small-vessel form, in which conventional vascular imaging appears normal despite biopsy-confirmed vasculitis affecting vessels too small to be resolved by even high-resolution angiographic techniques; recognizing that a normal angiogram does not exclude this diagnosis in a child with a compatible clinical presentation, applying the same imaging-limitation-awareness principle this book has emphasized throughout for other conditions where a specific modality's resolution limits its diagnostic yield, is essential to avoiding premature diagnostic exclusion in this specific small-vessel variant. The angiography-negative, small-vessel form typically presents with a more insidious, progressive clinical course than the more acute, stroke-like presentation characteristic of the angiography-positive form, and brain biopsy, while an invasive step not undertaken lightly, becomes the necessary diagnostic tool when this specific clinical pattern is present despite normal conventional and even advanced vessel wall imaging, since no imaging technique currently available can reliably resolve vasculitis at this smallest vessel scale.

Vessel Wall Imaging in Suspected CNS Vasculitis

Beyond conventional luminal angiographic techniques, dedicated vessel wall imaging, a specialized MRI technique directly visualizing the arterial wall itself rather than only the vessel lumen, offers a complementary tool for characterizing suspected vasculitis, since wall thickening and enhancement can be present even when luminal narrowing is subtle or absent on conventional angiographic sequences; this technique, increasingly available at specialized pediatric neurovascular imaging centers, exemplifies the ongoing evolution of imaging technology this book has noted throughout, in which techniques originally developed for adult neurovascular disease are increasingly adapted and validated for the distinct pediatric vasculitis population this section addresses. Vessel wall imaging further offers the potential to distinguish inflammatory vasculitis from the non-inflammatory vasculopathic mimics discussed later in this section based on the specific pattern of wall enhancement observed, concentric versus eccentric wall thickening in particular, an emerging application that, while not yet universally validated across every specific vasculopathy this distinction requires, represents a promising direction for improving the noninvasive discrimination this chapter has emphasized as a genuine, ongoing diagnostic challenge.

Secondary CNS Vasculitis

Secondary central nervous system vasculitis, arising in the context of an identifiable underlying systemic condition including systemic lupus erythematosus, other systemic autoimmune or rheumatologic diseases, and, less commonly in the pediatric population, an underlying infectious trigger such as varicella, requires evaluation extending beyond the central nervous system imaging emphasized throughout this section to actively identify and characterize the specific underlying systemic disease, since treatment in this circumstance addresses both the underlying systemic condition and its central nervous system vascular manifestation; a child presenting with imaging findings suggestive of vasculitis therefore warrants systematic screening for the systemic autoimmune and infectious triggers this section has named, rather than an assumption of the primary, CNS-confined form discussed above without this broader evaluation. Post-varicella arteriopathy specifically, in which a prior varicella infection, sometimes remote by many months, precedes the development of arterial narrowing and, at times, stroke, represents a well-documented, mechanistically distinct example of this secondary vasculitis category, and eliciting a careful, sometimes distant infectious history is a necessary component of the evaluation for a child presenting with a new arteriopathy of otherwise unclear etiology.

Neurosarcoidosis

Neurosarcoidosis, central nervous system involvement by the multisystem granulomatous disease sarcoidosis, though rare in the pediatric population, can produce leptomeningeal enhancement, cranial neuropathy from basal meningeal involvement, and, at times, a parenchymal mass-like presentation that can mimic a neoplasm, and recognizing this rare but important diagnostic possibility, particularly when accompanied by the pulmonary, ocular, or other systemic findings characteristic of sarcoidosis more broadly, prevents diagnostic delay in a child whose presentation might otherwise be pursued exclusively along an oncologic or infectious diagnostic pathway without this specific, rarer alternative being actively considered. Hypothalamic-pituitary involvement, producing central diabetes insipidus or other endocrine dysfunction from direct granulomatous infiltration of this region, is a further, specific presentation pattern worth recognizing, sharing some clinical overlap with the sellar and suprasellar entities discussed in Chapter 12 but distinguished by its underlying granulomatous, rather than neoplastic, pathology once biopsy or a compatible systemic evaluation confirms this diagnosis.

Hemophagocytic Lymphohistiocytosis and CNS Involvement

Hemophagocytic lymphohistiocytosis, a severe, life-threatening hyperinflammatory syndrome that can be primary, genetic, or secondary to an underlying infectious, oncologic, or autoimmune trigger, frequently involves the central nervous system, producing a range of imaging findings from diffuse white matter signal abnormality to focal, tumefactive lesions, and recognizing central nervous system involvement in a child with confirmed or suspected hemophagocytic lymphohistiocytosis carries direct implications for both the intensity of neurologic-specific treatment pursued and the overall prognosis this severe, multisystem diagnosis carries. Given the severity and rapid progression this condition typically demonstrates, prompt neuroimaging is warranted as soon as this diagnosis is confirmed or strongly suspected, even in the absence of an overt neurologic symptom, since subclinical central nervous system involvement identified early can meaningfully inform the overall treatment intensity selected for this life-threatening, multisystem hyperinflammatory process.

Integrating This Chapter's Framework Into Clinical Practice

Across every entity addressed in this chapter, from the monophasic-versus-relapsing distinction opening this chapter through the vasculitis and rarer inflammatory entities closing it, the recurring, unifying skill this chapter has developed is the ability to hold a broad, well-organized differential diagnosis for inflammatory and autoimmune central nervous system disease, correlate imaging findings tightly with clinical course and laboratory testing rather than any single data source in isolation, and recognize when normal or nonspecific imaging, far from excluding a diagnosis, is itself an expected, informative feature of a specific entity this chapter has named. This chapter's cumulative framework, holding a broad, well-organized differential and correlating imaging tightly with clinical and laboratory evidence, transfers directly to the acute vascular and traumatic presentations addressed in the remaining chapters of this book, where the same discipline of resisting premature diagnostic closure based on a single data source proves equally essential.

Distinguishing Vasculitis From Its Vasculopathic Mimics

A range of non-inflammatory vasculopathies, including the arteriopathy of childhood arterial ischemic stroke discussed in Chapter 18 and the moyamoya-pattern vasculopathy addressed in that same chapter, can produce arterial narrowing patterns superficially similar to the vasculitis this section has emphasized, and distinguishing a true inflammatory vasculitis from these non-inflammatory vasculopathic mimics depends on integrating the specific pattern and distribution of vascular involvement against the accompanying clinical presentation, inflammatory markers, and, where the distinction remains genuinely ambiguous, biopsy, rather than the angiographic appearance of arterial narrowing alone, which these different underlying mechanisms can each independently produce. Serial vascular imaging demonstrating progressive, worsening narrowing over time favors an active, ongoing inflammatory process over the more static, non-progressive pattern more typical of several non-inflammatory vasculopathies, a further, longitudinal distinguishing feature worth incorporating into this discrimination when the initial, single-timepoint evaluation leaves genuine diagnostic uncertainty.

Long-Term Outcome and Relapse Surveillance in CNS Vasculitis

Children with confirmed primary or secondary central nervous system vasculitis require structured, longitudinal surveillance extending well beyond the acute presentation this section has primarily addressed, incorporating serial vascular imaging to monitor for progression or, conversely, favorable regression of the arterial narrowing pattern initially identified, alongside ongoing clinical assessment for a new or recurrent neurologic symptom that might indicate disease relapse; this structured, longitudinal surveillance approach, applying the same serial-comparison principle this book has emphasized throughout for numerous other chronic conditions, provides the objective basis for decisions regarding immunosuppressive treatment duration and eventual, carefully monitored treatment discontinuation once sustained disease quiescence has been documented.

Figure 16.4: Focal Arterial Narrowing in Primary CNS Angiitis

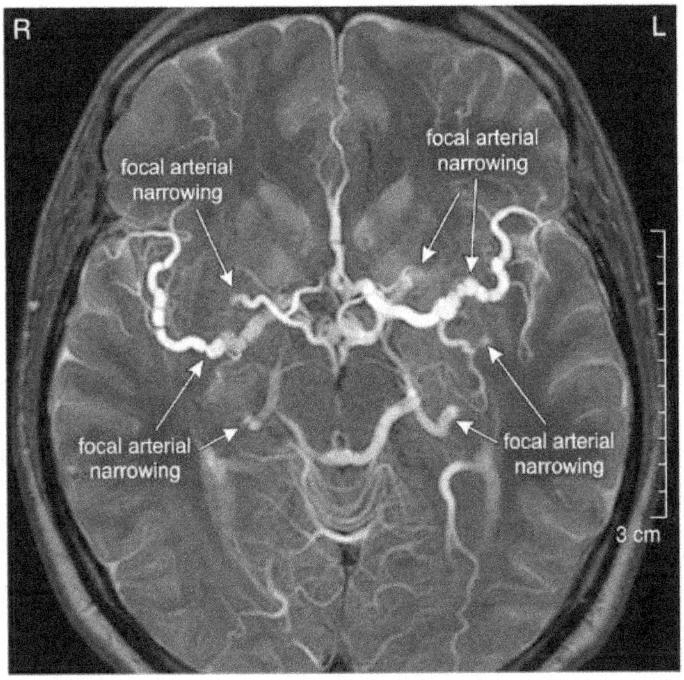

Case Presentation: MOG Antibody-Associated ADEM-Like Presentation

A five-year-old presents with encephalopathy, ataxia, and multifocal bilateral white matter and thalamic lesions on brain MRI following a recent upper respiratory illness, an initial clinical and imaging picture consistent with acute disseminated encephalomyelitis. Applying the reasoning developed in this chapter, MOG antibody testing is obtained as part of the initial evaluation given this specific ADEM-like presentation, and serum testing returns strongly positive, reclassifying the presentation as MOG antibody-associated disease rather than idiopathic acute disseminated encephalomyelitis. The family is counseled regarding the relapsing potential this specific antibody-defined diagnosis carries, distinct from the purely monophasic course idiopathic acute disseminated encephalomyelitis would imply, and structured clinical and antibody titer surveillance, applying the reasoning developed in this chapter, is established to monitor for the relapse risk this reclassified diagnosis specifically warrants. Follow-up MRI at six months demonstrates complete resolution of the original lesions without new lesion development, and MOG antibody titers, rechecked at this same interval, show a substantial decline, together supporting a favorable, lower-relapse-risk trajectory consistent with the titer-based prognostic framework this chapter has developed.

Case Presentation: Anti-NMDA Receptor Encephalitis With Normal Initial Imaging

A sixteen-year-old girl presents with two weeks of progressive behavioral change and new hallucinations, initially evaluated and treated as a primary psychiatric presentation, before developing orofacial dyskinesias and autonomic instability prompting neurology consultation. Applying the reasoning developed in this chapter, brain MRI is obtained and returns entirely normal, and, consistent with this section's discussion of frequently normal imaging in this specific diagnosis, the normal study does not deter further evaluation. Cerebrospinal fluid anti-NMDA receptor antibody testing returns positive, confirming the diagnosis, and pelvic ultrasound, applying the reasoning developed in this chapter, identifies a small ovarian teratoma, which is surgically removed alongside initiation of immunotherapy, illustrating thc complete, multi-step diagnostic and treatment pathway this chapter's autoimmune encephalitis framework has developed from an initially misleading psychiatric presentation through to a fully characterized, treatable underlying diagnosis. First-line immunotherapy combined with the teratoma removal produces substantial clinical improvement over the following six weeks, though residual short-term memory difficulty persists, prompting referral for the same structured neuropsychological support this chapter has emphasized for other conditions carrying a cognitive impact beyond their acute presenting symptoms.

THE CLINICAL-IMAGING CROSSWALK SYSTEM — Inflammatory and Autoimmune CNS Disease Recognition

Crossing 1 Recap: Intractable vomiting and hiccups without an identified gastrointestinal cause should prompt consideration of area postrema syndrome and dedicated dorsal medullary imaging, particularly in a child or adolescent.

Chapter Anchor: Inflammatory and autoimmune CNS disease diagnosis depends on integrating imaging pattern, clinical course, and serologic testing together rather than any single source in isolation; normal or nonspecific imaging, particularly in autoimmune encephalitis, is itself an expected, informative feature rather than evidence against the diagnosis, and correct serologic classification directly determines treatment selection and safety.

Summary and Key Concepts

ADEM is monophasic with encephalopathy and poorly demarcated, gray-matter-involving lesions; pediatric multiple sclerosis is relapsing with well-demarcated, perivenular (Dawson finger) lesions, and follow-up imaging at three to six months is often the definitive test distinguishing the two.

MOG antibody-associated disease shows longitudinally extensive optic nerve enhancement and can present as ADEM-like disease with relapsing potential; NMOSD, associated with aquaporin-4 antibodies, produces longitudinally extensive myelitis and area postrema syndrome, and correct serologic distinction from multiple sclerosis is essential since some MS therapies worsen NMOSD.

Anti-NMDA receptor encephalitis presents with a staged psychiatric-to-movement-to-autonomic clinical evolution and frequently normal or nonspecific imaging; cerebrospinal fluid antibody testing and pelvic imaging for ovarian teratoma are essential components of the diagnostic evaluation.

Primary CNS angiitis can be angiography-positive or angiography-negative (small-vessel), and a normal angiogram does not exclude the diagnosis; secondary vasculitis requires systematic screening for an underlying systemic autoimmune or infectious trigger.

Across this chapter, imaging is integrated tightly with clinical course, serologic testing, and treatment response rather than interpreted in isolation, and recognizing when normal imaging is itself an expected, diagnostically informative finding is a recurring, essential skill.

CHAPTER 17: METABOLIC AND NEURODEGENERATIVE DISEASE

Learning Objectives

1. Generate a white matter pattern-based differential diagnosis for suspected leukodystrophy and describe the imaging approach to its evaluation, including the role of imaging-directed genetic testing.
2. Recognize the imaging findings of the major mitochondrial and organic acid disorders, including MELAS and Leigh syndrome, and the role of magnetic resonance spectroscopy.
3. Distinguish the imaging patterns of the major pediatric neurodegenerative disorders based on regional atrophy and signal change, and distinguish progressive from static encephalopathy.
4. Recognize the characteristic imaging patterns of neonatal metabolic crisis and correlate them with the underlying metabolic category, prioritizing treatable causes in the acute evaluation.

Leukodystrophies and White Matter Disorders

Leukodystrophies, a heterogeneous group of genetic disorders primarily affecting white matter, present a diagnostic challenge given their individual rarity but collective frequency, and this section develops a systematic, pattern-based approach to generating a focused differential diagnosis from the specific distribution of white matter involvement rather than relying on rote memorization of each individual entity. Though collectively rare, this category as a whole is encountered with meaningful frequency across a career in pediatric neuroimaging, and the pattern-based reasoning skill this section develops, rather than an exhaustive named-entity catalog, is intended to remain durable and applicable even as new leukodystrophy entities continue to be characterized and added to the medical literature over time.

The Pattern-Recognition Approach to Leukodystrophy

Rather than approaching a suspected leukodystrophy by attempting to recall each named entity individually, a more reliable and durable diagnostic strategy involves systematically characterizing the specific pattern of white matter involvement, anterior-predominant versus posterior-predominant, symmetric versus asymmetric, confluent versus multifocal, and the presence or absence of contrast enhancement, cystic change, or calcification, and using this structured pattern description to generate a focused, narrowed differential diagnosis; this pattern-based approach, applied consistently across the specific entities this section addresses, exemplifies the same durable, transferable diagnostic reasoning this book has emphasized throughout, equipping the reader to reason through an unfamiliar or atypical leukodystrophy presentation using the same underlying logic rather than requiring exhaustive memorization of an ever-expanding list of named entities. Age of onset provides a further, complementary axis for narrowing this differential, since several leukodystrophies show a characteristic, though not absolute, association with either an infantile, childhood, or adolescent-to-adult onset pattern, and incorporating this age-based framework alongside the distributional pattern this section emphasizes further sharpens the resulting differential diagnosis before any genetic or biochemical testing is pursued.

X-Linked Adrenoleukodystrophy: The Posterior-Predominant Pattern

X-linked adrenoleukodystrophy, among the more common leukodystrophies and notable for its association with adrenal insufficiency, classically produces a posterior-predominant pattern of white matter involvement, beginning in the splenium of the corpus callosum and parieto-occipital white matter with a characteristic, though not universal, pattern of active, contrast-enhancing margins at the leading edge of disease progression, reflecting active inflammatory demyelination at this advancing border; this specific posterior-predominant, actively enhancing pattern, combined with the characteristic adrenal insufficiency this diagnosis carries, distinguishes it from several of the other leukodystrophies this section addresses and directs urgent evaluation given the availability of disease-modifying treatment, most effectively applied at the earliest, presymptomatic or minimally symptomatic disease stage. A structured severity scoring system, quantifying the extent of white matter involvement and the presence of contrast enhancement on a standardized numeric scale, is frequently applied to X-linked adrenoleukodystrophy surveillance imaging specifically to provide an objective, reproducible measure of disease extent and progression rate, supporting both individual treatment timing decisions and the broader outcomes research this severity scoring framework has enabled across affected populations.

Metachromatic Leukodystrophy and Krabbe Disease: Diffuse Symmetric Patterns

Metachromatic leukodystrophy, arising from arylsulfatase A deficiency, and Krabbe disease, arising from galactocerebrosidase deficiency, both produce a more diffuse, symmetric pattern of white matter involvement without the specific posterior predominance characteristic of X-linked adrenoleukodystrophy, and distinguishing between these two entities depends substantially on the specific clinical presentation, age of onset, and enzymatic or genetic confirmatory testing, since their imaging appearances share substantial overlap; a tigroid or leopard-skin pattern of alternating normal and abnormal white matter signal, while classically described for metachromatic leukodystrophy, is neither universally present nor entirely specific to this single entity, underscoring why imaging pattern recognition, while valuable for narrowing the differential, ultimately requires biochemical or genetic confirmation rather than serving as a standalone diagnostic endpoint. Krabbe disease in its infantile, most common presentation additionally shows characteristic thickening and enhancement of cranial nerves, particularly the optic and trigeminal nerves, reflecting direct infiltration of these structures by the abnormal storage material this disorder produces, a specific, complementary finding worth actively searching for when this diagnosis is suspected and one not shared by metachromatic leukodystrophy, providing a further discriminating feature between these two otherwise substantially overlapping entities.

Vanishing White Matter Disease

Vanishing white matter disease, a leukodystrophy characterized by progressive white matter rarefaction and cystic degeneration, produces a distinctive imaging appearance in which affected white matter progressively approaches and, in advanced disease, matches cerebrospinal fluid signal intensity on all sequences, reflecting near-complete tissue loss and replacement by fluid, and this specific radiographic signature, together with a characteristic clinical course of stepwise neurologic deterioration frequently triggered by febrile illness or minor head trauma, supports this diagnosis; recognizing this specific trigger-associated deterioration pattern, and counseling families to seek prompt medical attention for febrile illness given its potential to precipitate acute neurologic decline in this specific condition, is a practical, actionable component of comprehensive family education for this diagnosis. Radiating stripes of relatively preserved tissue traversing the otherwise rarefied, cystic white matter are a further, specific imaging feature described in this condition, best appreciated on FLAIR imaging, and this specific internal architectural pattern, while not required for diagnosis given the sufficiently characteristic overall appearance this section has already described, provides further supportive evidence when present alongside the primary, cerebrospinal-fluid-matching signal change this paragraph has emphasized.

Alexander Disease

Alexander disease, arising from mutation in the GFAP gene affecting astrocyte structural integrity, classically produces frontal-predominant white matter involvement, in contrast to the posterior-predominant pattern of X-linked adrenoleukodystrophy, together with a characteristic periventricular rim of abnormal signal and, at times, associated basal ganglia and brainstem involvement; recognizing this specific frontal-predominant distribution, essentially the anatomic inverse of the X-linked adrenoleukodystrophy pattern discussed earlier in this section, exemplifies how the same anterior-versus-posterior distributional framework this section has developed can be applied bidirectionally to narrow the differential toward one specific entity or its near-opposite distributional counterpart. Contrast enhancement in Alexander disease, when present, characteristically involves specific periventricular, ventricular, and certain deep gray matter structures in a pattern distinct from the leading-edge enhancement pattern of X-linked adrenoleukodystrophy discussed above, and this distinct enhancement distribution, considered alongside the frontal-predominant signal abnormality already discussed, provides a further complementary feature supporting this specific diagnosis when the overall clinical and imaging picture remains genuinely ambiguous between these two entities.

The Diagnostic Role of Genetic and Enzymatic Testing

While the pattern-based imaging approach this section has developed substantially narrows the leukodystrophy differential, definitive diagnosis for essentially every entity this section addresses ultimately depends on targeted genetic testing or, for several entities, enzymatic assay, and a structured, imaging-pattern-directed testing strategy, ordering the specific genetic or enzymatic test most consistent with the imaging pattern identified rather than a broad, undirected leukodystrophy gene panel, provides the most efficient path to diagnostic confirmation; this imaging-directed testing strategy exemplifies the same phenotype-directed testing principle developed in Chapter 7 for cortical malformations, applied here to the distinct diagnostic category of white matter disease.

Hematopoietic Stem Cell Transplantation for X-Linked Adrenoleukodystrophy

For X-linked adrenoleukodystrophy specifically, hematopoietic stem cell transplantation, when performed at an early, minimally symptomatic disease stage, can meaningfully halt or slow the progression of cerebral disease, making the specific imaging surveillance schedule this section has emphasized for presymptomatic, screening-identified boys a matter of direct, time-sensitive treatment eligibility rather than a purely observational monitoring exercise; a child identified with early, active cerebral disease on this surveillance imaging is referred promptly for transplant evaluation, since this treatment's effectiveness declines substantially once disease has progressed beyond this earliest, most treatable stage, reinforcing why the structured surveillance interval this section has developed carries genuine, time-critical clinical weight. Gene therapy approaches, an emerging alternative to traditional allogeneic hematopoietic stem cell transplantation that avoids the need for a matched donor, are increasingly available at specialized centers and offer a further, evolving treatment option for this specific, time-critical presymptomatic disease stage, extending the treatment landscape this section has described beyond transplantation alone.

Distinguishing True Leukodystrophy From Acquired White Matter Injury

Before pursuing the extensive genetic and biochemical evaluation this section has developed, actively excluding acquired causes of white matter signal abnormality, including the demyelinating and inflammatory conditions discussed in Chapter 16, the congenital infections discussed in Chapter 15, and the hypoxic-ischemic injury patterns discussed in Chapters 4 and 5, is an essential preliminary step, since these acquired entities can produce white matter signal changes that superficially resemble a genetic leukodystrophy without sharing its progressive, genetically determined course; correlating the specific clinical history, including gestational and birth history, infectious exposure, and the pace of symptom progression, against the imaging pattern identified helps distinguish a true, progressive genetic leukodystrophy from one of these acquired, non-progressive or differently-progressive mimics. Serial imaging demonstrating genuine, ongoing progression over a defined observation interval, applying the same progressive-versus-static distinction this chapter develops fully in its neurodegenerative disorders section, provides further, complementary support for a true, progressive leukodystrophy once these acquired mimics have been reasonably excluded through the clinical and historical correlation this paragraph has emphasized.

Figure 17.1: Anterior Versus Posterior Predominant Leukodystrophy Patterns

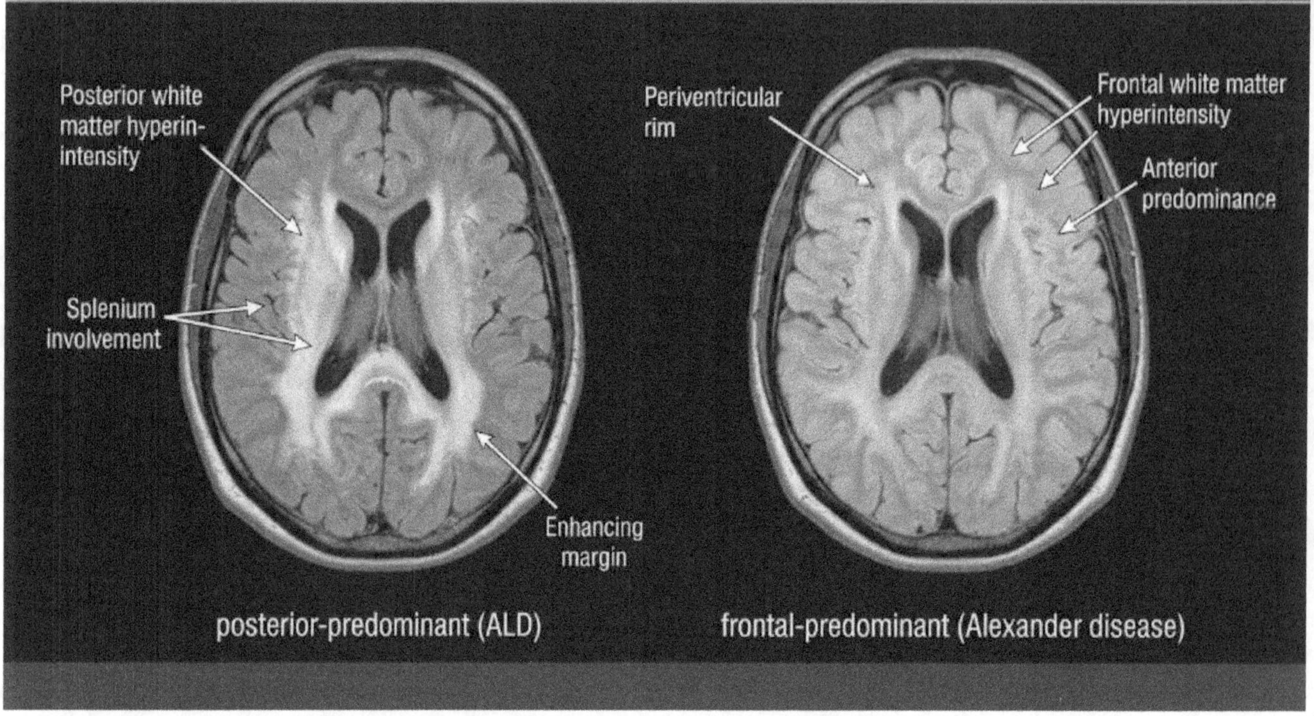

Entity	Distribution	Distinguishing Feature
X-linked adrenoleukodystrophy	Posterior-predominant, splenium	Enhancing leading edge, adrenal insufficiency
Metachromatic leukodystrophy	Diffuse, symmetric	Tigroid pattern (variable)
Vanishing white matter disease	Diffuse, progressive	CSF-signal-matching cystic degeneration
Alexander disease	Frontal-predominant	Periventricular rim, GFAP mutation

Mitochondrial and Organic Acid Disorders

Mitochondrial disorders and the related organic acidemias produce a distinct, energy-failure-driven pattern of brain injury that this section develops, with particular attention to Leigh syndrome and MELAS, the two most clinically and radiographically distinctive entities within this broader, biochemically heterogeneous category. The specific, symmetric, high-metabolic-demand-region pattern this section develops for these entities stands in useful contrast to the more distributionally variable, white-matter-predominant leukodystrophy patterns discussed in the preceding section, offering the reader a further, complementary anatomic reasoning framework, gray matter and brainstem energy-failure vulnerability rather than white matter tract-based distribution, to apply when generating a differential diagnosis for a child with suspected metabolic brain disease.

Leigh Syndrome: The Basal Ganglia and Brainstem Pattern

Leigh syndrome, a genetically heterogeneous mitochondrial disorder that can arise from mutation in either nuclear or mitochondrial DNA affecting oxidative phosphorylation, classically produces bilateral, symmetric T2/FLAIR signal abnormality within the basal ganglia, most characteristically the putamina, and brainstem, particularly the periaqueductal gray matter and dorsal brainstem, reflecting the high metabolic demand and correspondingly high vulnerability of these specific structures to the energy failure this disorder produces; recognizing this specific, symmetric basal ganglia and brainstem distribution, particularly in a young child with a compatible clinical presentation of developmental regression, hypotonia, and feeding difficulty, strongly supports this diagnosis and directs the specific metabolic and genetic testing this diagnosis requires. Lesion evolution in Leigh syndrome typically follows a relapsing-progressive course, with acute, often illness-triggered episodes of new or worsening signal abnormality superimposed on a background of gradually accumulating, permanent tissue injury, and serial imaging documenting this specific evolutionary pattern, applying the same structured, serial-comparison surveillance principle this book has emphasized throughout, provides both diagnostic support and a practical, objective measure of disease progression over a child's clinical course.

MELAS: Stroke-Like Episodes and Cortical Involvement

MELAS, an acronym denoting mitochondrial encephalomyopathy, lactic acidosis, and stroke-like episodes, produces a distinctive pattern of cortical and subcortical signal abnormality that characteristically does not conform to a single, discrete vascular territory, distinguishing these stroke-like episodes from the true arterial ischemic stroke discussed in Chapter 18, and this specific, non-vascular-territory-conforming pattern, together with elevated serum and cerebrospinal fluid lactate, supports this diagnosis in a child presenting with an acute, stroke-like clinical deficit; the posterior, occipital-predominant tendency of these lesions in MELAS specifically, together with their tendency to cross traditional vascular territorial boundaries, provides a further, specific imaging clue distinguishing this metabolic stroke-mimic from a true, vascular-territory-conforming arterial ischemic event. Serial imaging in MELAS frequently demonstrates migration or evolution of the stroke-like lesion pattern over time, with new lesions appearing in different locations on subsequent studies even as earlier lesions partially resolve, a dynamic, migratory pattern distinctly different from the fixed, permanent territorial infarct pattern characteristic of a true arterial ischemic event, further reinforcing the underlying metabolic, rather than purely vascular-occlusive, mechanism this specific stroke-like phenomenon reflects.

Magnetic Resonance Spectroscopy in Mitochondrial Disease

Magnetic resonance spectroscopy, introduced in Chapter 1 and applied throughout this book primarily in the oncologic context, offers a further, complementary diagnostic tool specifically valuable in suspected mitochondrial disease, since an elevated lactate peak, reflecting the impaired oxidative metabolism and resulting anaerobic glycolysis characteristic of these disorders, can be identified within affected brain regions even when conventional structural imaging findings remain ambiguous; this specific spectroscopic application exemplifies how a single advanced imaging technique introduced early in this book can be applied across dramatically different diagnostic contexts, oncologic tumor grading in Chapter 12 and metabolic disease characterization here, reinforcing the value of understanding a technique's underlying physical and biochemical principle rather than memorizing its application to a single, narrow clinical context alone. A lactate doublet identified even in apparently normal-appearing brain parenchyma, away from any region of overt structural signal abnormality, can be a subtle but genuinely informative early clue to an underlying mitochondrial disorder, worth actively searching for on spectroscopic sequences whenever this diagnostic category is under consideration, rather than restricting spectroscopic sampling only to the most visually abnormal-appearing regions on conventional imaging.

Organic Acidemias and Their Basal Ganglia Vulnerability

Several organic acidemias, including glutaric aciduria type 1, methylmalonic acidemia, and propionic acidemia, share a specific vulnerability of the basal ganglia, particularly the globus pallidus and, for glutaric aciduria type 1 specifically, the caudate and putamen, to acute metabolic decompensation, often precipitated by an intercurrent illness or catabolic stress; glutaric aciduria type 1 in particular produces a characteristic combination of bilateral basal ganglia injury following an acute encephalopathic crisis together with widened sylvian fissures and frontotemporal atrophy that may be apparent even before the first acute metabolic crisis occurs, making this specific, premorbid imaging pattern a potential clue to the underlying diagnosis that predates the first overt clinical decompensation. Subdural hemorrhage and, at times, retinal hemorrhage can occur in glutaric aciduria type 1 given this condition's associated vascular fragility, a finding that has, in the past, led to diagnostic confusion with abusive head trauma discussed in Chapter 19, underscoring why recognizing the specific, characteristic frontotemporal atrophy and widened sylvian fissure pattern this section has described is essential to correctly distinguishing this specific metabolic condition from a traumatic etiology when subdural hemorrhage is identified in an infant.

Newborn Screening and Presymptomatic Detection

Expanded newborn screening programs, incorporating tandem mass spectrometry capable of detecting a broad range of organic acid and other metabolic disorders, have transformed the clinical presentation of several conditions addressed in this section from an acute, often devastating metabolic crisis to a presymptomatic diagnosis allowing dietary and medical intervention before the first crisis occurs, and a child with a positive newborn screen result for one of these specific conditions warrants proactive baseline imaging and structured, anticipatory metabolic management rather than a wait-and-see approach pending the first clinical symptom, applying the same proactive, screening-driven surveillance principle this book has emphasized throughout for other conditions increasingly identified through structured screening programs. A positive newborn screen result, importantly, represents a screening flag rather than a definitive diagnosis, and prompt confirmatory biochemical and genetic testing, together with baseline clinical assessment, is required before a family is counseled regarding a confirmed diagnosis, since a meaningful proportion of positive newborn screen results, depending on the specific analyte and condition involved, ultimately prove to be false positives on confirmatory evaluation.

Acute Imaging During Metabolic Decompensation

A child with a known mitochondrial or organic acid disorder presenting with acute clinical decompensation, altered mental status, new movement abnormality, or a new focal deficit, warrants prompt imaging specifically to characterize the acute pattern and extent of metabolic injury, applying the diffusion-weighted and spectroscopic techniques this section has emphasized throughout, since this acute characterization directly informs both immediate metabolic management, including specific dietary and cofactor interventions tailored to the underlying biochemical defect, and longer-term prognostic counseling regarding the cumulative impact this specific decompensation episode is likely to carry.

Multisystem Involvement in Mitochondrial Disease

Mitochondrial disorders, given the near-universal cellular distribution of mitochondria and their essential role in energy production across every organ system, frequently produce multisystem manifestations extending well beyond the central nervous system findings this section has primarily emphasized, including cardiomyopathy, hearing loss, and gastrointestinal dysmotility, and comprehensive, coordinated multidisciplinary evaluation addressing each of these potentially affected systems, rather than a neurology-focused evaluation alone, reflects the genuinely multisystem nature of this diagnostic category, consistent with the coordinated, multisystem surveillance principle this book has applied to several other genetically defined conditions throughout its preceding chapters. Baseline cardiac and audiologic evaluation at the time of diagnosis, followed by structured periodic reassessment, allows early identification of these specific, treatable systemic manifestations before they progress to a more advanced, symptomatic stage, applying the same anticipatory, rather than purely reactive, surveillance philosophy this chapter has emphasized throughout its several constituent sections.

Muscle Biopsy and Additional Diagnostic Testing

Beyond the imaging and spectroscopic characterization this section has emphasized, definitive diagnosis of a suspected mitochondrial disorder frequently requires muscle biopsy for histochemical and biochemical analysis of mitochondrial respiratory chain function, alongside targeted or broad genetic testing given the substantial genetic heterogeneity, both nuclear and mitochondrial DNA-encoded, underlying this diagnostic category; this multimodal diagnostic approach, integrating imaging, spectroscopy, histopathology, and genetic testing together, exemplifies the same converging-evidence diagnostic philosophy this book has applied consistently throughout, particularly relevant given that no single test, imaging included, reliably establishes a mitochondrial disease diagnosis in isolation. Mitochondrial DNA testing specifically requires attention to the phenomenon of heteroplasmy, in which a variable proportion of an individual's mitochondrial DNA copies carry a given pathogenic variant, and this variable proportion, which can differ meaningfully between tissue types and even between affected family members carrying the same underlying variant, helps explain the substantial clinical variability this diagnostic category is well known to produce even among individuals sharing an identical genetic mutation.

Figure 17.2: Leigh Syndrome Basal Ganglia and Brainstem Involvement

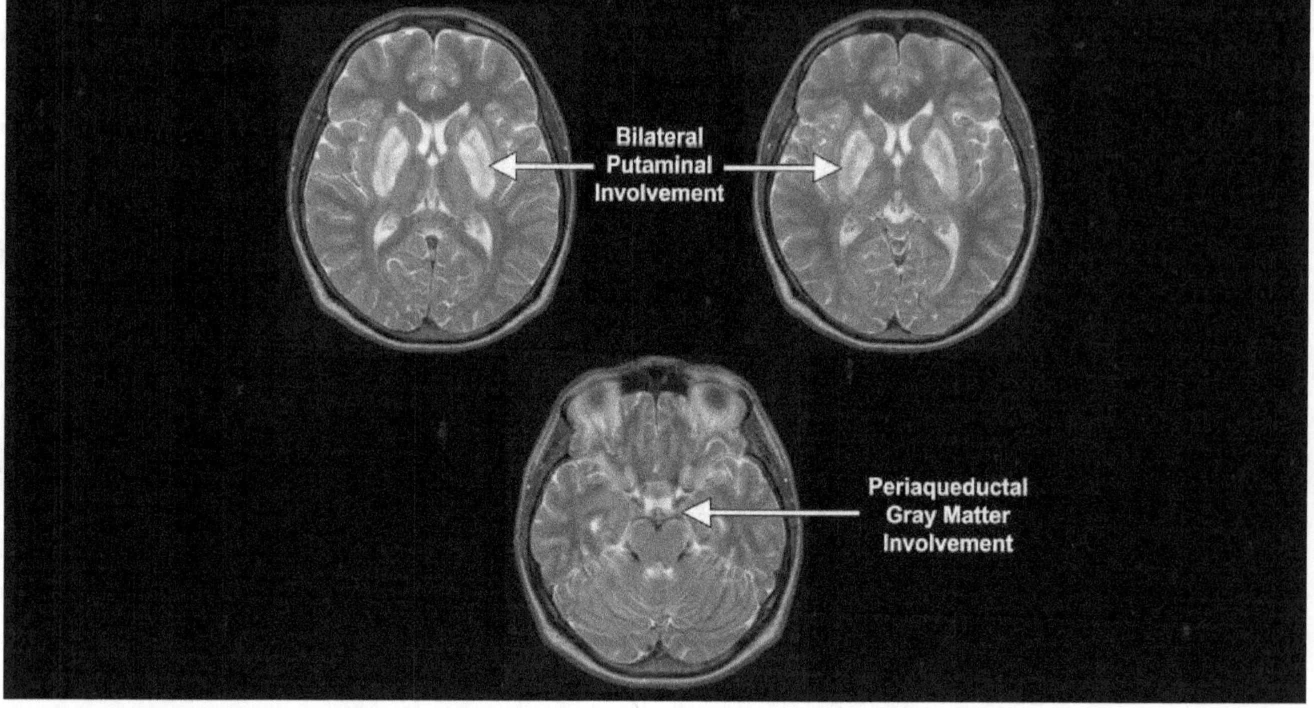

THE CLINICAL-IMAGING CROSSWALK SYSTEM — A Stroke-Like Lesion Not Respecting Vascular Territory

The Crossing: A fourteen-year-old presents with acute-onset visual disturbance and confusion, and brain MRI shows cortical and subcortical signal abnormality in the occipital and posterior temporal region that does not conform to the posterior cerebral artery territory.

Presentation Signature: An adolescent with an acute, stroke-like clinical deficit and an imaging lesion pattern that crosses or does not respect standard arterial vascular territorial boundaries.

Imaging Correlate: Serum and cerebrospinal fluid lactate are obtained given this atypical, non-vascular-territory-conforming pattern, both returning elevated, and magnetic resonance spectroscopy confirms an elevated lactate peak within the affected region, supporting a diagnosis of MELAS rather than a true arterial ischemic stroke.

Trap Logic: Pursuing an exclusively vascular stroke evaluation and treatment pathway, including consideration of thrombolysis, for a lesion pattern that does not conform to a vascular territory risks both an inappropriate, potentially harmful treatment for a non-thrombotic process and a missed opportunity to identify and appropriately manage the underlying mitochondrial disorder.

Crossing Anchor: A stroke-like lesion not conforming to a standard vascular territory should prompt lactate testing and consideration of MELAS rather than an exclusively vascular stroke evaluation pathway.

Neurodegenerative Disorders of Childhood

This section addresses the pediatric neurodegenerative disorders producing progressive, region-specific atrophy and signal change, developing the specific imaging patterns that distinguish the major entities within this heterogeneous, genetically diverse category of progressive childhood neurologic decline. Where the preceding sections of this chapter addressed white matter and gray-matter-and-brainstem energy-failure patterns respectively, this section shifts attention specifically to progressive volume loss and storage-related signal change as the primary imaging manifestations of the entities it addresses, a further, complementary pattern-recognition axis completing this chapter's overall framework for metabolic and neurodegenerative disease.

Neuronal Ceroid Lipofuscinosis

Neuronal ceroid lipofuscinosis, a group of lysosomal storage disorders producing progressive neurodegeneration with a characteristic combination of visual loss, seizures, and cognitive and motor decline, produces progressive, diffuse cerebral and cerebellar atrophy on imaging together with characteristic T2 hypointensity of the thalami, reflecting abnormal storage material accumulation within this specific structure; the specific age of onset and rate of progression vary across the several distinct genetic subtypes within this broader category, and correlating the specific clinical trajectory against the family's reported symptom onset and progression rate assists in narrowing the specific subtype even before genetic confirmation is available. Cerebellar atrophy in particular is frequently disproportionately severe relative to the degree of cerebral atrophy present in the earlier stages of several neuronal ceroid lipofuscinosis subtypes, a specific, quantifiable regional discrepancy worth actively assessing rather than simply characterizing the overall degree of atrophy as a single, undifferentiated global finding.

Rett Syndrome

Rett syndrome, predominantly affecting females and most commonly caused by mutation in the MECP2 gene, presents with a characteristic developmental regression occurring after a period of apparently normal early development, together with the distinctive clinical finding of stereotyped hand-wringing movements, and brain imaging, while frequently normal or showing only nonspecific, mild diffuse atrophy, serves primarily an exclusionary role in this diagnosis similar to the exclusionary imaging role this book has developed for several other primarily clinical and genetic diagnoses; recognizing that a normal or near-normal brain MRI does not exclude Rett syndrome in a child with the compatible, characteristic clinical presentation and developmental trajectory this section has described prevents inappropriate diagnostic delay pending a positive imaging finding that this specific diagnosis does not reliably produce. When mild atrophy is present in Rett syndrome, it tends to be diffuse and relatively nonspecific rather than the region-specific patterns this section has emphasized for the other neurodegenerative entities it addresses, further reinforcing the primarily clinical and genetic, rather than imaging-based, diagnostic pathway appropriate for this specific condition.

Pantothenate Kinase-Associated Neurodegeneration and Brain Iron Accumulation

Pantothenate kinase-associated neurodegeneration, the most common entity within the broader category of neurodegeneration with brain iron accumulation, produces a highly characteristic imaging finding termed the eye-of-the-tiger sign, central T2 hyperintensity within the globus pallidus surrounded by a rim of T2 hypointensity reflecting pathologic iron accumulation, a finding sufficiently distinctive that its recognition alone strongly supports this specific diagnosis; this sign is best appreciated on T2-weighted or susceptibility-sensitive sequences, and its presence in a child with a compatible clinical presentation of progressive dystonia, dysarthria, and cognitive decline should prompt targeted genetic testing for the PANK2 gene most commonly responsible for this specific condition. The eye-of-the-tiger sign, while highly characteristic, evolves over the disease course, with the central hyperintense component reflecting an early stage of tissue change that may become less conspicuous as iron accumulation progresses and increasingly dominates the imaging appearance in more advanced disease, meaning the absence of a fully developed, classic eye-of-the-tiger appearance at a single time point does not definitively exclude this diagnosis in a child at an earlier or later point along this specific disease's imaging evolution.

Distinguishing Progressive Neurodegeneration From a Static Encephalopathy

A critical, foundational distinction this section's entities require is separating a genuinely progressive neurodegenerative process, in which serial imaging demonstrates ongoing, worsening atrophy or signal change over time, from a static encephalopathy, discussed in relation to the hypoxic-ischemic and other acquired injury patterns addressed in Chapters 4 through 6, in which the underlying brain injury, while producing a fixed neurologic deficit, does not itself continue to progress; obtaining and carefully comparing serial imaging over a defined observation period, applying the same structured, quantitative serial-comparison principle this book has emphasized throughout, is frequently the most reliable way to make this distinction when the clinical trajectory alone leaves genuine diagnostic ambiguity between these two fundamentally different injury categories. A child whose developmental trajectory shows a plateau or slow, steady gain in skills, even if delayed relative to typical milestones, is more consistent with a static encephalopathy, while a child showing genuine loss of previously acquired skills over time is more consistent with a truly progressive process, and eliciting this specific developmental trajectory detail through careful history-taking is a necessary complement to the serial imaging comparison this paragraph has emphasized as the primary objective discriminator between these two categories.

Genetic Testing Strategy for Suspected Neurodegeneration

Given the extensive genetic heterogeneity underlying pediatric neurodegenerative disease, broad, next-generation sequencing-based testing approaches, including whole exome or genome sequencing, are increasingly favored over sequential, single-gene testing once a specific, highly characteristic imaging pattern such as the eye-of-the-tiger sign has not narrowed the differential sufficiently to direct targeted single-gene testing; this broader sequencing approach, applied when a specific imaging-directed testing strategy is not available or has not yielded a diagnosis, reflects the evolving genetic testing landscape this book has noted throughout, in which comprehensive sequencing increasingly complements, and at times supersedes, sequential single-gene testing for genetically heterogeneous conditions.

Palliative and Supportive Care Considerations

For the subset of pediatric neurodegenerative disorders carrying a progressive, ultimately life-limiting course, coordinated palliative care involvement, introduced proactively rather than only in a disease's final stages, supports the family through a diagnostic and disease trajectory that this chapter's imaging and genetic testing framework can characterize but not, for many of these entities, meaningfully alter; this proactive palliative care integration, applying the same honest, proportionate communication principle this book has emphasized throughout, allows a family to make informed decisions regarding the specific goals of care and quality-of-life priorities appropriate to their own values and their child's specific disease trajectory.

Family Genetic Counseling and Reproductive Planning

Once a specific genetic cause underlying a pediatric neurodegenerative disorder is confirmed, comprehensive family genetic counseling addressing inheritance pattern, recurrence risk for future pregnancies, and, where available, prenatal or preimplantation testing options, is an essential component of comprehensive care extending beyond the affected child alone; this genetic counseling conversation, ideally conducted by a genetics professional working in close coordination with the neurology team that established the underlying diagnosis, exemplifies the same multidisciplinary, family-centered care model this book has emphasized throughout for other genetically defined pediatric neurologic conditions.

Figure 17.3: Eye-of-the-Tiger Sign in Pantothenate Kinase-Associated Neurodegeneration

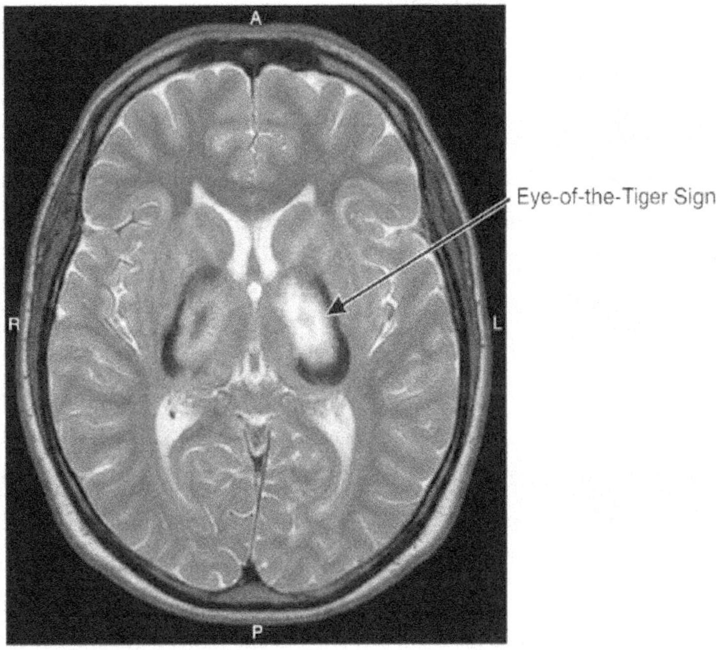

Neonatal Metabolic Crisis Imaging Patterns

This closing section addresses the specific imaging patterns accompanying acute neonatal metabolic crisis, a presentation requiring rapid, structured diagnostic reasoning given the time-sensitive nature of many treatable underlying metabolic conditions, extending this chapter's broader metabolic framework into the specific, urgent neonatal context. Unlike the three preceding sections, which primarily addressed chronic, progressive imaging patterns evaluated in a relatively less time-pressured setting, this closing section returns to the acute, emergency-department and neonatal-intensive-care-unit context this book has emphasized throughout for other time-critical presentations, requiring the reader to apply this chapter's metabolic imaging framework under genuine time pressure rather than in the more measured, longitudinal surveillance context the preceding sections have primarily emphasized.

The Clinical Presentation of Neonatal Metabolic Crisis

Neonatal metabolic crisis, presenting with a nonspecific but concerning constellation of poor feeding, lethargy, vomiting, and, in more severe cases, seizures or altered consciousness, requires urgent, parallel evaluation for both the acquired, structural causes addressed throughout the earlier chapters of this book, including hypoxic-ischemic injury discussed in Chapter 4 and infection discussed in Chapter 15, and the specific inborn errors of metabolism this section addresses, since these categories share substantial clinical overlap at initial presentation and their evaluation and management pathways diverge substantially once a specific cause is identified. A characteristic clinical clue supporting a metabolic, rather than acquired, etiology is a symptom-free interval following delivery, since many inborn errors of metabolism produce a period of apparent normalcy while maternal metabolic clearance mechanisms remain active before symptom onset once the newborn's own, deficient metabolic pathways become the primary route of clearance, a specific temporal pattern distinctly different from the immediate, at-birth presentation more typical of significant acute hypoxic-ischemic injury.

Urea Cycle Disorders and Hyperammonemia

Urea cycle disorders, producing acute hyperammonemia from impaired ammonia clearance, characteristically produce diffuse cerebral edema and, in the specific pattern most associated with severe hyperammonemia, relative sparing of the perirolandic cortex with more severe involvement of the remaining cortical mantle, a distinctive regional pattern worth recognizing since it distinguishes this specific metabolic crisis from the more diffuse, non-selective edema pattern characteristic of hypoxic-ischemic injury discussed in Chapter 4; recognizing this pattern, combined with the specific clinical and laboratory correlation of markedly elevated serum ammonia, directs urgent, specific treatment, including dialysis for severe hyperammonemia, that differs substantially from the supportive care approach appropriate for hypoxic-ischemic injury. The specific mechanism underlying this perirolandic sparing pattern remains incompletely understood, though it is hypothesized to relate to regional differences in glutamine synthetase activity and resulting astrocytic vulnerability to ammonia-induced cellular swelling across different cortical regions, a mechanistic detail worth noting for the reader seeking to understand why this specific, regionally selective pattern occurs rather than a uniform, non-selective pattern of injury.

Maple Syrup Urine Disease

Maple syrup urine disease, arising from impaired branched-chain amino acid metabolism, produces a characteristic pattern of diffusion restriction within the brainstem, cerebellar white matter, and posterior limb of the internal capsule, reflecting the specific regional vulnerability of these myelinated structures to the toxic accumulation of branched-chain amino acids and their metabolites this disorder produces; this specific, myelin-tract-predominant diffusion restriction pattern, together with the characteristic maple syrup odor this condition's name reflects, supports rapid clinical and laboratory confirmation and urgent initiation of dietary and, in severe cases, dialysis-based treatment given this disorder's rapid, potentially devastating progression if treatment is delayed. This myelinated-tract-selective vulnerability pattern reflects the specific biochemical mechanism underlying this disorder's tissue injury, in which the accumulated branched-chain amino acids and their toxic metabolites preferentially disrupt myelin lipid synthesis and structural integrity, explaining why actively myelinating or already myelinated white matter tracts bear the brunt of this specific metabolic insult rather than the gray matter structures more characteristically affected by several of the other metabolic crisis patterns this chapter addresses.

Nonketotic Hyperglycinemia

Nonketotic hyperglycinemia, arising from impaired glycine cleavage system function, produces a distinctive imaging pattern of diffusion restriction within the corpus callosum, particularly the genu and splenium, along with the dorsal brainstem, in a newborn presenting with severe encephalopathy, myoclonic seizures, and a burst-suppression pattern on electroencephalography; the corpus callosum involvement pattern this condition produces is worth distinguishing from the broader corpus callosum anomaly differential discussed in Chapter 8, since this specific signal abnormality reflects acute, toxic metabolic injury to an anatomically normal, previously fully formed structure rather than a primary developmental malformation of the callosum itself. Cerebrospinal fluid-to-plasma glycine ratio, rather than plasma glycine level alone, provides the definitive biochemical confirmation for this diagnosis, since plasma glycine elevation alone can occur in several other, unrelated metabolic contexts, and this specific ratio-based testing approach, correlated against the characteristic imaging pattern and burst-suppression electroencephalographic finding this paragraph has described, together establish this diagnosis with the same converging, multimodal evidence approach this chapter has applied consistently throughout its several constituent metabolic entities.

Prioritizing Treatable Causes in the Acute Evaluation

Given that several of the metabolic conditions this section addresses are directly treatable, dietary restriction, specific cofactor supplementation, or dialysis, when identified promptly, structuring the acute neonatal metabolic crisis evaluation to prioritize rapid identification of these specific, treatable entities, rather than proceeding through an unstructured, sequential differential diagnosis, reflects the same urgency-calibrated diagnostic approach this book has emphasized throughout for other acute, time-sensitive pediatric neurologic presentations; a structured, parallel evaluation incorporating immediate laboratory testing, ammonia, lactate, and amino acid and organic acid profiling, alongside the imaging characterization this section has developed, provides the most efficient path to identifying a treatable cause within the narrow therapeutic window several of these conditions require. Empiric treatment directed at the most likely or most immediately dangerous metabolic category, protein restriction and glucose infusion while awaiting definitive biochemical results, for example, is frequently initiated even before a specific diagnosis is confirmed, reflecting the same treat-first, confirm-second philosophy this book has emphasized for other time-critical pediatric neurologic emergencies, including the herpes simplex encephalitis management discussed in Chapter 15.

Long-Term Outcome Following Neonatal Metabolic Crisis

Even with prompt identification and appropriate acute treatment, a neonate surviving a severe metabolic crisis frequently carries a meaningful risk of long-term neurodevelopmental impairment reflecting the acute injury this crisis produced, and structured, longitudinal developmental surveillance, applying the same proactive, structured surveillance principle this book has emphasized throughout, is a standard, essential component of long-term care for this population, extending well beyond the acute metabolic stabilization this section has primarily addressed into the child's subsequent years of neurodevelopmental monitoring and support.

Coordinating Rapid Metabolic and Imaging Evaluation

Given the genuine time sensitivity several metabolic diagnoses this section addresses carry, institutional protocols ensuring rapid, parallel coordination between the laboratory metabolic evaluation and the imaging characterization this section has developed, rather than a sequential, one-after-the-other evaluation pathway, meaningfully shortens the time to diagnosis and treatment initiation for a critically ill neonate; a dedicated, rapid-response metabolic crisis protocol, specifying the specific laboratory tests, imaging sequences, and consultation pathways to be activated immediately upon clinical suspicion, reflects the same systems-level, protocol-driven urgency this book has emphasized for other acute, time-sensitive pediatric neurologic presentations addressed throughout its preceding chapters.

Family Support During the Acute Diagnostic Period

The acute, often rapidly evolving diagnostic period this section has described, in which a family confronts a critically ill newborn and a broad, initially undifferentiated differential diagnosis spanning both acquired and metabolic categories, represents one of the most acutely stressful clinical scenarios addressed throughout this book, and clear, honest, incremental communication regarding the evolving diagnostic picture, applying the honest, proportionate communication framework this book has emphasized throughout, supports the family through this acute uncertainty even before a specific, definitive diagnosis has been established.

Case Presentation: Presymptomatic X-Linked Adrenoleukodystrophy Identified Through Newborn Screening

A newborn boy's expanded newborn screen returns positive for X-linked adrenoleukodystrophy, and confirmatory genetic testing confirms the diagnosis in an otherwise clinically asymptomatic infant. Applying the reasoning developed in this chapter, baseline brain MRI is obtained and demonstrates a normal-appearing brain without the posterior-predominant white matter signal abnormality this chapter has described as characteristic of established disease, and coordinated endocrinology evaluation identifies early, subclinical adrenal insufficiency confirmed on laboratory testing. The family is counseled regarding the structured surveillance MRI schedule this presymptomatic diagnosis requires, typically every six months through early childhood, specifically to identify the earliest evidence of the posterior white matter involvement this chapter has described, since early identification of this transition from presymptomatic to active cerebral disease directly determines candidacy for disease-modifying treatment at the stage when it is most effective. Adrenal hormone replacement is initiated promptly given the confirmed subclinical insufficiency, addressing this specific, treatable manifestation proactively rather than waiting for an overt adrenal crisis to reveal it, illustrating the same anticipatory, screening-driven management philosophy this chapter has emphasized throughout for presymptomatically identified metabolic and neurodegenerative conditions.

Case Presentation: Acute Hyperammonemic Crisis in a Term Newborn

A previously well-appearing term newborn develops poor feeding, lethargy, and progressive encephalopathy on day of life three, and initial laboratory evaluation identifies markedly elevated serum ammonia. Applying the reasoning developed in this chapter, urgent brain MRI, obtained once the infant is stabilized enough for safe imaging, demonstrates diffuse cerebral edema with relative sparing of the perirolandic cortex, a pattern supporting the hyperammonemic mechanism already suggested by the laboratory findings rather than a primary hypoxic-ischemic process. Emergency dialysis is initiated alongside specific metabolic treatment targeting the underlying urea cycle disorder subsequently confirmed on expanded metabolic testing, and the family is counseled regarding both the acute treatment course and the structured, long-term developmental surveillance this chapter has emphasized as essential following any severe neonatal metabolic crisis, regardless of how successfully the acute presentation is managed. Genetic confirmation of the specific urea cycle enzyme defect responsible enables precise family counseling regarding recurrence risk, applying the family genetic counseling framework developed earlier in this chapter, for any future pregnancy the family may consider.

THE CLINICAL-IMAGING CROSSWALK SYSTEM — Metabolic and Neurodegenerative Disease Recognition

---

Crossing 1 Recap: A stroke-like lesion not conforming to a standard vascular territory should prompt lactate testing and consideration of MELAS rather than an exclusively vascular stroke evaluation pathway.

Chapter Anchor: Metabolic and neurodegenerative disease imaging depends on pattern-based reasoning, white matter distribution for leukodystrophy, symmetric basal ganglia and brainstem involvement for mitochondrial disease, region-specific atrophy or signal change for neurodegeneration, and myelinated-tract or hyperammonemic patterns for acute neonatal crisis, each directing targeted, imaging-guided genetic or biochemical confirmation rather than exhaustive, undirected testing. Presymptomatic detection through expanded newborn screening increasingly shifts this chapter's entities from reactive, crisis-driven diagnosis toward proactive, structured surveillance, mirroring the anticipatory care philosophy this book has developed across its full range of genetically and metabolically defined pediatric neurologic conditions.

Summary and Key Concepts

Leukodystrophy differential diagnosis is generated from the specific pattern of white matter involvement, anterior versus posterior predominance, symmetry, and enhancement; X-linked adrenoleukodystrophy shows posterior-predominant, enhancing disease while Alexander disease shows frontal-predominant involvement.

Leigh syndrome produces bilateral, symmetric basal ganglia and brainstem signal abnormality; MELAS produces stroke-like lesions not conforming to vascular territory with elevated lactate, distinguishing it from true arterial ischemic stroke.

Neuronal ceroid lipofuscinosis produces progressive atrophy with thalamic T2 hypointensity; Rett syndrome frequently shows normal imaging, and pantothenate kinase-associated neurodegeneration produces the pathognomonic eye-of-the-tiger sign.

Neonatal metabolic crisis requires parallel evaluation for acquired and metabolic causes; urea cycle disorders produce perirolandic-sparing edema, maple syrup urine disease produces myelinated-tract diffusion restriction, and nonketotic hyperglycinemia produces callosal and brainstem diffusion restriction.

Across this chapter, a structured, pattern-based imaging approach directs targeted genetic or biochemical confirmation, and presymptomatic detection through expanded newborn screening increasingly shifts several of these conditions from acute-crisis diagnosis to proactive, structured surveillance.

CHAPTER 18: CEREBROVASCULAR DISEASE AND PEDIATRIC STROKE

Learning Objectives

1. Describe the imaging protocol and differential diagnosis for suspected acute arterial ischemic stroke in a child.
2. Distinguish the major pediatric cerebral arteriopathies and recognize the imaging stages of moyamoya disease.
3. Distinguish arteriovenous malformation from cavernous malformation and describe the hemorrhage risk associated with each.
4. Recognize the imaging findings of cerebral sinovenous thrombosis and its risk factors in children.

Arterial Ischemic Stroke in Children

Pediatric arterial ischemic stroke, though far less common than in the adult population, carries a substantially broader and more heterogeneous underlying cause differential, and this section develops the specific imaging approach and evaluation strategy this distinct pediatric etiology spectrum requires. This etiologic breadth, spanning arteriopathy, cardiac disease, hematologic disorders, and vasculitis discussed throughout this chapter and cross-referenced against several of this book's preceding chapters, means a pediatric stroke evaluation cannot simply mirror an adult stroke protocol scaled down for smaller patients, but instead requires its own distinct, systematically comprehensive diagnostic framework this section develops from the ground up.

The Diagnostic Delay Challenge in Pediatric Stroke

Pediatric arterial ischemic stroke is well documented to carry a substantially longer average time to diagnosis than adult stroke, reflecting both the lower baseline clinical suspicion for this diagnosis in a child and the broader differential diagnosis, including the stroke mimics discussed throughout this book, that a child's acute focal neurologic presentation more often prompts; recognizing this well-documented diagnostic delay pattern and maintaining a proactively low threshold for urgent stroke imaging in a child presenting with an acute focal neurologic deficit, applying the same evidence-based imaging-ordering urgency this book has emphasized throughout, directly addresses this specific, well-characterized gap between adult and pediatric stroke recognition and treatment timelines. This diagnostic delay carries direct treatment implications, since time-sensitive interventions including thrombolysis and mechanical thrombectomy, established treatments in appropriately selected adult stroke, are similarly time-window-dependent when applied in the pediatric population, meaning each hour of diagnostic delay in a child potentially forecloses a treatment option that might otherwise have been available had the diagnosis been established more promptly.

Acute Stroke Imaging Protocol

Acute pediatric stroke imaging requires diffusion-weighted sequences as the primary, most sensitive tool for detecting acute ischemic injury, together with vascular imaging, most commonly MR angiography given its lack of radiation and ready incorporation into the same imaging session, to identify the specific vessel occlusion or narrowing responsible; this combination of diffusion and vascular imaging, obtained rapidly and without unnecessary delay, applies the same rapid, protocol-driven acute imaging approach this book has emphasized for other time-sensitive pediatric neurologic emergencies, including the status epilepticus imaging discussed in Chapter 11. Perfusion imaging, where obtained, offers a further, complementary characterization of the ischemic penumbra, the region of at-risk but not yet infarcted tissue that a time-sensitive intervention might still preserve, and incorporating this specific perfusion assessment into the acute protocol, where institutional resources and the child's clinical stability permit, provides additional information directly relevant to the thrombolysis and thrombectomy treatment decisions this section has discussed. A mismatch between the smaller region of restricted diffusion, representing already-infarcted core tissue, and a larger region of perfusion abnormality, representing the surrounding, still-salvageable penumbra, supports consideration of an intervention aimed at restoring flow to this specific, still-viable tissue, while a study showing little or no such mismatch suggests the opportunity for meaningful tissue salvage has largely passed, directly informing the urgency and expected benefit of any intervention considered.

Vascular Territory Recognition

Confirming that an area of restricted diffusion conforms to a recognized arterial vascular territory, applying the same vascular-territory reasoning developed in Chapter 17 for distinguishing MELAS stroke-like episodes from true arterial stroke, is an essential component of acute stroke characterization, since a lesion respecting a specific vascular territory boundary supports a true thromboembolic or vasculopathic arterial ischemic mechanism, while a lesion crossing multiple territories or following a non-vascular distribution should prompt reconsideration of the broader stroke-mimic differential this book has developed across several of its preceding chapters. This territorial confirmation, applied consistently as a deliberate, structured step rather than an implicit assumption, exemplifies the same disciplined pattern-verification habit this book has cultivated throughout, in which a presumptive diagnosis is actively checked against its expected anatomic signature rather than accepted on the basis of a superficially compatible clinical presentation alone.

The Broad Pediatric Stroke Etiology Differential

Unlike adult stroke, in which atherosclerotic and cardioembolic mechanisms predominate, pediatric arterial ischemic stroke arises from a substantially broader etiology spectrum including cerebral arteriopathy, discussed further in this chapter's next section, cardiac disease including congenital heart disease and cardiomyopathy, hematologic and prothrombotic conditions including sickle cell disease, and, less commonly, dissection and vasculitis discussed in Chapter 16; a comprehensive evaluation addressing each of these categories, rather than a narrow evaluation focused on the single most statistically common cause, is standard practice given this genuinely heterogeneous underlying etiology spectrum this specific pediatric population presents. Cervical arterial dissection specifically, whether spontaneous or related to minor trauma that the family may not initially recognize as clinically significant, warrants dedicated cervical vascular imaging extending the field of view beyond the intracranial circulation alone, applying the same field-of-view extension principle this book has emphasized throughout, since a dissection originating in the cervical vasculature may not be adequately characterized by intracranial vascular imaging confined to the circle of Willis and its immediate branches.

Sickle Cell Disease and Stroke Risk

Sickle cell disease carries a substantially elevated stroke risk related to both large-vessel vasculopathy, frequently producing the moyamoya pattern discussed in this chapter's next section, and microvascular occlusion from sickled erythrocytes, and transcranial Doppler ultrasound screening, identifying elevated flow velocities predictive of stroke risk, is a standard, structured surveillance tool for children with sickle cell disease, directing chronic transfusion therapy for those identified at highest risk before a first clinical stroke event occurs; this specific, validated screening and preventive treatment pathway represents one of the more successful examples of proactive, risk-stratified stroke prevention addressed throughout this book, meaningfully reducing first-stroke incidence in this specific, well-characterized high-risk population. Beyond overt clinical stroke, silent cerebral infarction, identified only on structural MRI surveillance rather than through an overt clinical event, occurs with meaningful frequency in children with sickle cell disease and carries its own independent association with cognitive impact, informing an increasingly recognized role for structured MRI surveillance alongside the transcranial Doppler screening this section has emphasized as the primary, most established preventive tool for this population.

Cardioembolic Stroke and Congenital Heart Disease

Children with congenital heart disease, particularly those with a right-to-left shunt allowing paradoxical embolization or those undergoing cardiac catheterization or surgery, carry an elevated stroke risk, and a child with known congenital heart disease presenting with an acute focal neurologic deficit warrants the same urgent stroke imaging protocol this section has developed, with particular attention to identifying a cardioembolic source through coordinated cardiology evaluation including echocardiography; recognizing this specific, cardiac-disease-associated stroke risk category reinforces the broader, multisystem etiology evaluation this section has emphasized throughout rather than a narrow, single-cause-focused diagnostic approach.

Perinatal Arterial Ischemic Stroke

Perinatal arterial ischemic stroke, occurring around the time of birth and frequently presenting with neonatal seizures rather than an overtly focal deficit given the limited motor repertoire available for a lateralizing examination finding in a newborn, represents a further distinct pediatric stroke category with its own characteristic risk factors, including placental pathology, perinatal complications, and neonatal prothrombotic states, and its own characteristic delayed clinical recognition pattern, since a diagnosis is often established only in retrospect once a later, hemiparetic presentation prompts imaging that reveals an established, chronic-appearing infarct rather than an acute one; recognizing this specific, delayed-recognition presentation pattern, unique to the perinatal stroke population relative to the older child stroke presentations this section has otherwise emphasized, is an important, distinct component of this chapter's comprehensive pediatric stroke framework. Perinatal stroke most commonly involves the middle cerebral artery territory, particularly its left-sided distribution, and early recognition through structured, proactive surveillance in an infant with an identified risk factor, rather than waiting for a later hemiparetic presentation, allows earlier initiation of the structured early intervention and rehabilitative therapy services this population benefits from, applying the same early-intervention philosophy this book has emphasized for other conditions carrying an established, fixed structural injury with an unfolding functional trajectory over subsequent infancy and childhood.

Secondary Stroke Prevention

Once an underlying stroke etiology is identified through the comprehensive evaluation this section has developed, secondary stroke prevention strategies, ranging from antiplatelet or anticoagulant therapy for a thromboembolic mechanism to the specific transfusion or revascularization approaches discussed elsewhere in this chapter for sickle cell disease and moyamoya disease respectively, are tailored precisely to the specific, confirmed underlying cause; this etiology-directed secondary prevention approach underscores why the comprehensive, multisystem evaluation this section has emphasized throughout is not merely an academic diagnostic exercise but the direct foundation for the specific, individualized secondary prevention strategy each child ultimately requires. Recurrent stroke risk varies substantially by underlying etiology, with an untreated progressive arteriopathy or an unaddressed high-risk cardiac lesion carrying a materially higher recurrence risk than a single, isolated thromboembolic event with no ongoing structural or hematologic risk factor, and communicating this etiology-specific recurrence risk honestly to a family, rather than a single, generic recurrence risk estimate applied uniformly regardless of cause, supports the family's understanding of why the specific secondary prevention strategy selected for their child carries the particular intensity and duration it does.

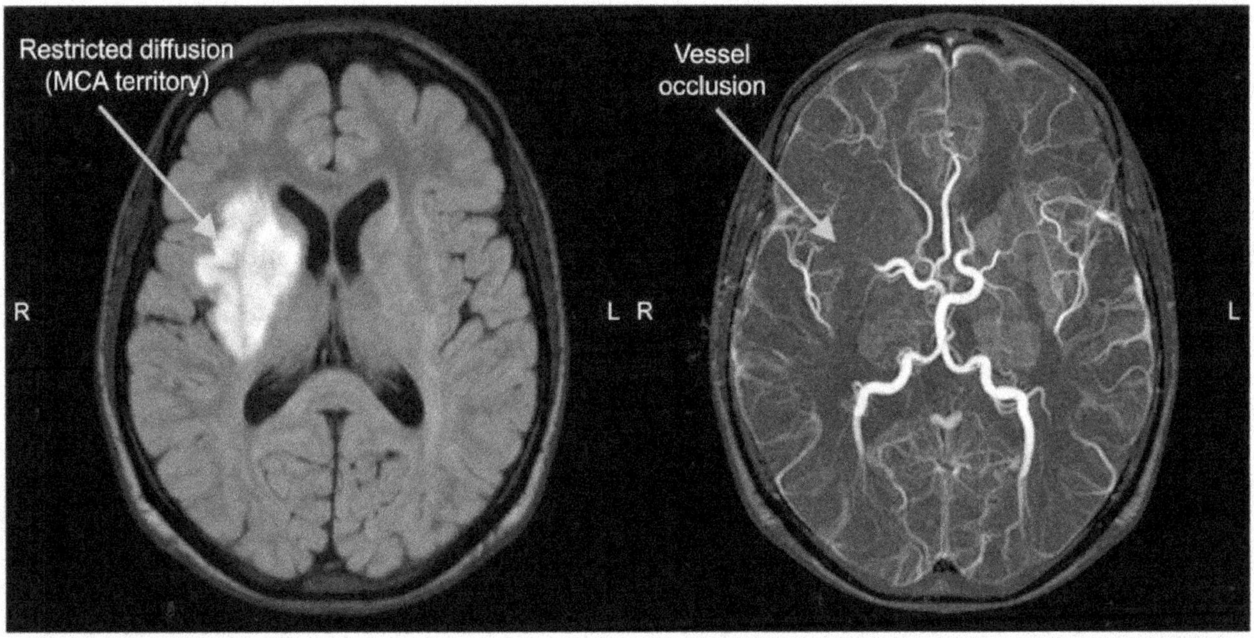

Figure 18.1: Pediatric Arterial Ischemic Stroke. Axial DWI (left) shows restricted diffusion in the right MCA territory (arrow). Corresponding TOF MRA source image (right) demonstrates occlusion of the right MCA (arrow).

Etiology Category	Example	Key Evaluation
Arteriopathy	Moyamoya, focal cerebral arteriopathy	Vascular imaging, serial follow-up
Cardiac	Congenital heart disease, cardiomyopathy	Echocardiography
Hematologic	Sickle cell disease, prothrombotic states	Hemoglobin electrophoresis, coagulation panel
Vasculitis/dissection	Primary CNS angiitis, cervical dissection	Vessel wall imaging, dedicated cervical vascular imaging

Cerebral Arteriopathies and Moyamoya

Cerebral arteriopathy represents the single most common identifiable cause of pediatric arterial ischemic stroke, and this section develops the specific imaging staging and recognition of moyamoya disease, the most distinctive and well-characterized entity within this broader arteriopathy category.

Focal Cerebral Arteriopathy of Childhood

Focal cerebral arteriopathy of childhood, a monophasic, self-limited arteriopathy typically affecting the distal internal carotid artery and proximal middle cerebral artery, is increasingly recognized as related to a preceding varicella infection in a substantial proportion of cases, applying the post-varicella arteriopathy mechanism introduced in Chapter 16; this specific arteriopathy characteristically shows focal, unilateral narrowing without the progressive, bilateral involvement characteristic of moyamoya disease discussed later in this section, and recognizing this monophasic, self-limited natural history, confirmed through serial vascular imaging demonstrating stability or improvement rather than progression, distinguishes it from the progressive arteriopathies this section addresses and informs a correspondingly time-limited, rather than indefinite, antithrombotic treatment duration. This entity was historically termed transient cerebral arteriopathy before its more precise, currently preferred nomenclature reflected growing recognition that the underlying arteriopathy, while monophasic, is not always fully transient in the sense of complete radiographic normalization, since a subset of children retain some residual, stable vessel irregularity even after the active, progressive phase of the arteriopathy has definitively resolved.

Moyamoya Disease: The Characteristic Angiographic Appearance

Moyamoya disease, a progressive arteriopathy characterized by bilateral stenosis or occlusion of the distal internal carotid arteries with compensatory development of an extensive network of fragile, abnormal collateral vessels, produces the characteristic angiographic appearance from which this condition derives its name, a hazy, puff-of-smoke pattern reflecting these numerous, fine collateral vessels; this progressive, bilateral pattern, evolving through recognized angiographic stages from initial stenosis through progressive collateral development to eventual occlusion, distinguishes moyamoya disease from the more focal, typically unilateral and self-limited arteriopathies discussed elsewhere in this section. This condition shows a distinct epidemiologic predilection for children of East Asian ancestry, though it occurs across all ethnic backgrounds, and a bimodal age distribution, with peaks in early childhood and again in the fourth decade of adulthood, epidemiologic features worth holding in mind alongside the specific angiographic pattern this paragraph has emphasized when generating a differential diagnosis for a child with bilateral distal internal carotid artery stenosis of uncertain etiology. The Suzuki staging system, describing six sequential angiographic stages from initial mild stenosis through progressive basal collateral proliferation to eventual disappearance of these collaterals as alternative, more distant collateral pathways take over, provides a standardized, structured framework for characterizing disease progression on serial imaging, and applying this staging system consistently, rather than a purely descriptive, unstructured account of each study, supports the same objective, reproducible longitudinal comparison this book has emphasized throughout for numerous other progressive conditions requiring structured serial surveillance.

Moyamoya Syndrome and Its Associated Conditions

This same characteristic angiographic pattern, when occurring secondary to an identifiable underlying condition rather than as an idiopathic, primary process, is termed moyamoya syndrome rather than moyamoya disease, and recognized associated conditions include sickle cell disease discussed earlier in this chapter, neurofibromatosis type 1 discussed in Chapter 14, and prior cranial radiation therapy, discussed in Chapter 12 as a recognized late effect of treatment for a primary brain tumor; distinguishing primary moyamoya disease from secondary moyamoya syndrome depends on actively screening for these specific, recognized associated conditions, since this distinction, while not altering the fundamental angiographic recognition and surgical management approach this section develops, carries direct implications for the broader evaluation and counseling a family receives. Down syndrome represents a further, less commonly recognized but well-documented association with this same moyamoya angiographic pattern, and a child with Down syndrome presenting with a new stroke or stroke-like presentation warrants the same dedicated vascular imaging this section has emphasized throughout, applying the specific syndrome-associated screening awareness this chapter has developed for each of its named associated conditions.

Advanced Imaging Techniques in Moyamoya Characterization

Beyond conventional angiographic characterization, perfusion imaging, quantifying cerebral blood flow and, particularly, cerebrovascular reserve, the brain's capacity to further increase blood flow in response to a vasodilatory challenge, provides essential physiologic information regarding hemodynamic compromise that structural angiographic staging alone cannot fully capture; a child with advanced angiographic staging but preserved cerebrovascular reserve may tolerate a more conservative, observation-focused management approach than a child with even earlier-stage angiographic findings but severely compromised reserve, illustrating why functional, physiologic characterization complements rather than duplicates the structural staging this section has emphasized throughout. Acetazolamide-challenge perfusion imaging, in which cerebral blood flow is measured before and after administration of this specific vasodilatory agent, is the most established technique for quantifying cerebrovascular reserve in this specific population, and a blunted or paradoxically decreased flow response to this vasodilatory challenge, termed a steal phenomenon, identifies the specific brain regions at greatest hemodynamic risk and most likely to benefit from the surgical revascularization this section discusses next.

Surgical Revascularization

Surgical revascularization, most commonly through indirect techniques such as pial synangiosis, in which a vascularized tissue flap is placed in direct contact with the brain surface to promote new collateral vessel ingrowth over subsequent months, represents the definitive treatment for moyamoya disease once significant hemodynamic compromise is identified, and precise preoperative imaging characterization of the specific vessels involved and the existing collateral pattern directly informs the surgical approach and expected revascularization territory; postoperative imaging, including both structural and perfusion-based assessment, confirms successful new collateral development over the months following surgery, applying the same structured, serial-comparison surveillance principle this book has emphasized throughout for other surgically treated conditions. Direct revascularization techniques, in which a scalp artery is directly anastomosed to a cortical vessel, offer an alternative or complementary approach to the indirect technique this paragraph has primarily described, generally favored in an older child or adolescent whose vessel caliber is more amenable to this technically more demanding direct anastomosis, while the indirect technique remains generally preferred in the younger child given both technical feasibility and this population's greater capacity for the gradual, angiogenic collateral formation this indirect approach depends upon. Bilateral disease, the more typical presentation this chapter has emphasized, generally requires staged, sequential surgical treatment of each hemisphere rather than a single combined procedure, and sequencing this staged approach to address the hemisphere with more severe hemodynamic compromise, as characterized by the acetazolamide-challenge perfusion imaging discussed above, first reflects the same risk-stratified, urgency-calibrated treatment sequencing principle this book has applied throughout to numerous other conditions requiring a staged, rather than single-step, treatment approach.

Hemorrhagic Presentation of Moyamoya

While moyamoya disease in children most commonly presents with ischemic symptoms related to the progressive arterial stenosis this section has emphasized, the fragile, abnormal collateral vessels this condition produces carry an independent hemorrhage risk, more classically recognized in the adult moyamoya population but occasionally encountered in children as well, and any child with known moyamoya disease presenting with acute headache or a new neurologic deficit warrants imaging evaluation for both possibilities, ischemic and hemorrhagic, rather than an assumption that the more common, ischemic presentation is automatically responsible for a new acute presentation in this specific population.

Bilateral Versus Unilateral Involvement at Presentation

A child presenting with unilateral moyamoya-pattern findings at initial imaging warrants careful, structured follow-up vascular imaging of the contralateral hemisphere, since a substantial proportion of children with apparently unilateral disease at presentation go on to develop contralateral involvement over subsequent years, meaning an initial unilateral finding does not reliably predict a persistently unilateral disease course; this specific, well-documented progression pattern from unilateral to bilateral involvement reinforces why moyamoya disease surveillance extends well beyond a single, reassuring initial evaluation into the structured, longitudinal imaging follow-up this section has emphasized throughout.

Cognitive Outcome in Moyamoya Disease

Beyond the overt ischemic and hemorrhagic stroke risk this section has emphasized, chronic, subclinical hemodynamic compromise in moyamoya disease carries a documented association with cognitive impact even in the absence of a clinically apparent stroke event, and structured neuropsychological baseline assessment and longitudinal monitoring, applying the same baseline-and-longitudinal-tracking principle developed in Chapter 11, is an increasingly recognized component of comprehensive moyamoya disease management extending beyond the vascular imaging and surgical revascularization this section has primarily addressed.

Figure 18.2 Progressive Moyamoya Angiographic Staging

Stage II: Early Stenosis and Collaterals

Stage IV: Extensive Moyamoya Network (Puff-of-Smoke)

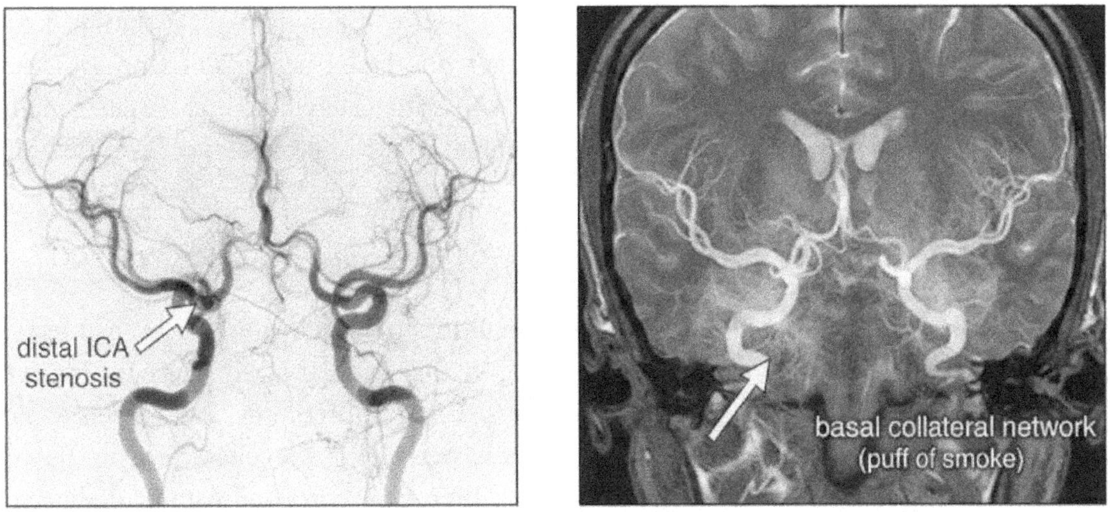

Stage IV: Extensive Moyamoya het collateral gata (puff-of-smoke)

THE CLINICAL-IMAGING CROSSWALK SYSTEM — Recurrent Transient Neurologic Symptoms in a Child With Neurofibromatosis Type 1

The Crossing: A nine-year-old with known neurofibromatosis type 1 presents with two episodes of transient left-hand weakness over the preceding month, each resolving within an hour.

Presentation Signature: A child with a known neurocutaneous syndrome and recurrent, transient focal neurologic symptoms suggestive of a vascular, rather than epileptic, mechanism.

Imaging Correlate: Dedicated vascular imaging is obtained given the recognized association between neurofibromatosis type 1 and moyamoya syndrome discussed in this chapter, demonstrating bilateral distal internal carotid artery stenosis with an early basal collateral network consistent with moyamoya syndrome.

Trap Logic: Attributing recurrent transient focal symptoms in a child with neurofibromatosis type 1 to a nonspecific or epileptic cause without considering this specific, well-documented vascular association risks delayed recognition of a progressive arteriopathy carrying genuine stroke risk if left unaddressed.

Crossing Anchor: Recurrent transient focal neurologic symptoms in a child with neurofibromatosis type 1 should prompt dedicated vascular imaging to evaluate for moyamoya syndrome, a recognized, specific association warranting active, rather than incidental, consideration.

Vascular Malformations: AVM and Cavernous Malformation

This section addresses arteriovenous malformation and cavernous malformation, two distinct vascular malformation categories each carrying its own characteristic imaging appearance, hemorrhage risk profile, and management approach this section develops in parallel to highlight their essential distinguishing features. Where the preceding sections of this chapter addressed acquired or progressive vascular pathology, arterial stroke and arteriopathy, this section shifts focus to congenital vascular malformations present from birth, extending this chapter's cerebrovascular framework to this further, structurally distinct category of pediatric vascular disease.

Arteriovenous Malformation: Structure and Imaging Appearance

Arteriovenous malformation, a congenital vascular malformation characterized by a direct, abnormal connection between arteries and veins without an intervening capillary bed, presents on imaging as a tangle of abnormal vessels, the nidus, fed by one or more enlarged arterial feeding vessels and drained by one or more enlarged, often tortuous draining veins, producing the characteristic flow voids on conventional MRI sequences that reflect this lesion's high-flow vascular nature; dedicated vascular imaging, whether MR angiography, CT angiography, or, for definitive presurgical characterization, conventional catheter angiography, precisely delineates this specific arterial feeder and venous drainage architecture, information essential to the treatment planning this section addresses. Unlike the arteriopathies discussed in this chapter's preceding section, which represent an acquired or progressive narrowing of otherwise normally formed vessels, arteriovenous malformation reflects a primary developmental error in vascular formation, present from birth even though clinical presentation, whether through hemorrhage, seizure, or an incidental finding, frequently occurs later in childhood or even adulthood once the lesion's specific presenting event occurs. A small minority of arteriovenous malformations, particularly those identified incidentally at a very young age, show apparent spontaneous regression on serial imaging, a genuinely uncommon but well-documented phenomenon worth holding in mind alongside the more typical, stable-or-growing natural history this section otherwise emphasizes, though this rare possibility does not by itself justify a purely observational approach for a lesion otherwise meeting the treatment criteria this section develops.

Hemorrhage Risk and the Spetzler-Martin Grading System

Arteriovenous malformation carries an ongoing, cumulative lifetime hemorrhage risk, and the Spetzler-Martin grading system, incorporating nidus size, eloquence of adjacent brain tissue, and venous drainage pattern, superficial versus deep, provides a structured, standardized framework for both hemorrhage risk stratification and surgical treatment planning; a higher Spetzler-Martin grade generally indicates both a technically more challenging surgical resection and, for some grading components, a distinct hemorrhage risk profile, and applying this standardized grading system consistently, rather than an unstructured qualitative impression, provides the objective, reproducible basis for the multidisciplinary treatment planning discussion this specific lesion category requires. A lesion presenting with hemorrhage carries a higher subsequent hemorrhage risk than an incidentally discovered, unruptured lesion of otherwise similar size and location, an important, specific risk-stratification detail beyond the Spetzler-Martin grade alone that should be incorporated into the overall risk assessment and family counseling conversation this section's broader framework has emphasized throughout.

Treatment Approaches for AVM

Treatment options for arteriovenous malformation include surgical resection, endovascular embolization, either as definitive treatment for smaller, favorably located lesions or as a preoperative adjunct reducing intraoperative blood loss for larger lesions, and stereotactic radiosurgery, particularly favored for smaller lesions in deep or eloquent locations where surgical resection carries prohibitive risk; the specific treatment approach or combination of approaches selected depends on the precise angioarchitecture this section's imaging characterization establishes, together with the lesion's size, location, and the Spetzler-Martin grade this section has discussed, reflecting the same individualized, imaging-informed treatment planning principle this book has applied throughout to numerous other conditions requiring a similarly tailored management approach. Stereotactic radiosurgery, unlike the more immediately effective surgical and embolization approaches this paragraph has also discussed, produces its therapeutic vascular obliteration gradually over a period of months to a few years following treatment, meaning a child undergoing this specific treatment modality continues to carry a meaningful, unaddressed hemorrhage risk throughout this latency period, a specific, important counseling point distinguishing this treatment's risk-benefit profile from the more immediately protective effect of successful surgical resection.

Cavernous Malformation: A Distinct Low-Flow Lesion

Cavernous malformation, in contrast to the high-flow arteriovenous malformation discussed above, is a low-flow vascular malformation composed of abnormal, thin-walled sinusoidal vascular channels without an intervening arterial feeder or the enlarged draining veins characteristic of arteriovenous malformation, producing a characteristic popcorn-ball appearance on MRI with mixed signal intensity reflecting blood products of varying age, surrounded by a complete, low-signal hemosiderin rim best appreciated on susceptibility-weighted or gradient-echo sequences; this specific imaging appearance, fundamentally distinct from the flow-void-predominant, high-flow appearance of arteriovenous malformation, reflects the different underlying vascular architecture and correspondingly different hemorrhage pattern, characteristically smaller-volume, recurrent microhemorrhage rather than the larger, single catastrophic hemorrhage risk more characteristic of arteriovenous malformation. Because cavernous malformation is angiographically occult, meaning it does not fill on conventional catheter angiography given its low-flow nature, MRI, rather than the catheter angiography favored for definitive arteriovenous malformation characterization, is both the primary detection and primary characterization tool for this specific lesion category, a modality distinction worth recognizing explicitly since it directly explains why the two entities this section addresses in parallel require genuinely different primary imaging approaches despite both falling under the broader vascular malformation category. Symptomatic hemorrhage from a cavernous malformation, when it occurs, is generally less catastrophic in immediate severity than a major arteriovenous malformation rupture given the comparatively lower pressure within this lesion's low-flow vascular channels, though a lesion located within eloquent brainstem or spinal cord parenchyma can nonetheless produce a clinically significant deficit even from a relatively small-volume hemorrhage, underscoring why lesion location, not hemorrhage volume alone, meaningfully shapes the clinical significance and treatment urgency a specific cavernous malformation warrants.

Familial Cavernous Malformation Syndrome

A subset of cavernous malformations occur in the context of a familial, autosomal dominant syndrome related to mutation in one of several recognized genes, characteristically producing multiple cavernous malformations throughout the brain and spinal cord rather than the single, isolated lesion more typical of sporadic disease, and identifying multiple cavernous malformations on a single study should prompt genetics referral and family screening applying the same multiplicity-as-diagnostic-clue reasoning developed in Chapter 14 for von Hippel-Lindau disease, since this specific familial pattern carries direct implications for both the affected child's own long-term surveillance and screening recommendations for at-risk family members.

Developmental Venous Anomaly as a Benign Mimic

Developmental venous anomaly, a benign, normal-variant venous drainage pattern with a characteristic caput medusae appearance, multiple small medullary veins converging into a single, larger draining vein, should not be mistaken for either of the two lesion categories this section has emphasized, since this specific finding, unlike arteriovenous malformation and cavernous malformation, carries essentially no independent hemorrhage risk and represents a normal, though anatomically atypical, venous drainage pathway rather than a true vascular malformation; recognizing this specific, benign entity and its characteristic imaging appearance prevents unnecessary alarm or intervention for what is, in the vast majority of cases, an incidental finding requiring no specific treatment or even routine surveillance imaging.

Mixed and Combined Vascular Malformations

A minority of children present with a mixed vascular malformation, most commonly a cavernous malformation occurring in direct association with an underlying developmental venous anomaly, and recognizing this specific combined pattern, rather than characterizing only the more clinically significant cavernous component in isolation, provides a complete anatomic picture that can inform surgical planning should intervention for the cavernous malformation component become necessary, since preserving the associated developmental venous anomaly's normal venous drainage function is an important surgical consideration given this structure's role in draining otherwise normal, adjacent brain tissue.

Figure 18.3 Arteriovenous Malformation Versus Cavernous Malformation

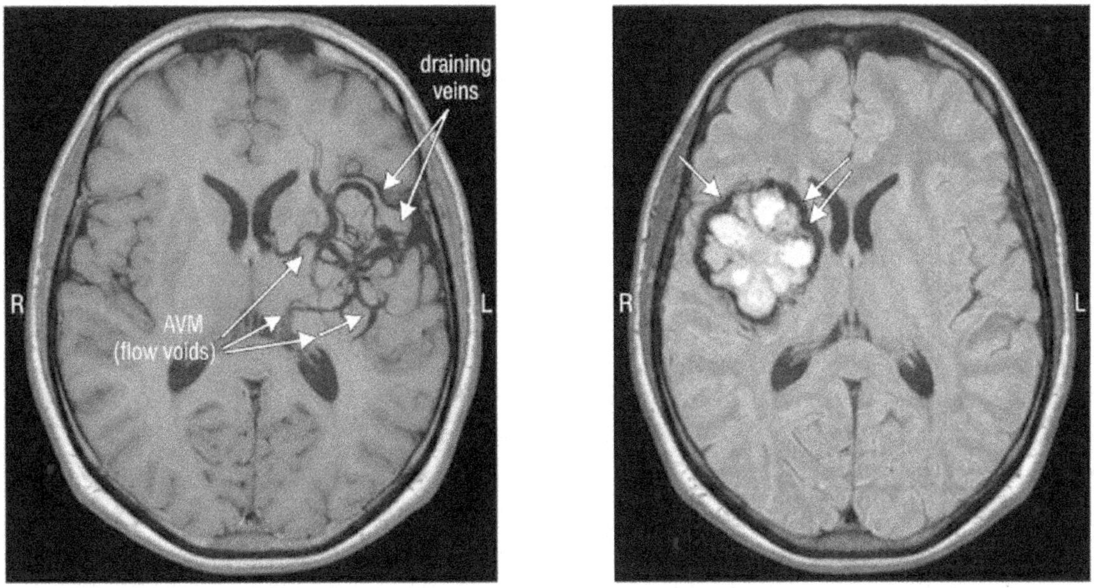

AVM (flow voids)

Cavernous malformation
(popcorn-ball, hemosiderin rim)

Sinovenous Thrombosis Revisited

This closing section returns to cerebral sinovenous thrombosis, introduced in its broader context in Chapter 6 and discussed as a specific complication of bacterial meningitis in Chapter 15, developing a comprehensive, standalone treatment of this entity's imaging findings, risk factors, and management within this chapter's broader cerebrovascular disease framework. Bringing this venous pathology together with the arterial stroke, arteriopathy, and vascular malformation entities addressed earlier in this chapter completes this chapter's comprehensive survey of the full pediatric cerebrovascular disease spectrum, arterial, venous, and malformative, equipping the reader with a unified, anatomically organized framework for approaching any pediatric cerebrovascular presentation regardless of which specific vascular compartment is ultimately implicated. This closing section's emphasis on temporal signal evolution, distinct from the vascular-territory and angioarchitecture reasoning emphasized throughout the rest of this chapter, introduces a further, complementary interpretive skill the reader carries forward into the remaining chapters of this book, in which recognizing an evolving, rather than static, imaging finding over a defined timeframe repeatedly proves as diagnostically consequential as the finding's spatial pattern alone.

Coordinating Multidisciplinary Cerebrovascular Care

Given the genuine breadth of this chapter's cerebrovascular disease spectrum, comprehensive care is best delivered through a dedicated, multidisciplinary pediatric stroke and cerebrovascular program bringing together neurology, neurosurgery, interventional neuroradiology, hematology, and, where relevant, cardiology and genetics, applying the same coordinated, multidisciplinary team principle this book has developed throughout for other complex, multisystem pediatric neurologic conditions; this team-based model ensures the specific, condition-appropriate evaluation and treatment pathway this chapter has developed for each of its constituent entities is applied consistently and coordinated effectively across a child's complete cerebrovascular care journey. Structured transition planning into adult-focused cerebrovascular care, applying the same transition-of-care principles this book has developed in several preceding chapters for other conditions requiring lifelong surveillance, becomes an increasingly relevant consideration as a child with a chronic cerebrovascular diagnosis, moyamoya disease or a familial cavernous malformation syndrome in particular, approaches adulthood and the ongoing, condition-specific surveillance this chapter has emphasized throughout must continue seamlessly into an adult care setting.

Risk Factors Across the Pediatric Age Spectrum

Cerebral sinovenous thrombosis risk factors vary meaningfully across the pediatric age spectrum, with the neonate carrying risk related to perinatal complications, dehydration, and maternal or neonatal prothrombotic conditions, while the older child and adolescent more often show risk factors including an underlying prothrombotic disorder, the infectious and inflammatory triggers discussed in Chapters 6 and 15, dehydration from an acute illness, and, in the adolescent specifically, oral contraceptive use; this age-dependent risk factor profile, similar to the age-dependent presentation patterns this book has noted for several other conditions, should inform the specific, targeted evaluation pursued once this diagnosis is identified or strongly suspected on imaging. A comprehensive prothrombotic evaluation, incorporating both inherited factors such as protein C, protein S, and antithrombin deficiency, and acquired factors such as antiphospholipid antibodies, is generally pursued for every child with confirmed sinovenous thrombosis regardless of whether a more immediately apparent precipitating factor, such as dehydration or a preceding infection, has already been identified, since more than one contributing risk factor is frequently present and each carries independent implications for anticoagulation duration and future recurrence risk counseling.

Imaging Recognition of Sinus Thrombosis

Cerebral sinovenous thrombosis is identified through absence of the normal flow signal within the affected dural venous sinus on venography, whether MR or CT-based, together with, on conventional MRI sequences, an evolving signal pattern within the thrombosed sinus itself that changes characteristically over the first one to two weeks following thrombus formation as the clot ages, transitioning through a sequence of signal changes on T1 and T2 sequences that parallels the blood product evolution discussed in Chapter 6 for parenchymal hemorrhage; recognizing this specific temporal signal evolution prevents mistaking a subacute, evolving thrombus for a normal, flowing sinus on a single, non-venographic sequence obtained without dedicated venous imaging technique. The empty delta sign, a specific finding on postcontrast CT or MRI in which the thrombosed superior sagittal sinus shows a triangular filling defect surrounded by a rim of enhancing dural collateral vessels, represents a further, classic though not universally present imaging sign worth recognizing specifically when this particular sinus is involved, complementing the dedicated venographic technique this section has emphasized as the primary, most reliable diagnostic approach.

Venous Infarction as a Complication

Venous infarction, a recognized complication of sinovenous thrombosis reflecting impaired venous drainage from the affected brain territory, characteristically does not respect a single arterial vascular territory boundary, instead crossing multiple arterial territories in a pattern corresponding to the specific venous drainage territory affected, and this specific, non-arterial-territory-conforming pattern, together with a disproportionately high rate of associated hemorrhagic transformation relative to typical arterial ischemic stroke, distinguishes venous from arterial infarction; recognizing this distinction directly shapes management, since anticoagulation, the standard treatment for sinovenous thrombosis, is generally continued even in the presence of hemorrhagic venous infarction, a management approach that would be markedly different, and generally contraindicated, in the setting of an equivalent hemorrhagic transformation following true arterial ischemic stroke. This specific, counterintuitive management approach, continuing rather than withholding anticoagulation despite visible hemorrhage, is worth explaining explicitly to a family and to any covering clinician unfamiliar with this specific condition's distinct management principles, since the instinct to withhold anticoagulation in the setting of any intracranial hemorrhage, while entirely appropriate for most other hemorrhagic presentations this book has addressed, does not apply in this specific venous infarction context given the underlying thrombotic process anticoagulation is specifically treating.

Anticoagulation Treatment and Monitoring

Anticoagulation represents the mainstay of treatment for confirmed cerebral sinovenous thrombosis in children, and structured, serial follow-up venous imaging, typically at defined intervals over the following months, documents the expected recanalization of the affected sinus over this treatment course, providing both confirmation of treatment response and the objective basis for determining anticoagulation treatment duration; a sinus failing to show expected recanalization on this serial follow-up imaging prompts reconsideration of the underlying prothrombotic evaluation and, at times, extended anticoagulation duration beyond the standard treatment course this section's typical management approach would otherwise recommend. Complete anatomic recanalization is not achieved in every case even with appropriate, adequately dosed anticoagulation, and a persistent, though non-progressive, area of residual sinus narrowing or occlusion on follow-up imaging, particularly when the child has returned to full clinical baseline, does not necessarily indicate treatment failure, since some degree of chronic, stable venous outflow compromise can be well tolerated once adequate collateral venous drainage has developed over the treatment course.

Long-Term Outcome and Recurrence Risk

Long-term outcome following cerebral sinovenous thrombosis correlates with the extent of venous infarction identified at presentation and the specific underlying risk factor or prothrombotic condition responsible, and children with a confirmed underlying prothrombotic disorder carry an elevated recurrence risk warranting structured, longitudinal hematologic follow-up extending well beyond the acute treatment period this section has primarily addressed, applying the same proactive, structured long-term surveillance principle this book has emphasized throughout for numerous other conditions carrying an ongoing, rather than purely acute, risk profile.

Neonatal Sinovenous Thrombosis

Sinovenous thrombosis in the neonate presents a distinct diagnostic and prognostic picture from the older child population this section has otherwise emphasized, often related to perinatal complications, dehydration, and maternal or neonatal prothrombotic states, and typically presenting with nonspecific findings including seizures rather than the more overt focal deficits characteristic of an older child's presentation; recognizing this age-specific presentation pattern, similar to the perinatal arterial stroke presentation discussed earlier in this chapter, ensures this specific neonatal risk factor and presentation profile is actively incorporated into the evaluation of a newborn presenting with unexplained seizures rather than assumed to reflect only the more commonly considered hypoxic-ischemic or infectious causes addressed elsewhere in this book.

Distinguishing True Thrombosis From Normal Anatomic Variation

A specific, well-recognized interpretive pitfall in sinovenous thrombosis evaluation involves normal anatomic variation in dural venous sinus size and configuration, including a hypoplastic or atretic transverse sinus, a common normal variant that can be mistaken for true thrombosis if the interpreting clinician is unfamiliar with this specific, benign anatomic possibility; correlating any apparent sinus flow signal abnormality against the specific sinus's expected caliber and against the contralateral side, together with the absence of the sinus signal evolution and clinical presentation this section has emphasized for true thrombosis, helps distinguish this benign anatomic variant from genuinely pathologic sinus thrombosis requiring the anticoagulation treatment this section has developed.

Figure 18.4: Cerebral Sinovenous Thrombosis With Venous Infarction

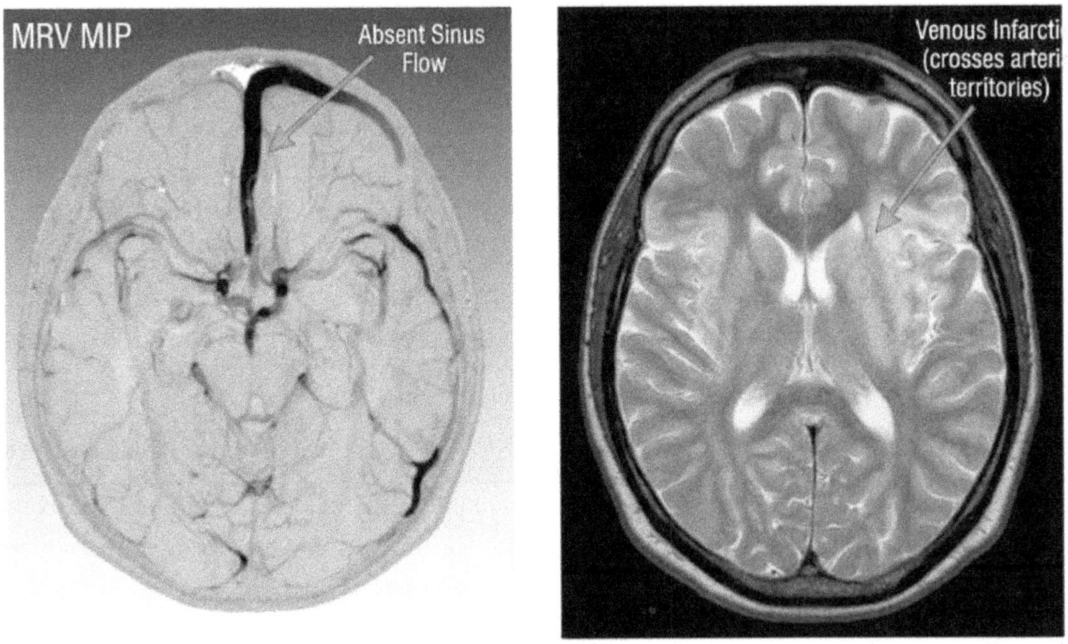

Figure 18.4: Cerebral Sinovenous Thrombosis With Venous Infarction

Case Presentation: Focal Cerebral Arteriopathy Following Varicella

A three-year-old presents with acute right hemiparesis six weeks after an uncomplicated varicella infection, and brain MRI demonstrates restricted diffusion in the left basal ganglia and internal capsule with corresponding focal narrowing of the distal left internal carotid and proximal middle cerebral artery on vascular imaging. Applying the reasoning developed in this chapter, the specific unilateral, focal arteriopathy pattern following a documented preceding varicella infection supports a diagnosis of focal cerebral arteriopathy of childhood rather than moyamoya disease, and antithrombotic therapy is initiated. Serial vascular imaging over the following twelve months demonstrates stability without the progressive, bilateral involvement that would instead suggest moyamoya disease, confirming the monophasic, self-limited natural history this chapter has described for this specific arteriopathy, and antithrombotic therapy is discontinued once this stable trajectory has been confirmed across the structured surveillance interval this chapter's framework has established. Structured neurorehabilitation, addressing the residual mild hemiparesis identified on discharge examination, is coordinated in parallel with this vascular surveillance, illustrating the same dual medical-and-functional follow-up approach this book has emphasized for other pediatric neurologic conditions carrying both an ongoing surveillance requirement and a residual functional deficit requiring dedicated rehabilitative support.

Case Presentation: Cavernous Malformation Multiplicity Identifying Familial Syndrome

A twelve-year-old presents with a new seizure, and brain MRI identifies a popcorn-ball lesion with a complete hemosiderin rim in the right temporal lobe consistent with cavernous malformation, and, on careful review of the full study, two additional smaller, similar lesions elsewhere in the brain. Applying the multiplicity reasoning developed in this chapter, this finding of multiple cavernous malformations prompts genetics referral rather than treating the seizure-associated lesion as an isolated, sporadic finding, and genetic testing confirms a familial cavernous malformation syndrome. The family is counseled regarding the autosomal dominant inheritance pattern this diagnosis carries, and cascade screening is offered to at-risk first-degree relatives, illustrating how the imaging-driven recognition of multiplicity this chapter has emphasized throughout directly triggered family-wide diagnostic and screening implications extending well beyond the originally presenting child. Spinal imaging, applying the same complete-anatomic-survey principle this chapter has emphasized for this specific familial syndrome, additionally identifies a small, asymptomatic thoracic spinal cord cavernous malformation, prompting baseline documentation and structured surveillance for this second, previously unrecognized lesion alongside the intracranial lesions already identified.

THE CLINICAL-IMAGING CROSSWALK SYSTEM — Cerebrovascular Disease Recognition

Crossing 1 Recap: Recurrent transient focal neurologic symptoms in a child with neurofibromatosis type 1 should prompt dedicated vascular imaging to evaluate for moyamoya syndrome, a recognized, specific association warranting active consideration.

Chapter Anchor: Pediatric cerebrovascular disease requires vascular-territory-conforming confirmation of arterial stroke, staged angiographic and physiologic characterization of arteriopathy, precise angioarchitecture and grading for vascular malformations, and temporal signal evolution recognition for sinovenous thrombosis, each directing a distinct, specific evaluation and treatment pathway integrated tightly with the child's broader clinical and risk-factor context.

Summary and Key Concepts

Pediatric arterial ischemic stroke carries a broader etiology differential than adult stroke and a well-documented diagnostic delay; confirming vascular-territory conformity distinguishes true stroke from stroke mimics, and sickle cell disease and congenital heart disease are important, specifically screened risk categories.

Focal cerebral arteriopathy of childhood is monophasic and often post-varicella, confirmed stable on serial imaging; moyamoya disease is progressive and bilateral, staged angiographically, and evaluated with perfusion imaging for hemodynamic compromise before surgical revascularization.

Arteriovenous malformation is a high-flow lesion graded by the Spetzler-Martin system for hemorrhage risk and treatment planning; cavernous malformation is a low-flow, popcorn-ball lesion with a hemosiderin rim, and multiplicity should prompt genetics referral for familial syndrome.

Cerebral sinovenous thrombosis shows absent sinus flow signal and an evolving thrombus signal pattern; venous infarction crosses arterial territorial boundaries and does not contraindicate continued anticoagulation despite hemorrhagic transformation.

Across this chapter, precise vascular characterization, territory, flow pattern, angiographic stage, and signal evolution, directs the specific evaluation, treatment, and family counseling pathway appropriate to each distinct cerebrovascular entity.

CHAPTER 19: TRAUMATIC BRAIN AND SPINE INJURY, INCLUDING ABUSIVE HEAD TRAUMA

Learning Objectives

1. Describe the acute imaging findings of pediatric traumatic brain injury and the criteria guiding imaging-ordering decisions.
2. Recognize the constellation of imaging findings supporting a diagnosis of abusive head trauma and describe the required skeletal and ophthalmologic evaluation.
3. Describe the imaging approach to pediatric spinal cord and spine trauma, including SCIWORA.
4. Distinguish expected postconcussive imaging findings from chronic traumatic imaging change requiring further evaluation.

Traumatic Brain Injury: Acute Imaging Findings

Pediatric traumatic brain injury spans a spectrum from mild, imaging-negative concussion through severe, life-threatening structural injury, and this section develops both the specific acute imaging findings this spectrum produces and the evidence-based decision rules that guide the imaging-ordering decision itself, a decision with direct radiation and sedation stewardship implications given this population's high injury frequency. Because head trauma represents one of the single most common reasons a child undergoes emergent neuroimaging, the evidence-based imaging-ordering framework this section develops carries outsized practical significance relative to several of the rarer conditions addressed elsewhere in this book, directly shaping daily practice in essentially every pediatric emergency care setting.

Clinical Decision Rules for Imaging After Head Trauma

Validated clinical decision rules, most notably the PECARN pediatric head trauma prediction rules, stratify children by age and specific clinical criteria, including the severity and mechanism of injury, the presence of a scalp hematoma, and the child's mental status, into risk categories guiding the decision to obtain CT, observe, or discharge without imaging, and applying these validated, evidence-based rules consistently, rather than an individually variable clinical gestalt, meaningfully reduces unnecessary CT radiation exposure in the very low-risk group while reliably identifying the small proportion of children harboring a clinically significant intracranial injury; this structured, rule-based approach exemplifies the evidence-based imaging-ordering discipline established in Chapter 3, applied here to one of the most common indications for pediatric neuroimaging encountered in acute care settings. These rules are specifically age-stratified, with distinct criteria applied to the infant younger than two years given this population's more limited capacity for reliable symptom reporting and the correspondingly greater reliance on objective examination findings, including the specific characteristics of any scalp hematoma present, and a clinician applying these rules should confirm they are using the age-appropriate criteria set rather than a single, undifferentiated rule applied uniformly across the full pediatric age range these validated tools actually stratify.

Epidural Hematoma

Epidural hematoma, classically arising from injury to the middle meningeal artery or an adjacent dural venous sinus, presents on imaging as a biconvex, lens-shaped extra-axial collection that characteristically does not cross cranial suture lines, since the dura remains firmly adherent to the skull at these specific suture locations, constraining the hematoma's shape as it expands; a child with an epidural hematoma classically, though not universally, presents with a lucid interval, a period of normal or near-normal consciousness following the initial injury before subsequent, sometimes rapid, deterioration as the hematoma expands, and recognizing both this specific imaging morphology and the classic though inconsistent clinical trajectory supports prompt neurosurgical evaluation given this lesion's potential for rapid, life-threatening expansion. The absence of a classic lucid interval, importantly, does not exclude epidural hematoma, since this specific clinical trajectory, while classic, is present in only a minority of confirmed cases, and a child presenting with persistent, unremitting altered consciousness following head trauma should not be excluded from this specific diagnostic consideration simply because the more textbook lucid-interval pattern is absent from their particular clinical course.

Subdural Hematoma

Subdural hematoma, arising from injury to the bridging veins traversing the subdural space, presents on imaging as a crescentic collection that, unlike epidural hematoma, does cross suture lines but does not cross the midline dural reflections, including the falx and tentorium, since these dural structures similarly constrain its spread; subdural hematoma is frequently associated with underlying parenchymal injury given the typically more diffuse, acceleration-deceleration mechanism producing this specific hemorrhage pattern, in contrast to the more focal, often isolated skull fracture mechanism more classically associated with epidural hematoma, and recognizing this associated parenchymal injury pattern is essential to accurately characterizing the full extent of a child's traumatic brain injury rather than reporting the subdural collection in isolation. A thin subdural collection identified incidentally, without an accompanying clinical history clearly explaining its presence, warrants the same careful correlation against the child's clinical history and developmental context this chapter has emphasized throughout, since this specific, incidental finding pattern can, in certain circumstances, itself represent the presenting sign of the abusive head trauma discussed in this chapter's next section rather than a truly isolated, mechanistically unexplained finding.

Diffuse Axonal Injury

Diffuse axonal injury, resulting from rotational acceleration-deceleration forces producing shearing injury at the interface between tissues of differing density, most characteristically the gray-white matter junction, corpus callosum, and dorsolateral brainstem, frequently shows a disproportionately severe clinical presentation relative to the sometimes subtle findings visible on conventional CT, and MRI, particularly susceptibility-weighted or gradient-echo sequences sensitive to the microhemorrhage this injury characteristically produces, and diffusion tensor imaging, are substantially more sensitive than CT for detecting this specific injury pattern; recognizing that a normal or near-normal CT does not exclude significant diffuse axonal injury in a child with a clinical presentation disproportionately severe relative to the CT findings should prompt MRI evaluation applying this more sensitive imaging approach, particularly once the child is stable enough to safely undergo this generally longer acquisition. The specific number, size, and location of microhemorrhagic foci identified on susceptibility-weighted imaging correlates broadly, though imperfectly, with injury severity and expected outcome, and quantifying this lesion burden using a structured, systematic count rather than a purely qualitative impression provides a more objective basis for both prognostic counseling and any research or outcomes-tracking application this specific imaging characterization might serve.

Skull Fracture Patterns and Their Clinical Significance

Skull fracture characterization, including whether a fracture is linear, depressed, or diastatic, and whether it crosses a vascular groove or dural venous sinus, carries direct clinical significance beyond the fracture itself, since a fracture crossing the middle meningeal artery groove or a major venous sinus carries an elevated risk of the epidural hematoma or venous sinus injury discussed elsewhere in this section, and a depressed fracture, particularly one depressed by more than the calvarial thickness, carries a distinct risk of direct cortical injury and, at times, warrants surgical elevation; three-dimensional reconstruction, applying the same technique discussed in Chapter 8 for craniosynostosis evaluation, assists in fully characterizing complex fracture patterns and their relationship to these specific adjacent vascular and dural structures. A diastatic fracture, in which the fracture line extends through and separates an adjacent cranial suture, carries particular relevance in the infant and young child given the open sutures characteristic of this age group, and recognizing this specific fracture pattern, together with its potential to widen further over time analogous in mechanism to the growing skull fracture phenomenon this section addresses next, supports the same structured follow-up imaging approach this section emphasizes for other fracture patterns carrying a delayed complication risk.

Growing Skull Fracture as a Delayed Complication

Growing skull fracture, a rare but well-recognized delayed complication occurring almost exclusively in a young infant with an associated dural tear at the time of the original fracture, results from progressive herniation of leptomeningeal and, at times, brain tissue through the dural defect, producing progressive widening of the fracture line on serial imaging over weeks to months following the initial injury; recognizing this specific, delayed complication in an infant with a skull fracture and, particularly, radiographic evidence of an associated dural tear at initial presentation supports the structured follow-up imaging this specific injury pattern warrants, since early surgical repair of the dural defect, once this complication is identified, prevents the further, progressive tissue herniation this condition would otherwise produce.

Diffuse Cerebral Edema and Herniation

Severe traumatic brain injury can produce diffuse cerebral edema and, in its most severe form, herniation across the falx, tentorium, or foramen magnum, findings requiring the same urgent recognition and communication this book has emphasized throughout for other acute, life-threatening intracranial processes; recognizing the specific pattern of herniation identified, subfalcine, uncal, or tonsillar, directly informs the specific, urgent neurosurgical intervention required, and communicating this finding immediately and directly to the treating team, applying the urgent-communication principle established in Chapter 1, takes clear precedence over the routine, asynchronous reporting workflow appropriate for a non-urgent finding.

Coordinating Trauma Imaging Within the Broader Resuscitation

Acute pediatric head trauma evaluation frequently occurs within the context of a broader trauma resuscitation addressing potential multisystem injury, and coordinating the specific timing and sequence of neuroimaging within this broader trauma evaluation, applying the same coordinated, multidisciplinary team principle this book has emphasized throughout, ensures that a child's neurologic evaluation proceeds efficiently alongside, rather than in unnecessary competition with, the evaluation of other potential injuries this specific trauma mechanism may have produced.

Figure 19.1: Epidural Versus Subdural Hematoma Morphology

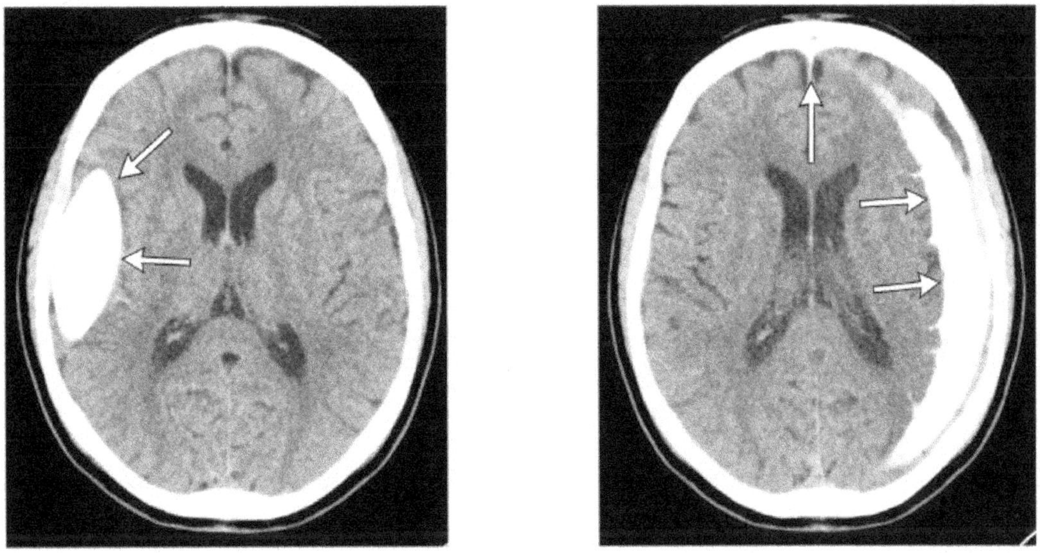

Epidural Hematoma
(biconvex, suture-limited)

Subdural Hematoma
(crescentic, midline-limited)

Feature	Epidural Hematoma	Subdural Hematoma
Shape	Biconvex (lens-shaped)	Crescentic
Crosses sutures	No	Yes

Crosses midline (falx/tentorium)	No	No
Associated parenchymal injury	Less common	More common

Abusive Head Trauma

Abusive head trauma represents one of the most consequential diagnoses this book addresses, carrying both severe, potentially fatal medical implications for the affected child and profound legal and child-protective implications, and this section develops the specific constellation of imaging findings, together with the required multidisciplinary evaluation, this diagnosis demands. Because the stakes of both under-diagnosis, leaving a child at risk of continued abuse, and over-diagnosis, wrongly implicating an innocent caregiver, are each so severe, this section places particular emphasis throughout on evidence-calibrated, appropriately bounded claims rather than overconfident pattern-recognition alone.

The Triad and Its Modern Reconceptualization

The classic triad historically associated with abusive head trauma, subdural hemorrhage, retinal hemorrhage, and encephalopathy, remains clinically relevant but is now understood within a broader, more nuanced framework incorporating the full constellation of findings this section develops, since the triad alone, considered in isolation from this broader clinical and radiographic context, is neither perfectly sensitive nor perfectly specific for abuse; a comprehensive, multidisciplinary evaluation integrating imaging findings, the specific pattern and stated mechanism of injury, developmental capability of the child, and the required skeletal and ophthalmologic evaluation this section addresses, rather than the triad in isolation, provides the most reliable basis for this significant diagnostic determination. This evolution in medical understanding, from a simple, checklist-style triad toward a comprehensive, integrated, multidisciplinary determination, reflects the same broader shift toward converging, multimodal evidence this book has emphasized across numerous other complex diagnostic categories, and a clinician who applies only the historical triad in isolation, without the fuller evaluation this section develops, risks both under- and over-diagnosis relative to the current, evidence-based standard of care.

Multifocal, Mixed-Age Subdural Hemorrhage

Multifocal subdural hemorrhage, particularly when bilateral, and hemorrhage of differing signal characteristics suggesting different ages, are findings carrying particular weight in the abusive head trauma evaluation, since these specific patterns are less well explained by a single, isolated accidental impact than by the repetitive or rotational acceleration-deceleration mechanism characteristic of abusive injury; interhemispheric subdural hemorrhage specifically, layering along the falx, is a further, characteristic finding in this context, and susceptibility-weighted imaging, applying the technique discussed throughout this book for its sensitivity to blood products, assists in fully characterizing the specific extent and apparent age distribution of hemorrhage this evaluation requires. Subdural hemorrhage of varying thickness across different intracranial locations, rather than a single, uniform collection, is a further pattern worth noting explicitly in the structured report, since this specific heterogeneity, considered alongside the mixed-signal-characteristic pattern already discussed, provides additional supportive detail for the comprehensive, multidisciplinary evaluation this section has emphasized throughout, though, consistent with the dating-limitation discussion that follows, this heterogeneity alone does not establish a precise injury timeline.

The Critical Limitation of Subdural Hemorrhage Dating

While the general concept of mixed-age hemorrhage carries diagnostic weight, precisely dating a specific subdural collection based on its signal characteristics alone carries substantial, well-documented uncertainty, since the imaging appearance of blood products depends on numerous factors beyond age alone, including hemorrhage volume, oxygenation, and the possibility of rebleeding into a chronic collection; this book's broader commitment to honest, evidence-calibrated communication requires the reader to resist over-interpreting subdural signal characteristics as providing a precise, narrow dating window, and instead characterizing findings using the more defensible, broader terminology, acute, subacute, or chronic, that the current evidence base genuinely supports, since overstating dating precision in this specific, legally consequential context carries genuine harm potential in either direction, wrongly implicating an innocent caregiver or wrongly exonerating a truly abusive one. This specific epistemic humility, resisting the temptation to offer a precise timeframe the underlying science cannot actually support, exemplifies the same evidence-calibrated communication discipline this book has emphasized throughout, applied here in a context where the consequences of overstatement are unusually severe and directly bear on legal determinations extending well beyond the medical record itself.

Parenchymal Injury Patterns in Abusive Head Trauma

Beyond the extra-axial hemorrhage emphasized above, abusive head trauma frequently produces a distinctive pattern of diffuse hypoxic-ischemic injury, applying the injury mechanism and imaging recognition developed in Chapter 4, believed to reflect a combination of direct impact, rotational shearing injury, and, in some cases, an associated apneic or hypoxic episode accompanying the abusive event; this specific, diffuse hypoxic-ischemic pattern, occurring in a young infant without the typical perinatal risk factors discussed in Chapter 4 that would otherwise explain this finding, should itself prompt active consideration of an abusive mechanism, extending this chapter's diagnostic reasoning beyond the hemorrhagic findings this section has primarily emphasized. Cervical spine and cervicomedullary junction injury, less commonly recognized than the intracranial findings this section has emphasized but increasingly appreciated as a component of the abusive head trauma injury spectrum, particularly in the context of violent shaking mechanisms, warrants dedicated evaluation of this specific anatomic region whenever abusive head trauma is suspected, applying the same complete, systematic anatomic survey principle this chapter has emphasized throughout for both the skeletal and now this additional spinal component of the comprehensive evaluation.

The Mandatory Skeletal Survey

A complete skeletal survey, a systematic series of radiographs imaging the entire skeleton according to a standardized protocol, is a mandatory, non-negotiable component of the evaluation for suspected abusive head trauma in an infant or young child, since occult fractures, particularly classic metaphyseal lesions and posterior rib fractures, both carrying high specificity for abusive mechanism, are frequently identified on this systematic survey despite an entirely unremarkable physical examination; a skeletal survey is never omitted based on an reassuring physical examination alone, and a follow-up skeletal survey two weeks after the initial study is standard practice given that some fractures, particularly subtle rib fractures, become more conspicuous as healing callus develops, improving detection sensitivity beyond the initial study alone. The classic metaphyseal lesion specifically, a distinctive fracture pattern through the metaphysis of a long bone reflecting a shearing or traction mechanism rather than a direct impact, is considered among the most specific individual skeletal findings for abusive mechanism in the published literature, and posterior rib fractures, believed to arise from squeezing compression of the chest, similarly carry high specificity given the substantial force and specific mechanism required to fracture a rib at this particular location in a young, still-elastic pediatric rib cage.

Ophthalmologic Evaluation for Retinal Hemorrhage

Dilated indirect ophthalmoscopic examination by an ophthalmologist experienced in pediatric retinal examination, rather than a non-specialist funduscopic examination alone, is a further mandatory component of the abusive head trauma evaluation, since retinal hemorrhage, particularly when extensive, multilayered, and extending to the peripheral retina, carries substantial diagnostic weight and is best characterized by this specific, detailed specialist examination rather than imaging; retinal hemorrhage from abusive head trauma classically differs in extent and pattern from the more limited retinal hemorrhage that can accompany a normal vaginal delivery or accidental trauma, and this specific, detailed characterization by an experienced pediatric ophthalmologist, rather than a general statement of retinal hemorrhage present, provides the diagnostically meaningful detail this evaluation requires. This ophthalmologic examination is most informative when performed promptly, ideally within the first several days following presentation, since retinal hemorrhage, similar to several of the other acute findings addressed throughout this book, resolves over time, and a delayed examination risks missing or understating the true initial extent of hemorrhage present, underscoring why this evaluation is coordinated urgently alongside, rather than deferred until after, the imaging and skeletal survey this section has otherwise emphasized.

The Multidisciplinary Child Protection Team

Given the profound medical, legal, and child-protective stakes this diagnosis carries, evaluation and determination regarding suspected abusive head trauma is conducted through a dedicated, multidisciplinary child protection team incorporating child abuse pediatrics, radiology, neurosurgery, ophthalmology, and social work, rather than a single clinician's independent determination, applying the same multidisciplinary, converging-evidence principle this book has emphasized throughout to this specific, uniquely consequential diagnostic context; this team-based approach ensures the full constellation of findings this section has developed, imaging, skeletal survey, ophthalmologic examination, and the specific clinical history and developmental context, is integrated systematically rather than any single component driving a premature, insufficiently supported conclusion in either direction.

Developmental Capability and Mechanism Plausibility

Correlating a child's specific developmental capability, whether the child could plausibly have accomplished the described mechanism independently, such as an infant who cannot yet roll independently reportedly having rolled off furniture, against the stated history is a further, essential component of the comprehensive determination this section has developed, and this specific developmental-plausibility assessment, typically established through careful history-taking and, where needed, direct developmental assessment, provides an additional, independent line of evidence beyond the imaging findings this section has otherwise emphasized; a stated mechanism requiring a developmental capability the child does not yet possess is a significant, specific inconsistency warranting the same careful, multidisciplinary scrutiny this chapter has applied to biomechanically implausible injury severity.

Documentation Standards in Suspected Abusive Head Trauma

Given the legal proceedings a confirmed abusive head trauma diagnosis frequently initiates, precise, structured, and objectively worded documentation of every imaging finding, using the specific descriptive terminology this section has developed rather than a conclusory or interpretive shorthand, supports both the immediate multidisciplinary determination process and any subsequent legal proceedings that may draw upon this documentation months or years after the original evaluation; a radiology report stating specifically what is seen, the location, extent, and specific signal characteristics of each hemorrhage identified, rather than a report that states only findings consistent with abuse without this underlying descriptive detail, provides the more defensible, clinically and legally useful documentation this specific diagnostic context requires.

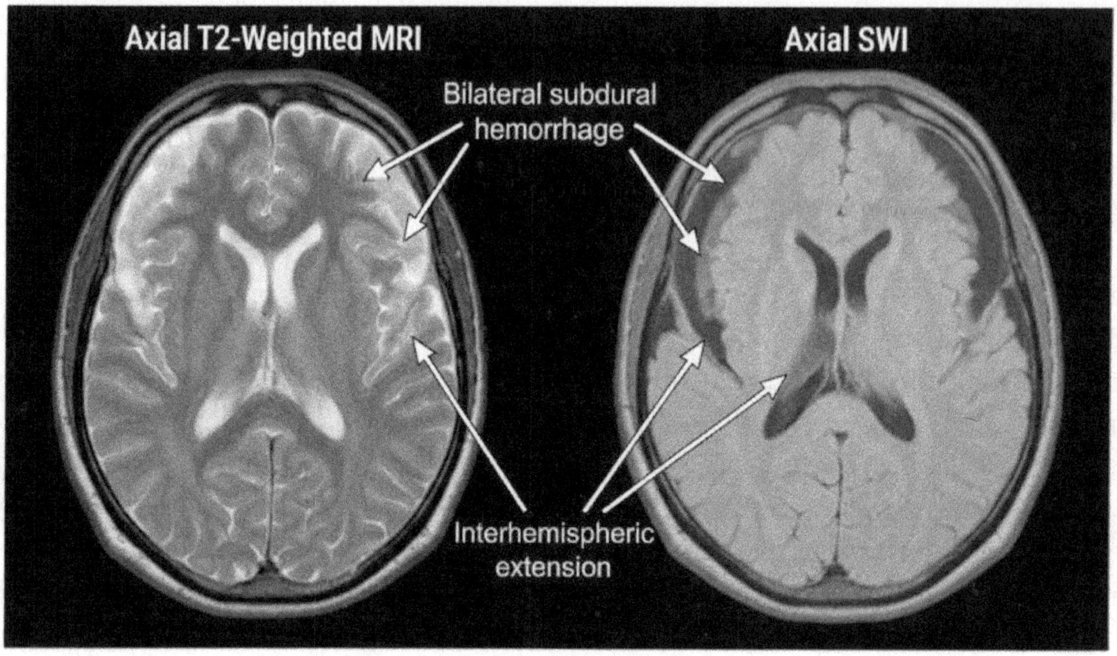

Figure 19.2: Mixed-Age Subdural Hemorrhage in Abusive Head Trauma

THE CLINICAL-IMAGING CROSSWALK SYSTEM — A Stated Mechanism Inconsistent With the Injury Severity

The Crossing: A four-month-old presents with lethargy and a bulging fontanelle, and the caregiver reports the infant rolled off a low couch, and brain MRI demonstrates extensive, mixed-age bilateral subdural hemorrhage with diffuse hypoxic-ischemic injury.

Presentation Signature: A young infant with severe intracranial findings disproportionate to a stated low-severity accidental mechanism.

Imaging Correlate: The multidisciplinary child protection team reviews the imaging alongside the stated mechanism, noting that a short fall of this described type is well documented in the biomechanical literature to rarely, if ever, produce this specific severity and pattern of injury, and the complete skeletal survey and dilated ophthalmologic examination this chapter has emphasized are obtained in parallel.

Trap Logic: Accepting a stated mechanism at face value without correlating it against the known biomechanical literature regarding the injury severity a given mechanism can plausibly produce risks overlooking a case of abusive head trauma, delaying the protective intervention this diagnosis, once appropriately supported, requires.

Crossing Anchor: A stated mechanism should be actively correlated against the known biomechanical plausibility of the resulting injury severity and pattern; a significant mismatch, considered alongside the full multidisciplinary evaluation this chapter has developed, is a component of the comprehensive determination process rather than dismissed in favor of the stated history alone.

Spinal Cord and Spine Trauma

This section addresses pediatric spinal cord and spine trauma, with particular attention to the distinct biomechanical vulnerability of the pediatric cervical spine and the specific phenomenon of spinal cord injury without radiographic abnormality, extending this chapter's traumatic injury framework into the spinal axis. The specific biomechanical reasoning this section develops, explaining why the pediatric spine responds to trauma differently than the adult spine, mirrors the same age-specific structural and developmental reasoning this book has applied throughout, from the fontanelle-mediated compensation discussed in Chapter 10 to the cervical spine considerations addressed here.

The Distinct Biomechanics of the Pediatric Cervical Spine

The pediatric cervical spine, particularly in the young child, differs biomechanically from the adult cervical spine in ways carrying direct injury-pattern implications, including a relatively large head-to-body ratio producing greater rotational and flexion-extension forces at the craniocervical junction, incompletely ossified vertebral bodies and ligamentous laxity permitting greater mobility without a corresponding bony fracture, and a fulcrum of maximal spinal mobility located more cranially, at the upper cervical spine, than the mid-to-lower cervical fulcrum more typical of the adult spine; these combined biomechanical differences explain why young children show a disproportionate predilection for upper cervical and craniocervical junction injury relative to the lower cervical injury pattern more typical of adolescents and adults, a distributional difference worth holding in mind when characterizing a pediatric spine trauma imaging study. This same fulcrum shift, migrating progressively caudally as a child grows and the cervical spine's proportions and ossification pattern increasingly approach the adult configuration, means the specific injury distribution pattern this section describes is itself age-dependent within the pediatric population, and an adolescent's cervical spine injury pattern more closely resembles the adult pattern than the young child's pattern this section has primarily emphasized, a further, specific age-stratification worth incorporating into the reader's overall diagnostic reasoning for this anatomic region.

Spinal Cord Injury Without Radiographic Abnormality

Spinal cord injury without radiographic abnormality, commonly termed SCIWORA, describes a clinical spinal cord injury occurring in the absence of a fracture or malalignment visible on plain radiography or CT, a phenomenon disproportionately affecting the pediatric population given the specific biomechanical properties discussed above, in which the elastic, incompletely ossified pediatric spinal column can transiently deform sufficiently to injure the enclosed, far less elastic spinal cord without sustaining a persistent, radiographically visible bony or ligamentous injury itself; MRI, rather than the radiography or CT that would appear falsely reassuring in this specific circumstance, is the essential diagnostic tool for characterizing the underlying cord injury in a child with a clinical presentation concerning for spinal cord injury and a nondiagnostic or normal plain radiographic and CT evaluation. A delayed or evolving neurologic deficit following spine trauma, presenting hours after the initial injury rather than immediately, is a further, specific presentation pattern associated with this phenomenon, believed to reflect ongoing microvascular or edematous injury evolution following the initial transient deformation, and this specific delayed-onset possibility should prompt a low threshold for MRI evaluation in a child with a concerning trauma mechanism even when an initial examination shortly after injury appears reassuringly normal.

MRI Characterization of Cord Injury Severity

MRI characterization of the spinal cord itself, assessing for cord edema, hemorrhage, and the specific length of cord signal abnormality, provides essential prognostic information beyond what the bony and ligamentous imaging this section has otherwise emphasized can offer, since the specific pattern and extent of cord signal change correlates meaningfully with expected functional outcome; cord hemorrhage specifically, visible as susceptibility artifact on gradient-echo or susceptibility-weighted sequences, generally carries a less favorable prognosis than isolated cord edema without hemorrhage, and communicating this specific, imaging-derived prognostic information honestly to a family, applying the honest, proportionate communication principle this book has emphasized throughout, supports informed family understanding and appropriate rehabilitation planning from the earliest stage of this child's recovery. The specific cranial-caudal length of cord signal abnormality similarly carries independent prognostic weight, with a longer segment of involved cord generally associated with more significant, persistent functional impairment than a shorter, more focal segment of signal change, and reporting this specific length measurement explicitly, rather than a qualitative description alone, provides the rehabilitation and neurosurgical teams with the precise, quantitative information this specific prognostic counseling depends upon.

Craniocervical Junction Injury

Craniocervical junction injury, including atlanto-occipital dissociation, a severe and frequently fatal injury reflecting complete ligamentous disruption between the skull base and upper cervical spine, carries particular relevance to the young child given the biomechanical predilection for upper cervical injury this section has discussed, and specific imaging measurements, including the Powers ratio and the basion-dens interval, provide objective, standardized criteria for identifying this specific, life-threatening injury pattern; recognizing the young child's specific vulnerability to this severe craniocervical injury pattern, and applying these standardized measurement criteria systematically rather than relying on subjective visual assessment of alignment alone, is essential given both this injury's severity and the subtlety with which it can present on imaging in a child who has, remarkably, survived the initial injury. Prevertebral soft tissue swelling at the craniocervical junction, while a nonspecific finding that can accompany numerous cervical spine injuries, is a further, complementary clue worth actively assessing when this severe injury pattern is suspected, since its presence, alongside the specific standardized measurements this section has emphasized, provides additional supportive evidence for a significant craniocervical junction injury even when the primary alignment measurements themselves fall in a borderline or ambiguous range.

Pediatric Spine Trauma Imaging Protocol

Imaging evaluation for suspected pediatric spine trauma is generally guided by validated clinical decision rules analogous to the head trauma decision rules discussed earlier in this chapter, with CT reserved for a child meeting specific high-risk criteria or one in whom plain radiography reveals or leaves genuine ambiguity regarding a bony injury, and MRI reserved for a child with a clinical presentation concerning for spinal cord injury regardless of the bony imaging findings, applying the SCIWORA reasoning this section has developed; this graduated, risk-stratified imaging approach, applying the same evidence-based imaging-ordering discipline this book has emphasized throughout, balances the genuine importance of not missing a significant spine injury against the radiation stewardship principle established in Chapter 1, particularly relevant given this population's cumulative lifetime radiation exposure risk.

Cervical Spine Immobilization Considerations During Imaging

A child undergoing spine trauma imaging requires appropriate cervical immobilization maintained throughout the imaging process, and the specific immobilization device used, whether a rigid collar or another stabilization approach, must accommodate the young child's proportionally larger head, since a standard, adult-proportioned immobilization device applied without this specific pediatric adaptation can itself produce inappropriate flexion or extension at the cervical spine, potentially confounding the imaging assessment or, in a genuinely unstable injury, worsening the underlying injury itself; coordinating this specific, pediatric-appropriate immobilization technique with the imaging team before and throughout image acquisition reflects the same careful, age-adapted technical attention this book has emphasized throughout for numerous other pediatric-specific imaging considerations.

Ligamentous Injury Without Fracture

Beyond the SCIWORA phenomenon addressing spinal cord injury specifically, the pediatric spine's inherent ligamentous laxity discussed earlier in this section similarly permits significant ligamentous injury to occur without an accompanying fracture, and dedicated MRI characterization of the paraspinal and interspinous ligaments, assessing for edema and discontinuity, is warranted when clinical suspicion for a significant ligamentous injury persists despite normal or equivocal bony imaging, since an unrecognized, unstable ligamentous injury carries its own distinct risk of delayed neurologic deterioration if not identified and appropriately managed, whether through external immobilization or surgical stabilization, at the time of initial evaluation.

Figure 19.3: Craniocervical Junction Measurement Criteria

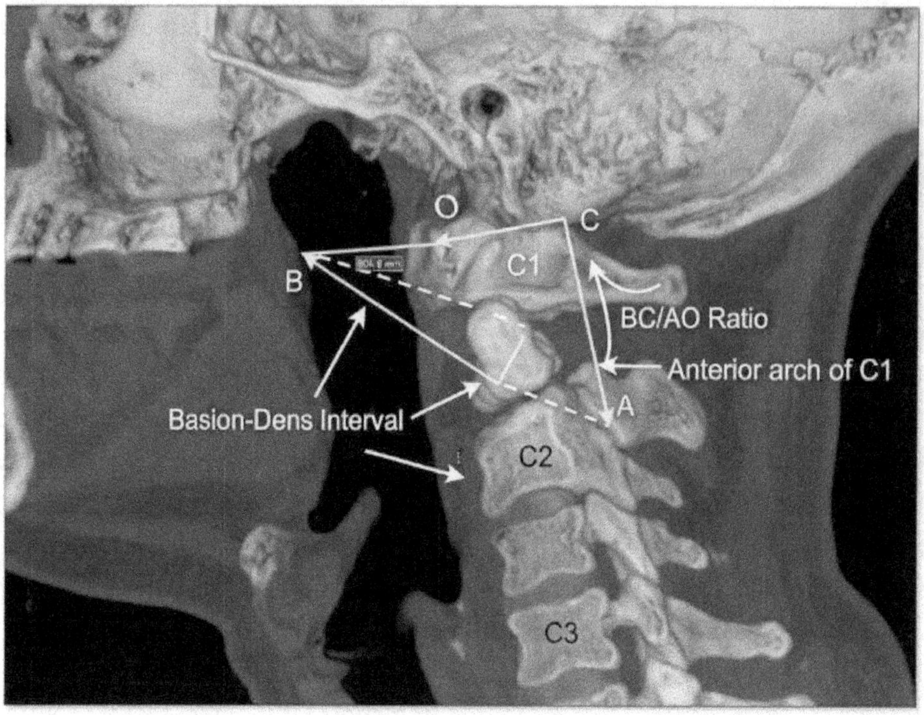

Postconcussive and Chronic Traumatic Findings

This closing section addresses the expected imaging trajectory following concussion and mild traumatic brain injury, together with the chronic imaging findings that can follow more severe injury, distinguishing expected, self-limited postconcussive findings from chronic change warranting further evaluation. This closing focus on distinguishing expected from concerning chronic change echoes the same interpretive discipline this book has cultivated across every preceding chapter, and its placement as this chapter's final section deliberately positions this durable, transferable skill as the reader's last, cumulative takeaway from this book's complete survey of pediatric neuroimaging.

Concussion as Primarily a Clinical Diagnosis

Concussion, or mild traumatic brain injury, is fundamentally a clinical diagnosis based on the specific constellation of symptoms following head trauma, and conventional structural imaging, when obtained, is expected to be normal in the great majority of cases, meaning a normal CT or MRI does not exclude a genuine, clinically significant concussion; applying the same exclusionary imaging role this book has developed for several other primarily clinical diagnoses, imaging in suspected concussion serves principally to exclude a more severe, structural injury requiring urgent intervention rather than to positively confirm the concussion diagnosis itself, and a family should be counseled clearly that a normal imaging result is an expected, reassuring finding in this specific context rather than evidence against the clinical diagnosis their child has received. The specific validated clinical decision rules discussed earlier in this chapter guide the decision regarding whether imaging is even warranted in a specific concussion presentation, and the great majority of children presenting with an isolated, uncomplicated concussion and no other red-flag clinical feature this chapter has developed do not require any structural imaging at all, reinforcing that the absence of imaging in this specific, common clinical scenario reflects appropriate, evidence-based practice rather than an incomplete evaluation.

Advanced Imaging in Research and Selected Clinical Contexts

Advanced imaging techniques, including diffusion tensor imaging and functional MRI, have identified subtle, statistically detectable white matter and functional connectivity changes following concussion in research settings, though these specific techniques remain investigational tools rather than validated, routine clinical diagnostic instruments for an individual child's concussion diagnosis or recovery monitoring; a family or clinician should understand this distinction clearly, since a normal conventional structural study, applying the standard clinical imaging approach this section has emphasized, remains the appropriate, validated clinical evaluation regardless of ongoing research interest in these more advanced, still-investigational techniques. This distinction between promising research findings and validated clinical practice, worth naming explicitly, mirrors a broader theme in medicine generally in which an active, evolving research literature does not automatically translate into an immediately actionable clinical tool, and this book's broader commitment to evidence-calibrated, honestly bounded claims applies with particular relevance to this specific, actively researched but not yet clinically validated application.

Encephalomalacia and Gliosis After Severe Injury

Following more severe traumatic brain injury, chronic imaging findings including focal encephalomalacia, volume loss with associated gliotic signal change reflecting the brain's chronic response to the original injury, and, at times, hemosiderin staining from prior hemorrhage, represent the expected, stable chronic sequelae of the original acute injury rather than an active, ongoing process requiring further evaluation; recognizing these findings as the anticipated chronic residua of a known prior injury, applying the same expected-versus-concerning chronic imaging change discrimination this book has developed for several other conditions with an established structural injury history, prevents unnecessary additional evaluation for a stable, well-explained chronic finding. Wallerian degeneration, a specific pattern of signal change along a white matter tract distal to the site of original axonal injury, reflecting the tract's gradual, predictable degeneration once its cell bodies or proximal axons have been disrupted, is a further, characteristic chronic finding worth recognizing explicitly as an expected downstream consequence of the original injury rather than evidence of an independent, ongoing pathologic process.

Post-Traumatic Epilepsy and Its Imaging Correlate

Post-traumatic epilepsy, a recognized long-term complication of moderate-to-severe traumatic brain injury, arises with particular frequency from injury involving the temporal lobe or from a region of chronic encephalomalacia and gliosis, applying the epileptogenic-lesion reasoning developed in Chapter 11 to this specific, trauma-related structural substrate, and a child with a known chronic post-traumatic structural change who develops new seizures warrants the dedicated epilepsy-protocol imaging discussed in Chapter 11, correlating the seizure semiology and electroencephalographic findings against the specific location of the known chronic traumatic change, applying the same clinical-imaging correlation principle this book's Crosswalk System embodies throughout. The latency period between the original traumatic injury and the eventual onset of post-traumatic epilepsy can extend from months to several years, meaning a family should be counseled regarding this delayed, ongoing risk at the time of the original injury rather than assuming the absence of early seizures indicates this specific long-term risk has been avoided, and structured, longitudinal neurologic follow up extending well beyond the acute and subacute recovery period this chapter has otherwise emphasized remains appropriate for a child with a significant traumatic brain injury history given this specific, delayed complication risk.

Distinguishing New Injury From Chronic Change on Repeat Imaging

A child with a known chronic traumatic brain injury presenting with a new, acute clinical change requires careful comparison of the current imaging study against the child's own established chronic baseline, applying the same baseline-comparison principle this book has emphasized throughout for numerous other conditions requiring longitudinal surveillance, since a new, acute finding superimposed on a stable chronic background carries fundamentally different clinical significance than an unchanged, expected chronic finding; obtaining and clearly documenting a stable baseline study once the acute injury has fully evolved provides the essential comparison reference this future evaluation depends upon, reinforcing why establishing this documented baseline is not merely an administrative formality but a genuine, forward-looking clinical investment in this child's future care.

Return-to-Play and Return-to-Learn Considerations

Following concussion, structured, graduated return-to-play and return-to-learn protocols, guiding a child's progressive return to physical and cognitive activity based on symptom resolution rather than a fixed, calendar-based timeline alone, represent the current evidence-based management standard, and imaging plays essentially no role in guiding this specific, symptom-based return-to-activity decision given the normal expected imaging appearance this section has emphasized throughout; a family seeking imaging-based clearance before a child returns to a specific activity should be counseled that this specific decision is appropriately guided by the structured clinical assessment this paragraph describes rather than a repeat imaging study, which would not be expected to add meaningful information to this specific return-to-activity determination.

Repetitive Head Injury and Second Impact Syndrome

Second impact syndrome, a rare but catastrophic phenomenon in which a second head injury sustained before full recovery from an initial concussion produces severe, rapidly progressive cerebral edema, underscores the genuine clinical importance of the structured, symptom-based return-to-activity protocols discussed above, and recognizing this rare but severe complication risk, while its precise underlying mechanism remains incompletely understood, has directly motivated the conservative, evidence-based return-to-play standards this section has emphasized throughout, protecting a child from repeat injury during the period of heightened vulnerability that follows an initial concussion.

Case Presentation: SCIWORA in a Young Child Following a Motor Vehicle Collision

A three-year-old restrained in an age-appropriate car seat presents with bilateral lower extremity weakness following a motor vehicle collision, and CT of the cervical spine demonstrates no fracture or malalignment. Applying the reasoning developed in this chapter, given the clinical presentation concerning for spinal cord injury despite the reassuring CT, dedicated spine MRI is obtained and demonstrates cord edema at the mid-thoracic level without associated hemorrhage, confirming spinal cord injury without radiographic abnormality. The family is counseled regarding the specific biomechanical vulnerability of the pediatric spine this chapter has developed, explaining why the normal CT does not exclude the confirmed cord injury now identified on MRI, and the absence of hemorrhage on the MRI is discussed as a relatively more favorable prognostic feature, applying the reasoning developed in this chapter, while acknowledging the genuine uncertainty regarding this child's ultimate functional recovery that remains despite this specific, favorable imaging feature. Structured, longitudinal rehabilitation is initiated promptly, and a documented baseline MRI is scheduled once the acute injury has stabilized, applying the same baseline-establishment principle this chapter has emphasized throughout, to serve as the reference study for any future evaluation this child may require.

Case Presentation: Multidisciplinary Evaluation Confirming Abusive Head Trauma

A two-month-old presents with seizures and lethargy, and brain MRI demonstrates bilateral, mixed-age subdural hemorrhage with interhemispheric extension and diffuse hypoxic-ischemic injury, without a history of significant trauma reported by the caregivers. Applying the reasoning developed in this chapter, the multidisciplinary child protection team is engaged, and a complete skeletal survey identifies healing posterior rib fractures and a classic metaphyseal lesion of the distal femur, findings not disclosed in the initial history and carrying high specificity for abusive mechanism. Dilated ophthalmologic examination confirms extensive, multilayered retinal hemorrhage extending to the periphery bilaterally. Applying the comprehensive, multidisciplinary determination framework developed in this chapter, the constellation of imaging, skeletal, and ophthalmologic findings, considered together and correlated against the absence of an adequate explanatory history, supports a determination of abusive head trauma, and the family is engaged with the child protection and legal systems this diagnosis requires, illustrating the complete, integrated evaluation pathway this chapter has developed for this uniquely consequential diagnostic category. A follow-up skeletal survey obtained two weeks later, applying the standard protocol this chapter has emphasized, identifies an additional, previously subtle healing rib fracture not clearly appreciated on the initial study, further reinforcing the diagnostic picture and the specific value of this structured, interval follow-up imaging component.

THE CLINICAL-IMAGING CROSSWALK SYSTEM — Traumatic Brain and Spine Injury Recognition

Crossing 1 Recap: A stated mechanism should be actively correlated against the known biomechanical plausibility of the resulting injury severity and pattern, considered alongside the full multidisciplinary evaluation rather than accepted or dismissed in isolation.

Chapter Anchor: Pediatric traumatic injury evaluation requires morphology-based hematoma discrimination, comprehensive multidisciplinary evaluation for suspected abuse, biomechanically informed spine injury recognition including SCIWORA, and confident distinction between expected chronic sequelae and new, acute change, each directing a distinct, evidence-based evaluation and communication pathway.

Summary and Key Concepts

Validated clinical decision rules guide pediatric head trauma imaging; epidural hematoma is biconvex and suture-limited while subdural hematoma is crescentic and midline-limited, and diffuse axonal injury requires MRI given its frequent CT-occult presentation despite severe clinical findings.

Abusive head trauma diagnosis depends on a comprehensive, multidisciplinary evaluation integrating multifocal mixed-age subdural hemorrhage, a mandatory skeletal survey, and dilated ophthalmologic examination, with subdural hemorrhage dating limited to broad, defensible categories rather than precise timeframes.

The pediatric cervical spine's distinct biomechanics predispose to upper cervical and craniocervical junction injury; SCIWORA requires MRI given normal radiography and CT, and cord hemorrhage carries a less favorable prognosis than isolated edema.

Concussion is a clinical diagnosis for which normal imaging is expected and reassuring rather than concerning; chronic encephalomalacia and gliosis after severe injury represent expected, stable sequelae serving as the baseline for detecting genuinely new, acute change.

Post-traumatic epilepsy arises from chronic structural injury, particularly temporal lobe involvement, applying the epileptogenic-lesion reasoning developed in Chapter 11; across this chapter, careful comparison against an established baseline distinguishes expected chronic findings from new, clinically significant change.

CHAPTER 20: HEADACHE, MACROCEPHALY, AND MICROCEPHALY

Learning Objectives

1. Apply evidence-based imaging-ordering criteria to a child presenting with headache, distinguishing red-flag features from low-yield presentations and recognizing when a prior negative evaluation warrants reconsideration.
2. Generate an age-appropriate differential diagnosis for macrocephaly and describe the evaluation this presentation warrants, including the distinction between stable and crossing-percentiles growth trajectories.
3. Generate a differential diagnosis for microcephaly based on its timing (congenital versus acquired) and associated imaging findings, and distinguish true microcephaly from craniosynostosis-related cranial restriction.
4. Synthesize the presentation-based, clinical-imaging correlation framework developed throughout this book into a unified approach applicable to any new pediatric neuroimaging presentation.

Headache: Imaging-Ordering Decisions

Headache is among the most common presenting complaints in pediatric neurology, and the overwhelming majority of pediatric headache reflects a primary headache disorder, migraine or tension-type headache, rather than an underlying structural lesion, making the central diagnostic task this section addresses the reliable identification of the small minority of children whose headache warrants neuroimaging. This section opens this book's final chapter deliberately, since headache exemplifies with particular clarity this book's central, recurring lesson, that confident, evidence-based restraint in the great majority of presentations is precisely what preserves the diagnostic urgency and clinical attention the genuinely concerning minority of presentations require.

Red-Flag Features Warranting Imaging

A defined set of red-flag clinical features, applying the same evidence-based imaging-ordering framework established in Chapter 3, meaningfully increases the likelihood of an underlying structural cause and should prompt neuroimaging: headache that wakes a child from sleep or is worse upon waking, headache accompanied by persistent vomiting without an alternative explanation, a focal neurologic deficit or papilledema on examination, headache in a child younger than six years given the lower baseline prevalence of primary headache disorders in this age group, a progressive, worsening headache pattern rather than a stable, recurrent one, and headache occurring in a child with a known risk factor discussed elsewhere in this book, including neurofibromatosis type 1 or a prior brain tumor history; the presence of any one of these specific features, rather than headache severity or frequency alone, is what should drive the imaging-ordering decision. A new, distinctly different headache pattern in a child with a pre-existing, well-characterized primary headache disorder is itself a further red-flag feature worth explicit recognition, since this specific change from an established baseline pattern, applying the same baseline-comparison principle this book has emphasized throughout, carries diagnostic weight independent of whether the new pattern individually meets any of the other criteria this paragraph has named.

The Low Yield of Imaging Without Red-Flag Features

A child with a stable, recurrent headache pattern consistent with migraine or tension-type headache, a normal neurologic examination, and none of the red-flag features this section has developed carries a very low likelihood of an underlying structural cause, and published evidence consistently demonstrates minimal diagnostic yield from neuroimaging in this specific, low-risk presentation; applying the evidence-based, low-yield-presentation reasoning developed in Chapter 3 to this specific, extremely common clinical scenario, and confidently reassuring a family regarding the appropriateness of forgoing imaging in this circumstance, exemplifies this book's broader commitment to imaging decisions grounded in evidence rather than reflexive anxiety-driven ordering. A detailed, structured headache history, systematically eliciting each of the red-flag features this section has developed rather than an open-ended, unstructured inquiry alone, is the essential clinical tool underlying this entire evaluation framework, and a clinician applying this structured approach consistently, rather than an intuitive impression alone, achieves the most reliable, reproducible application of the evidence-based criteria this section has established.

Migraine With Aura and Its Imaging Considerations

Migraine with aura, in which a child experiences transient visual, sensory, or, less commonly, motor symptoms preceding or accompanying the headache itself, occasionally raises diagnostic uncertainty given its symptomatic overlap with the stroke-like episodes discussed in Chapter 17 and the seizure semiology discussed in Chapter 11, and a first episode of aura, particularly one with an atypical feature such as prolonged duration or a clearly lateralizing motor component, warrants the same careful clinical correlation this book has emphasized throughout rather than an automatic assumption of a benign migrainous mechanism; once a child's specific aura pattern has been established as consistent and stereotyped across multiple episodes, however, this same pattern recurring in a subsequent episode does not require repeat imaging with each occurrence. Familial hemiplegic migraine, a specific, genetically defined migraine subtype producing prolonged, lateralizing motor aura, represents a particular diagnostic consideration when this specific motor aura pattern and a compatible family history are both present, and recognizing this specific entity, rather than presuming either a straightforward migrainous aura or an alternative structural or vascular process without this genetic consideration, exemplifies the same precise, mechanism-specific diagnostic reasoning this book has emphasized throughout even within the broad migraine category.

Headache Associated With a Specific Structural Diagnosis

Several of the structural diagnoses addressed throughout this book present with headache as a prominent or presenting symptom, including the hydrocephalus discussed in Chapter 10, the posterior fossa and other brain tumors discussed in Chapters 12 and 13, and the idiopathic intracranial hypertension discussed in

Chapter 10, and the specific accompanying features distinguishing each of these entities, morning-predominant timing and vomiting for hydrocephalus and posterior fossa tumors, transient visual obscurations and papilledema for idiopathic intracranial hypertension, are worth actively eliciting in the clinical history rather than treating headache as an undifferentiated single presenting symptom; this presentation-to-diagnosis reasoning exemplifies precisely the clinical-imaging correlation this book's Crosswalk System has developed throughout, now applied to headache as this chapter's organizing presenting symptom. Headache associated with the cerebral venous sinus thrombosis discussed in Chapter 6, and the cerebral sinovenous thrombosis discussed further in Chapter 18, represents a further, specific structural cause worth actively considering, particularly in an adolescent with additional risk factors such as oral contraceptive use or an underlying prothrombotic condition, since this specific presentation, headache accompanied by a recognized venous thrombosis risk factor, warrants the dedicated venous imaging evaluation this book has developed in those preceding chapters rather than the standard arterial-focused imaging protocol this section otherwise emphasizes.

Communicating a Negative Imaging Result

When imaging is obtained for headache and returns normal, clearly communicating this reassuring result to the family, while continuing to address the child's headache management through the appropriate primary headache disorder treatment pathway, prevents a family from either dismissing a genuinely reassuring result or, conversely, assuming a normal study means the headache itself is not real or does not warrant continued clinical attention; this specific communication task, ensuring a normal structural study is understood as reassuring regarding the specific, feared structural cause without implying dismissal of the child's genuine, ongoing symptom burden, reflects the honest, proportionate communication principle this book has emphasized throughout applied to this chapter's presenting complaint. Coordinating referral to headache-focused primary care or neurology follow-up once a structural cause has been confidently excluded ensures the child's ongoing symptom burden continues to receive dedicated clinical attention through the appropriate, condition-specific treatment pathway, rather than the family experiencing the normal imaging result as an unsatisfying conclusion to their evaluation with no further, actionable next step offered.

Repeat Imaging for Evolving Headache Presentations

A child with a previously normal headache evaluation whose symptom pattern subsequently evolves to include a new red-flag feature, a change in headache character, or a new examination finding, warrants reconsideration of imaging rather than an assumption that the prior negative evaluation remains permanently applicable regardless of subsequent clinical evolution; applying the same principle this book has emphasized throughout that an unexpected or evolving clinical trajectory should prompt active reassessment, a family and treating clinician should understand that a prior normal headache evaluation reflects the clinical picture at that specific time rather than a permanent, unconditional exclusion of a structural cause for any future headache presentation. This specific principle, that a prior negative evaluation describes a moment in time rather than a permanent guarantee, has recurred throughout this book in various forms, from the serial imaging surveillance this book has emphasized for tuberous sclerosis complex in Chapter 14 to the repeat skeletal survey this book has emphasized for suspected abusive head trauma in Chapter 19, and its restatement here, in this book's final chapter, underscores its status as one of this framework's most broadly applicable diagnostic principles.

Headache in the Context of a Known Chronic Neurologic Condition

A child with a known chronic neurologic condition addressed elsewhere in this book, including a treated brain tumor discussed in Chapter 12, a ventricular shunt discussed in Chapter 10, or Sturge-Weber syndrome discussed in Chapter 14, presenting with a new or changed headache pattern warrants evaluation calibrated specifically to that child's known underlying condition and its recognized complication spectrum, applying the condition-specific reasoning this book has developed throughout, rather than the generic, undifferentiated headache evaluation framework this section has otherwise developed for a child without this specific, relevant prior history. This condition-specific calibration, tailoring the evaluation to the child's own individual medical history rather than applying a single, generic protocol uniformly, exemplifies the same individualized, whole-child approach this book has modeled throughout its complete twenty-chapter survey, treating each child not as an interchangeable instance of a named diagnostic category but as a specific individual whose own particular history and risk profile should directly shape the evaluation pursued.

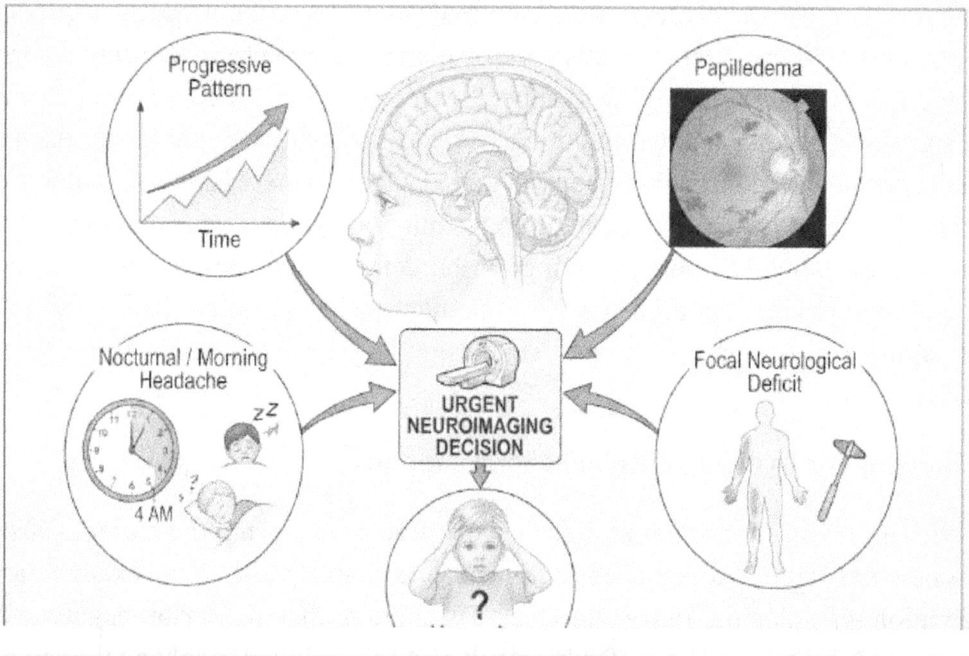

Feature	Increases Structural Likelihood	Reassuring Pattern
Timing	Nocturnal, morning-predominant	Any time of day, stable pattern
Progression	Worsening over weeks to months	Stable frequency and severity

Examination	Papilledema, focal deficit	Entirely normal
Age	Younger than 6 years	Older child or adolescent

Macrocephaly: Differential Diagnosis and Evaluation

Macrocephaly, head circumference exceeding the 97th percentile or, more precisely, more than two standard deviations above the age- and sex-adjusted mean, carries a broad differential diagnosis this section organizes into benign and pathologic categories, extending the head circumference reasoning introduced in Chapter 2 into this chapter's dedicated, presentation-focused framework. Head circumference, a single, simple measurement obtainable at every well-child visit, functions throughout this book as a recurring gateway sign, and this section's systematic organization of its differential diagnosis exemplifies how a single, accessible clinical measurement can direct the reader toward the full range of diagnostic reasoning this book has developed across its preceding chapters, from the benign variant recognition of Chapter 2 through the hydrocephalus framework of Chapter 10 to the neurocutaneous and metabolic disease categories addressed later in this book.

Benign Familial Macrocephaly

Benign familial macrocephaly, the most common cause of macrocephaly overall, describes a pattern of large head size, generally with a parallel, appropriately tracking growth curve rather than a crossing-percentiles pattern, in a developmentally normal child, frequently with one or both parents sharing this same large head size; confirming this specific, reassuring pattern, a stable percentile tracking rather than progressive crossing, normal developmental trajectory, and a positive family history of similarly large head size, applying the same evidence-based, low-yield-presentation reasoning this book has emphasized throughout, supports clinical observation without imaging in this specific, common, benign presentation. Benign familial macrocephaly is understood to reflect a genetic tendency toward a larger, though structurally entirely normal, brain volume rather than any pathologic process, and when imaging has been obtained for another reason in a child ultimately found to have this benign pattern, the structural study characteristically shows a normal brain and ventricular system proportionally enlarged along with the overall skull size, without the ventriculomegaly, extra-axial fluid excess, or other structural abnormality that would instead indicate one of the pathologic causes this section addresses next.

Benign Enlargement of the Subarachnoid Spaces

Benign enlargement of the subarachnoid spaces, introduced in Chapter 2 as a common cause of macrocephaly in infancy, presents with prominent frontal subarachnoid fluid spaces and mildly enlarged ventricles without the specific findings of true hydrocephalus discussed in Chapter 10, and this specific, characteristic imaging pattern, correlated against the developmentally normal, appropriately growing infant this condition typically affects, distinguishes it from the pathologic macrocephaly causes this section addresses; recognizing this pattern confidently, applying the reasoning developed in Chapter 2, prevents both unnecessary additional evaluation and inappropriate parental alarm regarding a benign, generally self-resolving finding. This condition typically resolves spontaneously over the first two to three years of life as the expanded subarachnoid spaces gradually normalize alongside the infant's overall brain growth, and a family can be counseled with genuine confidence regarding this expected, favorable natural history once the specific, characteristic imaging pattern this section has described has been confirmed, distinguishing this reassuring counseling conversation from the more measured, uncertainty-acknowledging counseling this book has emphasized for several of the less favorable conditions addressed in its preceding chapters.

Hydrocephalus as a Pathologic Cause

Hydrocephalus, discussed comprehensively in Chapter 10, represents one of the more common pathologic causes of macrocephaly, and distinguishing progressive, pathologic ventricular enlargement from the benign extra-axial fluid pattern discussed above depends on the specific ventricular and extra-axial space characterization this book has developed throughout, together with the growth trajectory, a rapidly crossing-percentiles head circumference pattern favoring a pathologic, rather than benign, process; a macrocephalic infant showing this specific, concerning growth trajectory warrants the structured hydrocephalus evaluation developed in Chapter 10 rather than the observational approach appropriate for the benign macrocephaly patterns this section has otherwise emphasized. The specific accompanying clinical features discussed in Chapter 10, a bulging fontanelle, split sutures, and prominent scalp veins, provide further, complementary examination-based support for a hydrocephalus diagnosis beyond the head circumference growth trajectory and imaging characterization this section has primarily emphasized, and eliciting these specific findings on physical examination, rather than relying on head circumference measurement alone, strengthens the overall clinical picture supporting this specific, pathologic diagnosis.

Macrocephaly-Associated Genetic Syndromes

Beyond benign familial macrocephaly and hydrocephalus, several genetic syndromes addressed throughout this book, including several of the neurocutaneous syndromes discussed in Chapter 14 and certain overgrowth syndromes, carry macrocephaly as a recognized feature, and a macrocephalic child with additional syndromic features on examination, disproportionate body overgrowth, characteristic facial features, or the cutaneous findings developed in Chapter 14, warrants the syndrome-specific evaluation this book has developed for each named entity rather than an assumption that macrocephaly, however severe, reflects the benign familial pattern this section has primarily emphasized. Neurofibromatosis type 1 specifically, discussed in Chapter 14, carries macrocephaly as a recognized, though not universal, feature, and this specific association is worth holding in mind when evaluating a macrocephalic child, particularly one with any of the additional cutaneous or clinical findings this book's Chapter 14 has developed as diagnostic criteria for this specific, common neurocutaneous syndrome.

Structured Evaluation Algorithm for Macrocephaly

A structured evaluation algorithm for macrocephaly, beginning with careful growth curve and family history assessment, proceeding to neurologic examination for any accompanying red-flag feature, and reserving imaging for a child showing a concerning growth trajectory, an abnormal examination, or additional syndromic features, applies the same evidence-based, risk-stratified imaging approach this book has developed throughout to this specific, common presenting sign; a family of a macrocephalic infant benefits directly from this structured, transparent reasoning, understanding clearly why their specific child either does or does not require imaging based on the concrete, named criteria this algorithm applies rather than an unexplained, seemingly arbitrary determination. This same structured, criteria-based approach, rather than an intuitive or purely experience-based clinical impression, ensures consistent, reproducible decision-making across different clinicians evaluating a similar macrocephalic presentation, applying the same evidence-based standardization principle this book has emphasized throughout for numerous other clinical decision points spanning its full twenty-chapter scope.

Parental Head Circumference Measurement

Directly measuring parental head circumference, rather than relying solely on a family's subjective report of a large head size, provides objective, quantitative support for a suspected benign familial macrocephaly diagnosis, and this simple, low-cost measurement, incorporated into the structured evaluation algorithm this section has developed, strengthens the evidentiary basis for a decision to forgo imaging in a way that a family's unquantified verbal report alone cannot fully provide, particularly valuable when a specific family's history is uncertain or a parent is not readily available for direct examination. This same measurement discipline, quantifying an objective finding rather than relying on subjective report alone wherever feasible, echoes the same evidence-based rigor this book has applied throughout to numerous other clinical determinations, from the standardized ventricular measurements developed in Chapter 5 to the structured severity scoring systems addressed in Chapter 17, reinforcing that precise, quantitative characterization, wherever practically achievable, consistently strengthens the diagnostic and counseling conversation that follows.

Macrocephaly With Developmental Delay

A macrocephalic child showing developmental delay, in contrast to the developmentally normal trajectory characteristic of benign familial macrocephaly, warrants a substantially broader evaluation incorporating both the structural imaging this section has emphasized and the genetic and metabolic evaluation frameworks developed in Chapters 7 and 17, since this specific combination, large head size accompanied by developmental impairment, meaningfully shifts the differential away from the benign, isolated macrocephaly patterns this section has primarily addressed toward the broader, more consequential neurodevelopmental and metabolic disease categories this book's preceding chapters have developed in detail. This specific combination of findings, macrocephaly plus developmental delay, functions as a further, distinct red-flag pattern in its own right, analogous to the headache red-flag features developed earlier in this chapter, and a clinician evaluating a macrocephalic child should actively assess developmental status as a core, integral component of the structured evaluation algorithm this section has developed rather than an optional or secondary consideration appended after the primary growth curve and imaging assessment.

Figure 20.2: Macrocephaly Evaluation Algorithm

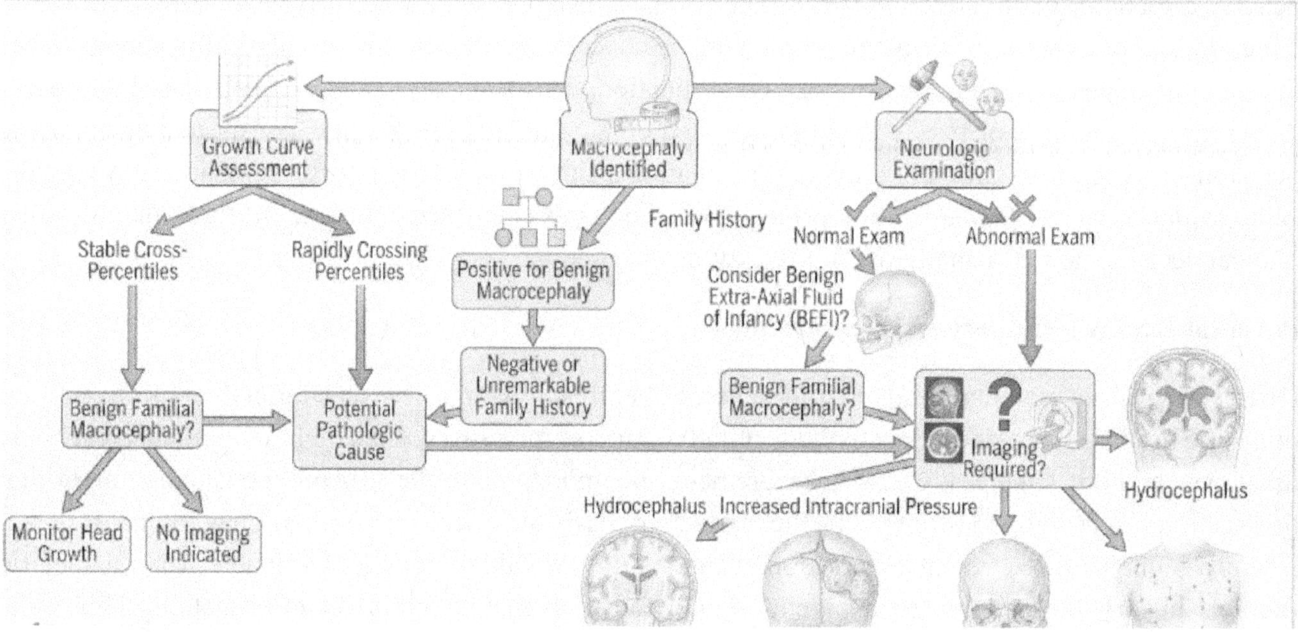

THE CLINICAL-IMAGING CROSSWALK SYSTEM — Macrocephaly With a Crossing-Percentiles Growth Trajectory

The Crossing: A four-month-old with head circumference tracking at the 50th percentile at birth now measures above the 99th percentile, a clear crossing-percentiles pattern, without a family history of large head size.

Presentation Signature: An infant with a rapidly crossing-percentiles head circumference growth trajectory, distinct from the stably tracking pattern characteristic of benign familial macrocephaly.

Imaging Correlate: Brain ultrasound, applying the age-appropriate imaging modality reasoning developed in Chapter 1, demonstrates progressive ventriculomegaly without the specific frontal-predominant extra-axial fluid pattern of benign enlargement of the subarachnoid spaces, supporting a diagnosis of hydrocephalus.

Trap Logic: Attributing this specific, crossing-percentiles growth pattern to benign familial macrocephaly without correlating it against the growth trajectory criterion this chapter has developed, or without obtaining imaging given this specific, concerning trajectory, risks a delayed diagnosis of a treatable, pathologic hydrocephalus that could otherwise have been identified and addressed at a substantially earlier, less advanced stage.

Crossing Anchor: A crossing-percentiles head circumference growth trajectory, distinct from a stably tracking large head size, is a specific red-flag feature warranting imaging evaluation rather than reassurance based on head size alone, regardless of how large or small the absolute head circumference measurement itself appears at any single time point.

Microcephaly: Differential Diagnosis and Evaluation

Microcephaly, head circumference falling more than two standard deviations below the age- and sex-adjusted mean, carries a differential diagnosis this section organizes by timing of onset, congenital versus acquired, or postnatally progressive, drawing together entities addressed across numerous preceding chapters of this book into a single, presentation-focused framework. This section's organization by timing, rather than by isolated etiologic category, mirrors the same gestational-timing framework this book developed explicitly in Chapter 15 for congenital infection, reinforcing across this book's final content chapters that precisely when, developmentally, an insult or disruption occurs is often as diagnostically informative as what specific insult occurred, a principle this chapter now applies one final time to its closing presenting sign.

Congenital Microcephaly: Primary Versus Secondary

Congenital microcephaly, present from birth, is further subdivided into primary microcephaly, reflecting a primary genetic disruption of neuronal proliferation discussed in relation to the malformations of cortical development addressed in Chapter 7, and secondary microcephaly, reflecting an extrinsic insult during gestation, most commonly the congenital infections discussed in Chapter 15, disrupting an otherwise genetically normal proliferative and migratory process; distinguishing these two congenital categories depends substantially on the specific imaging pattern identified, a simplified gyral pattern and reduced cortical volume without the destructive calcification and encephaloclastic findings of congenital infection favoring primary microcephaly, while the specific calcification patterns and destructive changes discussed in Chapter 15 favor a secondary, infectious or other extrinsic cause. Maternal exposure history, including the teratogenic exposures and specific infectious risk factors discussed in Chapter 15, together with maternal serologic testing where indicated, complements the imaging characterization this section has emphasized, and a comprehensive congenital microcephaly evaluation integrates this maternal and gestational history alongside the specific structural imaging pattern rather than relying on imaging characterization in isolation to establish the primary-versus-secondary distinction this section has developed.

Postnatally Progressive Microcephaly

Postnatally progressive microcephaly, in which head circumference is normal at birth but progressively falls across percentiles over subsequent months, carries a distinct differential from the congenital microcephaly discussed above, including Rett syndrome discussed in Chapter 17, several of the leukodystrophies and neurodegenerative disorders addressed in that same chapter, and severe global hypoxic-ischemic or other acquired brain injury sufficiently severe to impair subsequent brain growth; this specific postnatal onset and progressive pattern, rather than a congenitally small head size from birth, should prompt the specific neurodegenerative and metabolic evaluation developed in Chapter 17 applied to this chapter's presenting sign of progressively declining head circumference. Serial head circumference measurement, plotted against the same standardized growth curve at each visit, is essential to reliably distinguishing this specific, postnatally progressive pattern from a congenital microcephaly that was simply under-recognized or inconsistently measured at the earliest newborn visits, and this measurement precision, discussed further later in this section, is the foundational technical requirement upon which the entire timing-based differential this section has developed actually depends.

Craniosynostosis as a Microcephaly Mimic

Craniosynostosis, discussed comprehensively in Chapter 8, can produce an apparent microcephaly, or more precisely a restricted cranial vault growth, distinct from the primary brain growth disorders this section has otherwise emphasized, and distinguishing this specific, skull-growth-restriction mechanism from a true, primary brain growth disorder depends on the specific suture and skull shape characterization developed in Chapter 8, together with brain volume assessment confirming whether the brain itself, as opposed to the skull housing it, is disproportionately small; this distinction carries direct management implications, since craniosynostosis-related cranial restriction may warrant the surgical cranial vault expansion discussed in Chapter 8, an intervention not applicable to the primary brain growth disorders this section's remaining differential addresses. Multi-suture, syndromic craniosynostosis in particular carries an elevated risk of this specific cranial restriction mechanism producing functionally significant microcephaly, applying the specific syndromic craniosynostosis reasoning developed in Chapter 8, and a child presenting with apparent microcephaly and any suture or skull shape abnormality on examination warrants the same dedicated craniofacial evaluation this book's Chapter 8 has developed rather than proceeding directly to the brain-growth-disorder evaluation this section otherwise emphasizes.

Genetic Evaluation for Microcephaly

Given the substantial genetic heterogeneity underlying primary congenital microcephaly, broad genetic testing, incorporating chromosomal microarray and, increasingly, exome or genome sequencing, is a standard component of the evaluation once the imaging characterization this section has developed narrows the differential toward a primary, rather than secondary or postnatally acquired, mechanism, applying the same phenotype-directed genetic testing principle this book has developed throughout for numerous other structurally and imaging-defined categories of pediatric neurologic disease. Primary microcephaly overlaps substantially with the malformations of cortical development addressed in Chapter 7, since disrupted neuronal proliferation, the specific mechanism underlying most primary microcephaly, represents one component of the broader proliferation-migration-organization framework that chapter developed, and applying that same embryologic framework here, asking specifically which stage of cortical development was disrupted, provides a further, complementary diagnostic lens beyond the head-circumference-focused framework this chapter's presentation-based organization has primarily emphasized.

Developmental Surveillance in Microcephaly

Regardless of the specific underlying cause ultimately identified, structured, longitudinal developmental surveillance is a standard, essential component of comprehensive care for a child with confirmed microcephaly, applying the same proactive, structured surveillance principle this book has emphasized throughout, since the degree of microcephaly correlates broadly, though imperfectly, with expected developmental outcome, and early, structured developmental support services benefit this population regardless of the ultimate, specific etiologic diagnosis this section's evaluation framework identifies.

Serial Head Circumference Measurement in Surveillance

Precise, structured serial head circumference measurement, using consistent technique and plotted against the same standardized growth curve at each measurement, is the essential foundation upon which this section's entire timing-based differential diagnosis framework depends, and inconsistent measurement technique or infrequent measurement intervals can obscure the specific growth trajectory pattern, congenital, progressive, or stable, that this chapter's diagnostic reasoning requires; this measurement precision, while seemingly a basic technical detail, directly determines whether the specific, evidence-based differential diagnosis this section has developed can even be reliably applied to a given child's presentation. Documenting head circumference at every well-child visit, using the same standardized measurement technique regardless of which specific clinician performs the measurement, ensures the growth curve this section's diagnostic reasoning depends upon remains complete and internally consistent over time, and a gap in this longitudinal measurement record, whether from missed visits or inconsistent technique, can meaningfully limit the reliability of the timing-based differential diagnosis this section has otherwise developed with considerable precision.

Family Genetic Counseling for Primary Microcephaly

Once a specific genetic cause underlying primary congenital microcephaly is confirmed through the testing strategy this section has developed, comprehensive family genetic counseling addressing inheritance pattern and recurrence risk for future pregnancies, applying the same family counseling framework this book has developed throughout for other genetically confirmed pediatric neurologic conditions, is an essential component of comprehensive care extending beyond the affected child alone to the family's broader reproductive planning. This closing genetic counseling step, appearing here in this book's final content chapter as it has across numerous preceding chapters, from the neurocutaneous syndrome counseling of Chapter 14 to the leukodystrophy and neurodegenerative disease counseling of Chapter 17, reinforces one final time that a precise, confirmed diagnosis in pediatric neuroimaging is never merely an academic endpoint but the direct foundation for the specific, actionable family counseling and reproductive planning conversation that follows.

Figure 20.3: Congenital Versus Postnatally Progressive Microcephaly

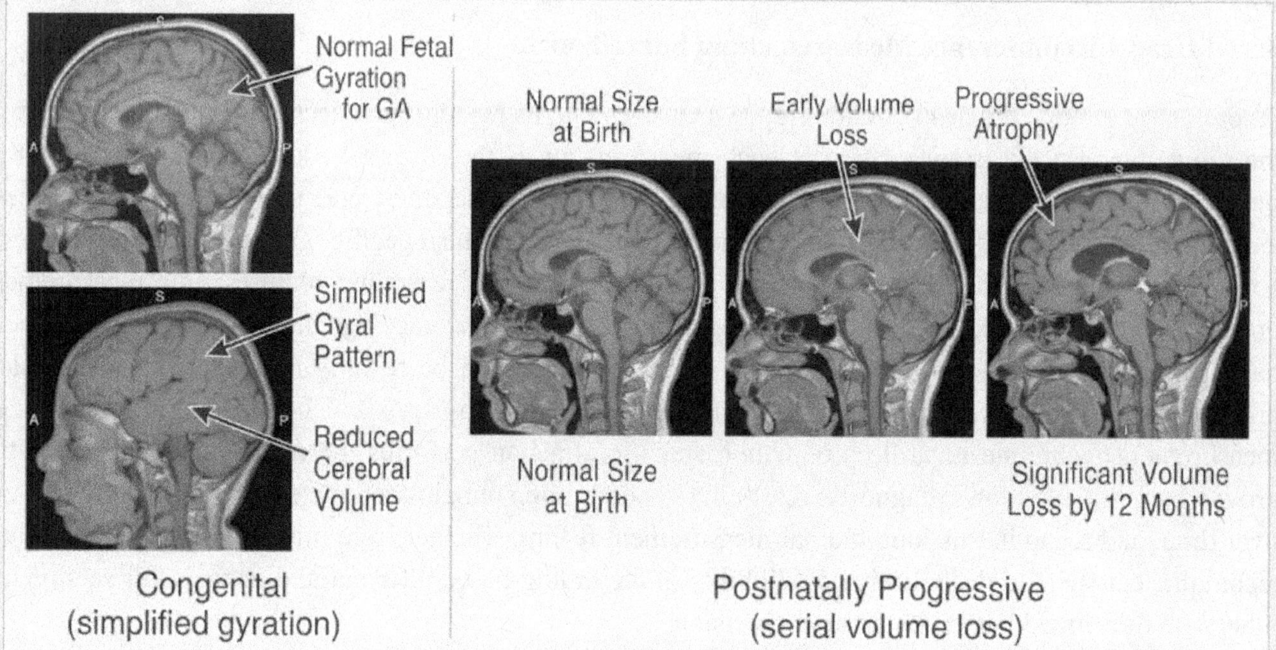

Integrating Presentation-Based Reasoning Across This Book

This closing section draws together the presentation-based diagnostic reasoning this final chapter has applied to headache, macrocephaly, and microcephaly into a single, generalizable framework, synthesizing the clinical-imaging correlation principle this book's Crosswalk System has developed across its full twenty-chapter survey of pediatric neuroimaging. Positioned deliberately as this book's final section before its dedicated Anchor reference, this synthesis serves both as a genuine, substantive conclusion to the presentation-based reasoning this specific chapter has developed and as a bridge connecting this chapter's specific content to the complete, twenty-chapter body of clinical-imaging reasoning this book has built.

From Presenting Sign to Precise Diagnosis

Across this entire book, the recurring, foundational skill this reader has developed is the ability to translate a presenting clinical sign, whether headache, macrocephaly, microcephaly, or any of the numerous other presentations addressed throughout this book's preceding chapters, into a precise, evidence-based imaging strategy and a correspondingly narrowed, well-organized differential diagnosis, rather than proceeding from an undifferentiated clinical complaint directly to an unfocused, exhaustive imaging evaluation; this presentation-to-diagnosis translation skill, rather than the memorization of any single named entity in isolation, is the durable, transferable clinical capability this book has aimed to build throughout its complete survey of pediatric neuroimaging. This same translation skill has been modeled explicitly across every one of this book's preceding chapters, from seizure semiology directing epilepsy-protocol imaging in Chapter 11, to cutaneous findings directing neurocutaneous syndrome surveillance in Chapter 14, to the specific red-flag features this closing chapter has developed for headache, macrocephaly, and microcephaly, each instance reinforcing the same underlying, generalizable diagnostic reasoning process.

The Recurring Themes of This Book

Several specific, recurring themes have appeared across this book's twenty chapters and warrant explicit, final restatement: age-specific interpretation, since a finding's significance depends critically on the child's developmental stage, from the neonatal ventricular measurements of Chapter 5 to the pubertal pituitary enlargement of Chapter 2; evidence-based imaging thresholds, resisting reflexive imaging for low-yield presentations while maintaining a low threshold for red-flag features, developed explicitly in Chapter 3 and applied throughout every subsequent chapter; precise anatomic and mechanistic characterization over generic labeling, distinguishing malformation from injury, benign variant from pathology, and expected chronic change from new, concerning findings; and honest, proportionate, uncertainty-acknowledging communication, particularly in the highest-stakes diagnostic contexts this book has addressed, including the abusive head trauma discussed in Chapter 19 and the severe, life-limiting diagnoses addressed in Chapters 12, 13, and 17. A fifth, cross-cutting theme worth naming explicitly in this closing restatement is the value of active, systematic multisystem and multidisciplinary evaluation, resisting the temptation to conclude an evaluation upon identifying a single, satisfying finding when a coexisting second finding, an associated systemic manifestation, or a coordinated specialist evaluation carries independent diagnostic or management significance, a discipline this book has applied from the dual-pathology reasoning of Chapter 11 through the comprehensive, multidisciplinary abusive head trauma evaluation of Chapter 19.

The Named Feature's Cumulative Function

The Clinical-Imaging Crosswalk System, this book's named proprietary feature, has appeared in every preceding chapter specifically to model this presentation-to-diagnosis translation skill in a structured, repeatable format, and the reader who has engaged with each of these Crossings across this book's full survey now carries a internalized template, presentation signature, imaging correlate, trap logic, and crossing anchor, that transfers directly to any new, unfamiliar presentation this book has not specifically named, exemplifying the durable, generalizable clinical reasoning this entire framework has been constructed to teach. Each individual Crossing, considered in isolation, addressed a single, specific diagnostic pitfall, an incidental finding requiring context, a subtle imaging sign easily overlooked, or a stated history requiring active correlation against known biomechanical or clinical plausibility; considered together, across this book's complete twenty-chapter arc, these Crossings collectively demonstrate that the same five-part reasoning structure applies with equal validity regardless of the specific anatomic region, developmental stage, or disease category involved, the deepest, most consequential lesson this book's named feature has aimed to convey.

Applying This Framework to an Unfamiliar Presentation

When this book's reader eventually encounters a presenting sign or imaging finding not specifically addressed across its preceding chapters, the same underlying reasoning process this book has modeled repeatedly, correlating the specific clinical presentation against the anatomic region and developmental stage involved, generating a structured differential organized by mechanism rather than an unstructured list, and applying evidence-based criteria to the imaging-ordering and further-evaluation decisions that follow, remains fully applicable regardless of the specific, unfamiliar entity ultimately identified; this transferability is the final, cumulative measure of this book's success as a teaching framework, extending well beyond the specific named entities its twenty chapters have individually addressed. A reader confronting a genuinely novel presentation, one this book's twenty chapters have not directly named, is therefore not without a path forward, but rather equipped with the same systematic questions this book has repeatedly modeled, what anatomic structures are involved, what developmental stage does this child occupy, what mechanism, malformative, destructive, neoplastic, infectious, inflammatory, metabolic, vascular, or traumatic, best explains the pattern observed, and what specific imaging or laboratory evaluation would most efficiently distinguish among the resulting candidate diagnoses.

Closing Synthesis

From the foundational imaging principles and age-specific developmental framework established in this book's opening chapters, through the systematic survey of congenital malformation, acquired injury, neoplastic, infectious, inflammatory, metabolic, vascular, and traumatic disease addressed across its subsequent chapters, to this closing chapter's presentation-based synthesis, this book has aimed to equip its reader with both the specific, evidence-based knowledge pediatric neuroimaging requires and the durable, transferable diagnostic reasoning that outlasts any single fact this book has presented, preparing the reader for the full, evolving scope of pediatric neuroimaging practice this field will continue to present. The specific diseases, imaging signs, and clinical thresholds this book has named will continue to be refined as the underlying medical evidence base evolves, new imaging techniques mature from investigational to clinical tools, and molecular and genetic classification systems continue their ongoing evolution, and the reader who has internalized this book's underlying reasoning framework, rather than only its current, specific factual content, is best positioned to incorporate this ongoing evolution into their own continuing clinical practice.

The Anchor Section as a Continuing Reference

The Pediatric Neuroimaging Crosswalk Atlas, this book's dedicated Anchor Section following this final chapter, consolidates every Crossing introduced across these twenty chapters into a single, dual-indexed reference organized by both presenting complaint and imaging pattern, allowing the reader to navigate directly to the relevant reasoning developed throughout this book regardless of which starting point, a clinical presentation or an imaging finding, their future practice happens to present first; this closing chapter's synthesis and the Atlas that follows it together complete this book's dual-layer proprietary structure, the chapter-integrated Rhythm reasoning and this consolidated Anchor reference, each reinforcing the other toward the same underlying goal of durable, transferable clinical competence in pediatric neuroimaging. A reader encountering an unfamiliar clinical scenario in future practice can consult this Atlas as a rapid, structured starting point, locating the specific Crossing most closely analogous to their current situation and drawing on its underlying reasoning structure even when the precise, presenting details differ from the exact scenario originally described, extending this book's teaching function well beyond a single, cover-to-cover reading into an ongoing, practical clinical reference resource.

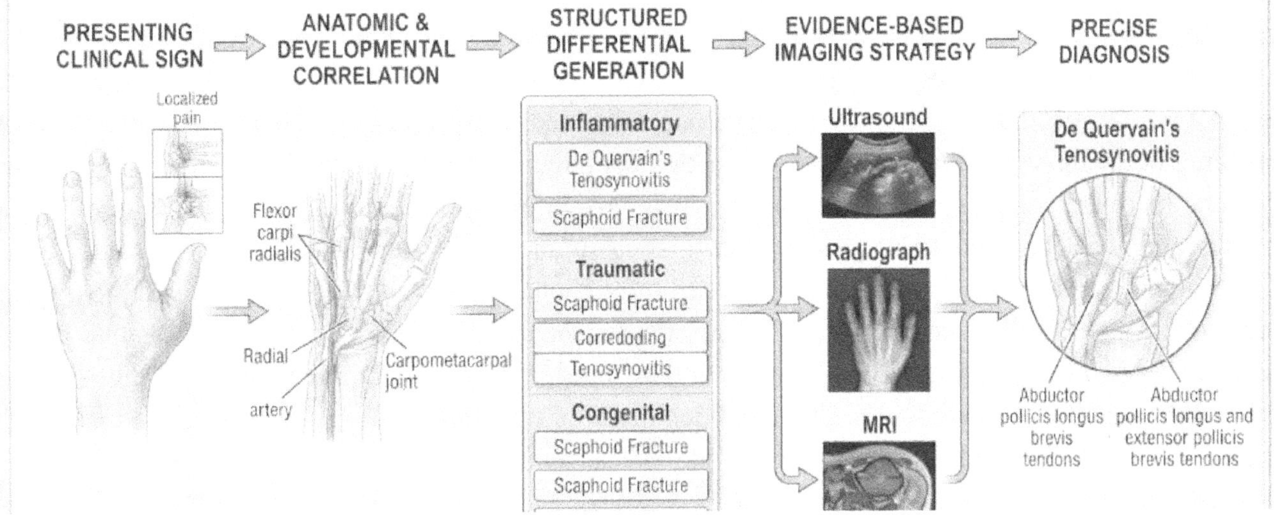

Figure 20.4: The Presentation-to-Diagnosis Translation Framework

Case Presentation: Headache With a Red-Flag Feature Identifying Hydrocephalus

An eight-year-old presents with a two-month history of headache that has progressively worsened and now regularly wakes him from sleep, accompanied by morning vomiting. Applying the reasoning developed in this chapter, this specific combination of red-flag features, progressive course, nocturnal timing, and morning vomiting, prompts brain MRI despite the absence of a focal deficit on examination, and the study identifies a posterior fossa mass with associated obstructive hydrocephalus, applying the reasoning developed in Chapters 10 and 13. The family is counseled regarding the specific features that appropriately triggered this imaging evaluation, reinforcing the evidence-based framework this chapter has developed, and the child proceeds to the coordinated neurosurgical and oncologic evaluation this specific finding requires, illustrating how this chapter's headache red-flag framework functioned as the essential first step directing this child toward a timely, ultimately consequential diagnosis. This case, positioned deliberately as this book's final full clinical illustration, exemplifies the complete presentation-to-diagnosis arc this entire framework has been constructed to teach, beginning with a common, usually benign presenting complaint and, through structured, evidence-based reasoning rather than reflexive imaging or reflexive reassurance, arriving at a precise, consequential, and ultimately treatable diagnosis. The subsequent surgical resection, applying the extent-of-resection and postoperative imaging surveillance framework developed in Chapters 12 and 13, proceeds according to this book's established, structured surgical and surveillance pathway, and the family's engagement with the coordinated multidisciplinary neuro-oncology team this book has emphasized throughout continues across the child's subsequent treatment course.

Case Presentation: Reassuring Benign Familial Macrocephaly

A six-month-old presents with a head circumference at the 98th percentile, and the family reports the father has an unusually large head as well. Applying the reasoning developed in this chapter, careful review of the growth curve confirms a stably tracking, rather than crossing-percentiles, pattern since birth, and the infant's developmental examination is entirely normal. Direct measurement of the father's head circumference, applying the specific technique discussed in this chapter, confirms an objectively large head size consistent with the reported family history. Applying the structured evaluation algorithm developed in this chapter, the family is counseled confidently that this presentation is consistent with benign familial macrocephaly, and imaging is not obtained, illustrating this chapter's evidence-based reasoning in the more common, reassuring direction complementing the concerning, imaging-warranting presentation of the preceding case. The family is offered a brief explanation of the specific criteria, stable tracking and normal development, that support this reassurance, consistent with the transparent, criteria-based communication this chapter has emphasized throughout, and routine well-child growth monitoring continues without further specific intervention. This second, deliberately paired case closes this book's complete clinical narrative on a note of confident reassurance rather than intervention, illustrating that the same rigorous, evidence-based reasoning this book has applied throughout serves the reader equally well whether its ultimate conclusion is urgent action or, as in this final case, thoughtful, well-supported restraint.

THE CLINICAL-IMAGING CROSSWALK SYSTEM — Presentation-Based Reasoning Across Headache, Macrocephaly, and Microcephaly

---

Crossing 1 Recap: A crossing-percentiles head circumference growth trajectory, distinct from a stably tracking large head size, is a specific red-flag feature warranting imaging evaluation rather than reassurance based on head size alone.

Book-Closing Anchor: Across every chapter of this book, translating a presenting clinical sign into a precise, evidence-based imaging strategy through age-specific, anatomically precise, mechanism-based reasoning, rather than memorizing isolated named entities, is the durable, transferable skill this framework has aimed to build, applicable to any future presentation this book's twenty chapters have not specifically addressed. This same skill, practiced across headache, macrocephaly, and microcephaly in this closing chapter and across every named entity in the nineteen chapters preceding it, is this book's complete, cumulative teaching legacy, carried forward by the reader into their own continuing clinical practice.

Summary and Key Concepts

The great majority of pediatric headache reflects a primary headache disorder; red-flag features (nocturnal or morning timing, progressive course, papilledema, focal deficit, young age, or a known risk factor) rather than headache severity alone should guide the imaging-ordering decision, and an evolving symptom pattern warrants reconsideration even after a prior negative evaluation.

Macrocephaly differential diagnosis is organized by growth trajectory: stably tracking large head size with normal development supports benign familial macrocephaly, while a crossing-percentiles pattern or accompanying developmental delay warrants evaluation for hydrocephalus, a genetic syndrome, or another pathologic cause.

Microcephaly differential diagnosis is organized by timing: congenital microcephaly is subdivided into primary (proliferative) and secondary (destructive/infectious) categories by imaging pattern, while postnatally progressive microcephaly warrants the neurodegenerative and metabolic evaluation developed in Chapter 17.

Craniosynostosis can mimic microcephaly through restricted cranial vault growth rather than a primary brain growth disorder, requiring the suture-specific characterization developed in Chapter 8 to distinguish these mechanisms; precise serial measurement technique underlies the reliability of this entire timing-based framework.

Across this book, translating a presenting clinical sign into a precise, evidence-based imaging strategy through age-specific, anatomically precise, mechanism-based reasoning is the central, durable skill this framework has developed, transferable to any future presentation not specifically named across its twenty chapters and consolidated in the Anchor Section that follows.

THE PEDIATRIC NEUROIMAGING CROSSWALK ATLAS

The Pediatric Neuroimaging Crosswalk Atlas consolidates every Clinical-Imaging Crosswalk introduced across this book's twenty chapters into a single, structured reference, indexed twice, once by presenting complaint and once by imaging pattern, so the reader can navigate directly to the relevant reasoning regardless of which starting point, a clinical presentation encountered in clinic or on call, or an imaging finding encountered at the workstation, their own practice happens to present first. This dual-indexing structure reflects a deliberate design choice: clinical practice does not always begin with a tidy, pre-categorized question, and a resident on call may find themselves starting from either end, a family's description of symptoms or an unexpected finding already on the screen, and this Atlas is built to serve both starting points equally well.

Each entry that follows carries four fixed components: the Pattern Name naming the specific diagnostic pitfall or reasoning pattern the Crossing addresses; the Stem Signature summarizing the clinical presentation in which this pattern arises; the Decision Anchor stating the durable, transferable rule the reader should carry forward; and the Trap Logic Key naming the specific error this pattern is designed to prevent. Every entry cites the chapter in which its full clinical reasoning and supporting evidence were originally developed, and the reader is encouraged to return to that chapter for the complete discussion whenever an Atlas entry alone does not fully resolve the clinical question at hand. This four-part structure deliberately mirrors, in condensed form, the five-part Crossing structure used throughout the body of this book, omitting only the specific narrative Imaging Correlate detail in favor of the more universally applicable Decision Anchor and Trap Logic Key, the two components most directly useful for rapid clinical orientation.

This Atlas is a structured, indexed reference, not a substitute for the reasoning developed across this book's full twenty chapters, and it is deliberately question-free throughout, containing no quizzes, drills, or self-assessment items of any kind; its function is to consolidate, cross-reference, and make rapidly navigable the pattern-recognition reasoning this book has already taught, scanned during clinic, on call, or before rotation, rather than to test the reader's recall of that reasoning. The twenty-seven entries collected here span every major category this book has addressed, congenital malformation, acquired perinatal and neonatal injury, epilepsy, neoplasm, neurocutaneous disease, infection, inflammatory and autoimmune disorders, metabolic and neurodegenerative disease, cerebrovascular disease, trauma, and presentation-based reasoning, and together they represent this book's complete diagnostic reasoning framework in its most concentrated, immediately actionable form.

Index by Presenting Complaint

This index organizes every Atlas entry by the clinical presentation or referral context in which the underlying reasoning pattern arises, allowing the reader to navigate directly from a patient's presenting complaint to the relevant entry.

Asymptomatic toddler, sacral dimple, borderline conus	16. Borderline Conus Position With Normal Filum	Ch. 9
Shunted child, symptomatic, unchanged ventricles	17. Unchanged Ventricles in a Symptomatic Shunt	Ch. 10
Presurgical epilepsy evaluation, discordant postprocessing	18. Flagged Region Without Visual/EEG Correlation	Ch. 11
Adolescent, diabetes insipidus, suprasellar mass	19. Suprasellar Mass With Elevated Tumor Markers	Ch. 12
Delayed mutism after posterior fossa surgery	20. Posterior Fossa Syndrome, Not New Complication	Ch. 13
Tuberous sclerosis, surveillance imaging	21. Growing Subependymal Nodule Near Foramen of Monro	Ch. 14
Fever, altered mental status, early normal MRI	22. Normal Early MRI in Suspected HSV Encephalitis	Ch. 15
Adolescent, intractable vomiting and hiccups	23. Intractable Vomiting as a Neurologic Presentation	Ch. 16
Adolescent, acute stroke-like deficit	24. Stroke-Like Lesion Not Respecting Vascular Territory	Ch. 17
NF1, recurrent transient focal symptoms	25. Transient Symptoms in NF1 Suggesting Moyamoya	Ch. 18
Infant, severe findings, minor stated mechanism	26. Stated Mechanism Inconsistent With Injury Severity	Ch. 19
Infant, rapidly crossing-percentiles head growth	27. Macrocephaly With a Crossing-Percentiles Trajectory	Ch. 20

Index by Imaging Pattern

This second index organizes every Atlas entry by the specific imaging finding or pattern involved, allowing the reader to navigate directly from an observation at the workstation back to the clinical reasoning this book has developed for that specific pattern.

Imaging Pattern	Entry	Chapter
Isolated diffusion-weighted signal without structural correlate	3. Motion Artifact Mimicking Restricted Diffusion	Ch. 1

Normal-appearing white matter myelination	4. Myelination Status Against Corrected Age	Ch. 2
FLAIR-suppressing basal ganglia lesions	5. Perivascular Spaces Mistaken for Cystic Disease	Ch. 2
Enlarged sphenoid sinus relative to prior study	6. Pubertal Sinus Pneumatization Mistaken for Lesion	Ch. 2
Full-thickness cerebral cleft	14. Schizencephaly Versus Porencephalic Cyst	Ch. 7
Cerebellar tonsillar descent	15. Chiari I Malformation Discovered Incidentally	Ch. 8
Low conus medullaris position	16. Borderline Conus Position With Normal Filum	Ch. 9
Chronically small, slit-like ventricles	17. Unchanged Ventricles in a Symptomatic Shunt	Ch. 10
Postprocessing-flagged cortical region	18. Flagged Region Without Visual/EEG Correlation	Ch. 11
Homogeneously enhancing suprasellar mass	19. Suprasellar Mass With Elevated Tumor Markers	Ch. 12
Normal postoperative resection cavity	20. Posterior Fossa Syndrome, Not New Complication	Ch. 13
Enlarging periventricular nodule	21. Growing Subependymal Nodule Near Foramen of Monro	Ch. 14
Normal conventional MRI, abnormal DWI	22. Normal Early MRI in Suspected HSV Encephalitis	Ch. 15
Small dorsal medullary (area postrema) lesion	23. Intractable Vomiting as a Neurologic Presentation	Ch. 16
Cortical/subcortical signal crossing vascular territories	24. Stroke-Like Lesion Not Respecting Vascular Territory	Ch. 17
Bilateral distal ICA stenosis with basal collaterals	25. Transient Symptoms in NF1 Suggesting Moyamoya	Ch. 18
Extensive, mixed-age subdural hemorrhage	26. Stated Mechanism Inconsistent With Injury Severity	Ch. 19
Progressive ventriculomegaly on serial imaging	27. Macrocephaly With a Crossing-Percentiles Trajectory	Ch, 20

Asymmetric, fan-shaped periventricular echogenicity	11. Grade 4 Hemorrhage as Venous Infarction	Ch. 5
Reassuring discharge cranial ultrasound in a very preterm infant	12. Diffuse PVL Requiring MRI Despite Normal Ultrasound	Ch. 5
Hemorrhagic lesion crossing arterial boundaries	13. Hemorrhage Not Fitting an Arterial Territory	Ch. 6
Diffusion-weighted imaging in the day 5-10 HIE window	10. Diffusion Pseudonormalization in HIE	Ch. 4

Index by Reasoning Pattern

Beyond the two indices above, a third, complementary organizing view groups every entry by the underlying type of diagnostic reasoning error it guards against, rather than by clinical presentation or imaging finding. This view is most useful not for locating a specific entry during a live clinical encounter, but for recognizing, in retrospect or during structured teaching, that a small number of recurring cognitive patterns account for the great majority of the pitfalls this book has addressed across its full twenty-chapter survey.

Reasoning Pattern	Entries
Normal or reassuring imaging does not exclude the diagnosis	3, 4, 8, 12, 17, 22
A finding requires correlation against age or developmental stage	4, 5, 6
Serial or comparison imaging is required for a reliable conclusion	6, 14, 17, 21, 27
A stated history or mechanism requires active, independent verification	9, 26
An isolated imaging finding requires correlation with another data source	3, 18, 19, 22, 23, 24
A benign, common finding is mistaken for a pathologic one	5, 6, 15, 16
A recognized syndrome-specific association is not actively considered	9, 19, 25

The imaging-ordering decision itself, not only technique, requires evidence-based scrutiny	1, 2, 7, 8
A distributional or territorial pattern is the key discriminating feature	13, 14, 24
A delayed or unexpected clinical course is mistaken for a new complication	20

A reader who studies this reasoning-pattern index will notice that several entries appear under more than one pattern, since a single clinical scenario frequently tests more than one type of diagnostic discipline simultaneously; Entry 22, for example, tests both the normal-imaging-does-not-exclude pattern and the isolated-finding-requires-correlation pattern, since the diagnosis ultimately depends on integrating a subtle diffusion finding with the compatible clinical presentation and the cerebrospinal fluid testing that follows. This overlap is not a flaw in the classification but a genuine, accurate reflection of how real diagnostic reasoning actually proceeds, rarely through the application of a single, isolated rule but through the simultaneous, integrated application of several complementary reasoning disciplines at once, precisely the multimodal, converging-evidence approach this book has modeled throughout its full twenty-chapter survey. A reader building their own future teaching material, whether a brief case conference presentation or a longer structured teaching session, may find this reasoning-pattern index particularly useful as an organizing scaffold, since grouping several entries under a shared underlying cognitive pattern, rather than presenting them as an unconnected list of isolated facts, more effectively conveys the transferable, generalizable nature of the reasoning this book has aimed to teach throughout.

The entries in this and the following sections are presented in the order their originating chapters appear across this book, from the foundational imaging principles of Chapter 1 through the presentation-based synthesis of Chapter 20.

Atlas Entries: Chapters 1-5

The entries in this and the following sections are presented in the order their originating chapters appear across this book, from the foundational imaging principles of Chapter 1 through the presentation-based synthesis of Chapter 20. This first cluster of entries, drawn from the book's foundational and earliest developmental and perinatal chapters, is weighted toward the imaging-ordering and modality-selection discipline established in Chapters 1 and 3 and the age-specific interpretive discipline established in Chapter 2, reflecting the foundational, front-loaded position these specific reasoning skills occupy in this book's overall teaching sequence.

1. Epilepsy-Protocol Sequencing for First Seizure (Chapter 1)

Stem Signature: A child with new-onset focal seizure and a normal general neurologic examination, referred for a routine brain MRI without further protocol specification. Decision Anchor: Any new-onset focal seizure with a normal examination should trigger a dedicated epilepsy MRI protocol, not a routine brain protocol, whenever epilepsy is a genuine diagnostic consideration. Trap Logic Key: A standard protocol ordered without epilepsy-specific sequencing may read as falsely normal, delaying recognition of subtle cortical dysplasia that only the dedicated, hippocampus- and gray-white-junction-optimized protocol reliably detects.

2. Deferring Sedation Until Indication Is Confirmed (Chapter 1)

Stem Signature: A toddler with a single, classically stereotyped breath-holding spell, referred directly for sedated MRI without first revisiting whether imaging is indicated. Decision Anchor: The imaging-ordering decision always precedes the imaging-technique decision; a child should never be scheduled for sedation before the underlying indication for imaging has been explicitly reassessed. Trap Logic Key: Proceeding directly to sedation scheduling exposes the child to unnecessary anesthetic risk for a low-yield presentation and normalizes skipping the imaging-ordering step this book's evidence-based framework requires.

3. Motion Artifact Mimicking Restricted Diffusion (Chapter 1)

Stem Signature: A motion-degraded study in a young or incompletely sedated child shows apparent diffusion restriction without a corroborating structural correlate or a clinical picture fitting acute ischemia. Decision Anchor: Any diffusion-weighted finding lacking a directly corresponding, vascular-territory-concordant signal change on paired structural sequences should be treated as motion-suspect until reproducibility across diffusion directions is confirmed. Trap Logic Key: Accepting an isolated, artifact-degraded diffusion finding at face value risks a false stroke diagnosis and unnecessary downstream hematologic and cardiac workup.

4. Myelination Status Against Corrected Age (Chapter 2)

Stem Signature: A term neonate referred because an outside report described white matter as showing delayed myelination for age. Decision Anchor: Myelination status must always be interpreted against the specific structures expected to be myelinated at the child's exact corrected age, never against a generic adult-pattern expectation. Trap Logic Key: A term neonate's largely unmyelinated cerebral white matter is the normal, expected pattern; labeling it delayed rather than age-appropriate generates unwarranted parental alarm and unnecessary additional evaluation.

5. Perivascular Spaces Mistaken for Cystic Disease (Chapter 2)

Stem Signature: An asymptomatic child with incidental, small, round, symmetric basal ganglia lesions identified on a study obtained for an unrelated indication. Decision Anchor: Any small, round, symmetric basal ganglia or centrum semiovale lesion that fully suppresses on FLAIR and follows cerebrospinal fluid signal on every sequence is a perivascular space until proven otherwise. Trap Logic Key: Failing to confirm complete FLAIR suppression, the single most reliable discriminating feature, risks mistaking this benign, near-universal finding for pathologic cystic disease and triggering an unnecessary metabolic or neurodegenerative workup.

6. Pubertal Sinus Pneumatization Mistaken for Lesion (Chapter 2)

Stem Signature: An adolescent's current study shows a sphenoid sinus dramatically larger than a pre-pubertal comparison study, prompting concern for an interval skull base lesion. Decision Anchor: Any interval skull base or sinus change identified when comparing a pre-pubertal study to a later adolescent study should be evaluated first against expected pubertal pneumatization before any additional workup is pursued. Trap Logic Key: Comparing across a pubertal interval without accounting for expected pneumatization risks describing a normal developmental process as a concerning interval finding.

7. Fastest Adequate Modality in Instability (Chapter 3)

Stem Signature: A child with a known ventriculoperitoneal shunt presents with vomiting, lethargy, and signs of rising intracranial pressure, and the on-call team must select between an immediate CT and a delayed, sedated MRI. Decision Anchor: In an acutely deteriorating child, modality selection is governed first by acquisition speed and availability, not by which modality would be preferred under nonurgent circumstances. Trap Logic Key: Waiting for the theoretically preferred modality in an acutely deteriorating child risks a diagnostic delay in a genuine surgical emergency. This entry generalizes beyond its specific shunt-malfunction stem signature to any acute pediatric neurologic deterioration in which the modality-selection reasoning developed across this book's early chapters, and applied repeatedly in the acute stroke, status epilepticus, and metabolic crisis contexts addressed in later chapters, converges on the same underlying principle: speed and availability, not theoretical modality preference, govern the acute imaging decision.

8. Recognizing When Imaging Is Not the Next Step (Chapter 3)

Stem Signature: A neurodevelopmentally normal toddler with a classic simple febrile seizure and a family requesting an MRI to be safe despite the absence of a clinical indication. Decision Anchor: A true simple febrile seizure in a neurodevelopmentally normal child is not an indication for neuroimaging; the correct response is evidence-based, family-centered reassurance. Trap Logic Key: Ordering an MRI in response to parental anxiety alone exposes the child to unnecessary sedation risk for a study with well-documented negligible yield in this specific, common presentation.

9. Family History Shifting an Imaging Threshold (Chapter 3)

Stem Signature: A new, otherwise low-yield headache presentation in a child whose family history includes a hereditary vascular malformation syndrome carrying an elevated cavernous malformation risk. Decision Anchor: A relevant family history of a hereditary structural or vascular neurologic condition shifts an individual child's imaging threshold even when the presenting complaint alone would otherwise fall into the low-yield category. Trap Logic Key: Applying the general population-level low-yield threshold without eliciting this specific family history would miss the individualized, elevated risk this particular child actually carries.

10. Diffusion Pseudonormalization in HIE (Chapter 4)

Stem Signature: A term neonate with moderate hypoxic-ischemic encephalopathy imaged on day seven of life shows deceptively unremarkable diffusion-weighted imaging. Decision Anchor: Diffusion-weighted imaging obtained between approximately day five and day ten of life should never be interpreted in isolation; conventional T1 and T2 sequences and the established clinical severity staging are more reliable in this specific window. Trap Logic Key: Interpreting normal-appearing diffusion in this pseudonormalization window as evidence of mild or resolved injury, without scrutinizing conventional sequences, risks substantially underestimating true injury extent.

11. Grade 4 Hemorrhage as Venous Infarction (Chapter 5)

Stem Signature: A preterm infant with an established grade 3 intraventricular hemorrhage develops a new, asymmetric, fan-shaped area of periventricular echogenicity on follow-up ultrasound. Decision Anchor: A new asymmetric, fan-shaped parenchymal lesion adjacent to a graded intraventricular hemorrhage represents periventricular hemorrhagic venous infarction, a distinct mechanism with a distinct, more guarded prognosis. Trap Logic Key: Describing this finding simply as extension or progression of the intraventricular hemorrhage obscures the distinct venous mechanism and its correspondingly different prognostic and counseling implications.

12. Diffuse PVL Requiring MRI Despite Normal Ultrasound (Chapter 5)

Stem Signature: A former twenty-six-week preterm infant has a reassuring discharge cranial ultrasound without cystic change, and the family asks whether term-equivalent MRI adds anything further. Decision Anchor: A reassuring cranial ultrasound in a very preterm infant does not exclude diffuse periventricular leukomalacia or punctate white matter lesions; term-equivalent MRI is the appropriate study for full white matter injury characterization. Trap Logic Key: A normal ultrasound reassures only against the classic cystic pattern; the more common, diffuse, noncystic contemporary pattern requires MRI for reliable detection.

Atlas Entries: Chapters 6-13

This second cluster of entries spans the congenital malformation chapters, the CSF dynamics and epilepsy chapters, and the neuro-oncology chapters, and it is weighted toward two recurring reasoning patterns this book has emphasized throughout this span: the necessity of correlating an imaging finding against a specific, named lining, position, or physiologic marker rather than accepting a superficially similar appearance at face value, and the necessity of correlating a finding against additional laboratory or physiologic data before committing to a single, most-statistically-common diagnosis.

13. Hemorrhage Not Fitting an Arterial Territory (Chapter 6)

Stem Signature: A young infant with a recent febrile illness and new lethargy shows a hemorrhagic parenchymal lesion that does not conform to a single recognizable arterial territory. Decision Anchor: A hemorrhagic parenchymal lesion that does not conform to a recognizable arterial territory should prompt dedicated venous-phase imaging to evaluate for underlying cerebral sinovenous thrombosis before any other mechanism is presumed. Trap Logic Key: Interpreting an atypically distributed hemorrhagic lesion as a primary hemorrhage or unusual arterial infarct without obtaining venous imaging risks missing the underlying, treatable venous thrombosis.

14. Schizencephaly Versus Porencephalic Cyst (Chapter 7)

Stem Signature: An infant with hemiparesis shows a full-thickness cerebral cleft extending from the cortical surface to the ventricle, with an uncertain history regarding a documented perinatal vascular event. Decision Anchor: A full-thickness cerebral cleft is characterized as schizencephaly only when its margins are lined by dysplastic, polymicrogyric gray matter; gliotic white matter lining instead indicates an acquired porencephalic cyst. Trap Logic Key: Both entities can appear grossly similar as a fluid-containing cleft on cursory review; failing to specifically characterize the cleft lining conflates a true malformation with an acquired lesion carrying different recurrence-risk and counseling implications.

15. Chiari I Malformation Discovered Incidentally (Chapter 8)

Stem Signature: A child imaged for headache incidentally shows cerebellar tonsillar descent of six millimeters below the foramen magnum, with no other neurologic symptom. Decision Anchor: Incidental tonsillar ectopia should be evaluated for an associated syrinx and correlated against Chiari-specific red-flag symptoms before being presumed causally related to a presenting headache. Trap Logic Key: Mild, asymptomatic tonsillar ectopia is a common incidental finding; reflexively attributing an unrelated headache to it risks both mismanaging the true headache etiology and generating unwarranted anxiety.

16. Borderline Conus Position With Normal Filum (Chapter 9)

Stem Signature: An asymptomatic toddler imaged for a sacral dimple shows a conus terminating at a borderline position relative to the normal age-adjusted range. Decision Anchor: A borderline conus position is interpreted alongside filum thickness and signal, not in isolation; a normal filum and absence of progressive symptoms support conservative observation rather than surgical referral. Trap Logic Key: Recommending surgical intervention based on conus position alone, without the corroborating filum assessment, risks an unnecessary surgical referral for a borderline normal variant.

17. Unchanged Ventricles in a Symptomatic Shunt (Chapter 10)

Stem Signature: A shunted child with symptoms consistent with malfunction shows ventricles essentially unchanged from a prior study, in the context of a known chronic slit-ventricle pattern. Decision Anchor: In a child with known chronically small, slit-like ventricles, unchanged ventricular size does not exclude shunt malfunction; clinical presentation and shunt series findings are weighted more heavily than ventricular size change alone in this specific population. Trap Logic Key: Assuming unchanged ventricular size excludes malfunction, without recognizing the child's chronic slit-ventricle pattern, risks a falsely reassuring interpretation and a missed, genuine malfunction. This entry pairs naturally with Entry 7, since both address acute decision-making in a shunted child; where Entry 7 addresses the speed of imaging acquisition, this entry addresses the correct interpretation of the resulting images once obtained, together spanning this specific population's complete acute evaluation pathway from ordering through interpretation.

18. Flagged Region Without Visual/EEG Correlation (Chapter 11)

Stem Signature: Voxel-based morphometry postprocessing flags a region discordant with the clinical and electrographic lateralization already established in a child undergoing presurgical epilepsy evaluation. Decision Anchor: A postprocessing-flagged region without visual imaging correlation or electroencephalographic concordance should not be accepted as the surgical target; postprocessing serves as an adjunct to, not a replacement for, correlated assessment. Trap Logic Key: Accepting a discordant postprocessing flag as the surgical target without visual or electrographic corroboration risks directing surgical planning toward an incorrect, non-epileptogenic region.

19. Suprasellar Mass With Elevated Tumor Markers (Chapter 12)

Stem Signature: A school-age or adolescent child presents with diabetes insipidus, a suprasellar mass, and a mildly elevated serum tumor marker. Decision Anchor: A suprasellar mass with diabetes insipidus warrants serum and cerebrospinal fluid tumor marker assessment before presuming craniopharyngioma; elevated markers should prompt dedicated pineal region imaging to evaluate for bifocal germinoma. Trap Logic Key: Attributing a suprasellar mass with diabetes insipidus reflexively to craniopharyngioma without first assessing tumor markers risks missing a germ cell tumor with a distinct treatment pathway.

20. Posterior Fossa Syndrome, Not New Complication (Chapter 13)

Stem Signature: A child develops delayed-onset mutism, emotional lability, and worsened ataxia on postoperative day two following apparently uncomplicated posterior fossa tumor resection. Decision Anchor: Delayed-onset mutism and emotional lability following posterior fossa tumor resection, in the absence of a new structural finding on imaging, is characteristic of posterior fossa syndrome; supportive management and family counseling regarding the generally favorable recovery trajectory is the appropriate response. Trap Logic Key: The delayed onset of this syndrome can be mistaken for a new, acute surgical complication requiring urgent additional intervention if the clinician is unfamiliar with its typical timeline.

Atlas Entries: Chapters 14-20

This final cluster of entries spans the neurocutaneous syndrome chapter, the acquired and inflammatory disease chapters, the vascular and traumatic disease chapters, and the closing presentation-based synthesis chapter, and it is weighted toward the theme that recurs most heavily across this book's later, more clinically complex chapters: that normal or unremarkable-appearing imaging, far from excluding a serious diagnosis, is frequently the expected, informative finding for several of this book's most time-sensitive and highest-stakes diagnostic categories, and that recognizing this pattern, rather than being falsely reassured by it, is essential to avoiding diagnostic delay in exactly the clinical scenarios where delay carries the greatest cost.

21. Growing Subependymal Nodule Near Foramen of Monro (Chapter 14)

Stem Signature: A child with known tuberous sclerosis complex shows interval enlargement of a subependymal nodule near the foramen of Monro compared to a study obtained eighteen months earlier. Decision Anchor: A subependymal nodule near the foramen of Monro is reclassified as a giant cell astrocytoma based on demonstrated interval growth on serial, quantitatively compared surveillance imaging, not appearance at a single time point alone. Trap Logic Key: Evaluating this nodule at a single time point without reference to the prior comparison study would miss the growth that is the specific, defining reclassification criterion.

22. Normal Early MRI in Suspected HSV Encephalitis (Chapter 15)

Stem Signature: A child with fever, altered mental status, and new focal seizures shows a grossly unremarkable conventional T2 and FLAIR MRI obtained within twelve hours of symptom onset. Decision Anchor: A normal conventional MRI does not exclude early herpes simplex encephalitis; diffusion-weighted imaging is the most sensitive early sequence, and empiric antiviral treatment, once clinically initiated, continues pending cerebrospinal fluid confirmation regardless of an equivocal imaging appearance. Trap Logic Key: Interpreting a normal-appearing conventional MRI as evidence against this diagnosis, and withholding or discontinuing empiric antiviral therapy on this basis, risks a severe, potentially preventable outcome. This entry is among the most time-sensitive in this entire Atlas, since herpes simplex encephalitis is one of the few pediatric neurologic emergencies in which treatment is deliberately initiated before, rather than after, imaging or laboratory confirmation, and a reader encountering this specific clinical picture should treat the absence of confirmatory imaging as no reason to delay or withhold the antiviral treatment already underway.

23. Intractable Vomiting as a Neurologic Presentation (Chapter 16)

Stem Signature: A school-age or adolescent child presents with prolonged, otherwise unexplained intractable vomiting and hiccups following an extensive, unrevealing gastroenterology evaluation. Decision Anchor: Intractable vomiting and hiccups without an identified gastrointestinal cause should prompt consideration of area postrema syndrome and dedicated dorsal medullary imaging, particularly in a child or adolescent, rather than an exclusively gastrointestinal diagnostic pathway. Trap Logic Key: Pursuing an exclusively gastroenterology-focused evaluation without considering this specific neurologic syndrome risks a substantial, harmful delay in recognizing and treating NMOSD.

24. Stroke-Like Lesion Not Respecting Vascular Territory (Chapter 17)

Stem Signature: An adolescent with an acute-onset visual disturbance and confusion shows cortical and subcortical signal abnormality that does not conform to a single arterial vascular territory. Decision Anchor: A stroke-like lesion not conforming to a standard vascular territory should prompt lactate testing and consideration of MELAS rather than an exclusively vascular stroke evaluation pathway. Trap Logic Key: Pursuing an exclusively vascular stroke evaluation and treatment pathway, including thrombolysis consideration, for a non-territory-conforming lesion risks an inappropriate treatment and a missed underlying mitochondrial disorder. This entry shares its core discriminating principle, vascular-territory conformity as the key distinguishing feature between a true arterial event and its metabolic mimic, with Entry 3 from this book's opening chapter, illustrating how the same fundamental anatomic verification habit recurs from this book's earliest imaging-technique reasoning through its most advanced metabolic disease reasoning.

25. Transient Symptoms in NF1 Suggesting Moyamoya (Chapter 18)

Stem Signature: A child with known neurofibromatosis type 1 presents with recurrent, transient focal neurologic symptoms suggestive of a vascular, rather than epileptic, mechanism. Decision Anchor: Recurrent transient focal neurologic symptoms in a child with neurofibromatosis type 1 should prompt dedicated vascular imaging to evaluate for moyamoya syndrome, a recognized, specific association warranting active, rather than incidental, consideration. Trap Logic Key: Attributing recurrent transient focal symptoms in this population to a nonspecific or epileptic cause without considering this well-documented vascular association risks delayed recognition of a progressive, treatable arteriopathy.

26. Stated Mechanism Inconsistent With Injury Severity (Chapter 19)

Stem Signature: A young infant presents with severe intracranial findings, including extensive mixed-age bilateral subdural hemorrhage, disproportionate to a caregiver-reported, low-severity accidental mechanism. Decision Anchor: A stated mechanism should be actively correlated against the known biomechanical plausibility of the resulting injury severity and pattern; a significant mismatch, considered alongside the full multidisciplinary evaluation, is a component of the comprehensive determination process rather than dismissed in favor of the stated history alone. Trap Logic Key: Accepting a stated mechanism at face value without this correlation risks overlooking a case of abusive head trauma, delaying the protective intervention this diagnosis, once appropriately supported, requires. This entry, given the severity of its subject matter, is presented with particular care: the specific determination it describes is never made from imaging or mechanism correlation alone but always through the complete, multidisciplinary evaluation this book's Chapter 19 develops in full, including the mandatory skeletal survey and dilated ophthalmologic examination that evaluation requires.

27. Macrocephaly With a Crossing-Percentiles Trajectory (Chapter 20)

Stem Signature: An infant with head circumference tracking at the 50th percentile at birth now measures above the 99th percentile, without a family history of large head size. Decision Anchor: A crossing-percentiles head circumference growth trajectory, distinct from a stably tracking large head size, is a specific red-flag feature warranting imaging evaluation rather than reassurance based on head size alone. Trap Logic Key: Attributing this specific, crossing-percentiles growth pattern to benign familial macrocephaly without correlating it against the growth trajectory criterion risks a delayed diagnosis of a treatable, pathologic hydrocephalus. As this Atlas's final numbered entry, this Crossing closes the same loop it opened with Entry 1, moving from this book's earliest sequence-selection reasoning for a first seizure through nineteen intervening entries spanning this book's complete diagnostic scope, back to a single, simple growth curve measurement, illustrating that the same underlying discipline, correlating the specific pattern observed against the correct comparative standard, applies with equal force whether the standard in question is an MRI protocol, a vascular territory, or a growth percentile curve.

Using This Atlas in Practice

This Atlas is designed for three specific, recurring uses reflecting the practical circumstances under which a busy clinician most needs rapid, reliable access to this book's reasoning: during an active clinic visit, when a presenting complaint prompts the reader to consult the Index by Presenting Complaint and navigate directly to the relevant entry without re-reading the full originating chapter; while on call, when an unexpected or ambiguous imaging finding prompts the reader to consult the Index by Imaging Pattern for the same rapid orientation; and before beginning a new clinical rotation or assignment, when a reader benefits from scanning the complete set of twenty-seven entries in sequence as a structured, comprehensive refresher of this book's full diagnostic reasoning framework. A fourth, less immediate but equally valuable use is as a teaching tool in its own right, since a supervising clinician can direct a trainee to a specific Atlas entry as a concise, focused starting point for a teaching conversation built around a real case, using the entry's compressed structure as scaffolding for a more extended discussion drawing on the full chapter this entry summarizes.

Each Atlas entry is deliberately self-contained, providing enough context to be genuinely useful without requiring the reader to return to the originating chapter for basic orientation, while still directing the reader back to that chapter's full discussion whenever a specific clinical scenario requires the complete evidentiary and mechanistic detail an entry's necessarily brief format cannot fully capture. A reader who has worked through this book's twenty chapters in sequence will recognize each entry immediately; a reader consulting this Atlas as a standalone reference, without having read the originating chapter in full, will still find each entry sufficient to orient an initial clinical response, with the chapter citation provided as the clear next step whenever deeper engagement with the underlying evidence and reasoning is warranted. This dual accessibility, useful both to the reader who has completed this book cover to cover and to the reader consulting a single entry in isolation during a genuine clinical moment, reflects this Atlas's design intent as a living, standalone reference rather than merely an appendix summarizing content available only in full elsewhere.

This Atlas, like every chapter preceding it, is question-free by design: it contains no practice items, no quizzes, no self-assessment exercises, and no answer keys of any kind. Its twenty-seven entries are pattern references, not test items, and its value to the reader lies entirely in the speed and reliability with which it connects a real clinical or imaging encounter back to this book's underlying, evidence-based reasoning, the same Clinical-Imaging Crosswalk System that has organized every chapter of this book from its opening pages through this closing, consolidated reference. As new editions of this book incorporate evolving evidence, refined imaging techniques, and updated diagnostic criteria, this Atlas is intended to be updated in parallel, preserving its function as a current, reliable index into this book's complete diagnostic reasoning framework rather than a static, time-limited artifact of any single edition.